Medical Intelligence Unit

Current Controversy in Parathyroid Operation and Reoperation

Göran Åkerström

University Hospital
Uppsala, Sweden

R.G. Landes Company
Austin

Medical Intelligence Unit

CURRENT CONTROVERSY IN PARATHYROID OPERATION AND REOPERATION

R.G. LANDES COMPANY
Austin

CRC Press is the exclusive worldwide distributor of publications of the Medical Intelligence Unit.
CRC Press, 2000 Corporate Blvd., NW, Boca Raton, FL 33431. Phone: 407/994-0555.

Submitted: August 1994
Published: December 1994

Please address all inquiries to the Publisher:
R.G. Landes Company, 909 Pine Street, Georgetown, TX 78626
or
P.O. Box 4858, Austin, TX 78765
Phone: 512/ 863 7762; FAX: 512/ 863 0081

ISBN 1-57059-086-9
CATALOG # LN9086

Library of Congress Cataloging-in-Publication Data

Current controvery in parathyroid operation and reoperation - [edited
by] Göran Åkerström, Claes Juhlin, Jonas Rastad.
p. cm. -- (Medical intelligence unit)
Includes bibliographical references and indexes.
ISBN 1-57059-086-9
1. Parathyroid glands-Surgery. 2. Parathyroid glands-
-Reoperation. 3. Parazthyroid glands--Diseases. I. Åkerström,
Göran. II. Juhlin, Claes. III. Rastad, Jonas. IV. Series.
[DNLM: 1. Hyperparathyroidism--surgery. 2. Parathyroid Glands-
-surgery. 3. Reoperation--methods. 4.Surgery, Operative--methods.
WK 300 C9755 1994]
RD599.5.P37C87 1994
617.5'39--dc20
DNLM/DLC
for Library of Congress 94-39604
CIP

While the authors, editors and publisher believe that drug selection and dosage and the specifications and usage of equipment and devices, as set forth in this book, are in accord with current recommendations and practice at the time of publication, they make no warranty, expressed or implied, with respect to material described in this book. In view of the ongoing research, equipment development, changes in governmental regulations and the rapid accumulation of information relating to the biomedical sciences, the reader is urged to carefully review and evaluate the information provided herein.

To Our Readers

R.G. Landes Company publishes four book series: *Medical Intelligence Unit, Molecular Biology Intelligence Unit, Neuroscience Intelligence Unit,* and *Biotechnology Intelligence Unit.* Our goal is to publish the most recent information in biomedical science for sophisticated researchers and physicians.

To achieve this goal we have accelerated our publishing program to conform to the fast pace in which information grows in biomedical science. Most of our books are published within 90 to 120 days of receipt of the manuscript.

As you might expect, this causes a few problems for us; sometimes it makes our office more like a big city newspaper than a scholarly publisher. So as you look through this book you may see something that isn't just right. Please let us know. Or if you have an idea for improving our books, we'd like very much to hear from you. If the problem you describe hasn't already been discovered or if your idea is provocative enough to promote a discussion here, we'll give you a free book of your choice. Just list three titles in order of preference and we'll send you one, based on availability—with our thanks. Our address is printed on the copyright page of each of our books.

Carol Harwell
Publications Director
R.G. Landes Company

Dedication

This book is dedicated to retired Professor Henry Johannsson, with whom the great interest in parathyroid surgery was firmly rooted in Uppsala, and who trained us in the discipline of Endocrine Surgery and patient care.

CONTENTS

EDITORS

Göran Åkerström, M.D.
Professor of Endocrine Surgery
Department of Surgery
University Hospital
Uppsala, Sweden
Chapters 2, 3, 4, 6, 7, 8, 9, 10

Claes Juhlin, M.D.
Associate Professor
Department of Surgery
University Hospital
Uppsala, Sweden
Chapters 2, 6, 8, 10

Jonas Rastad, M.D.
Associate Professor
Department of Surgery
University Hospital
Uppsala, Sweden
Chapters 2, 5, 6, 7, 9

CONTRIBUTORS

Lars Grimelius, Professor
Department of Pathology
University Hospital
Uppsala, Sweden
Chapter 3

Per Hellman, M.D.
Department of Surgery
University Hospital
Uppsala, Sweden
Chapter 2

Henry Johansson, Professor
Department of Surgery
University Hospital
Uppsala, Sweden
Chapters 1, 10

Sverker Ljunghall, Professor
Department of Internal Medicine
University Hospital
Uppsala, Sweden
Chapter 6

Peter Ridefelt, M.D.
Department of Clinical Chemistry
University Hospital
Uppsala, Sweden
Chapter 2

Britt Skogseid
Associate Professor
Department of Internal Medicine
University Hospital
Uppsala, Sweden
Chapter 7

INTRODUCTION

Many of the first patients subjected to surgery for hyperparathyroidism (HPT) at the beginning of this century had to undergo several operations, yet some still had persistent disease. The history of parathyroid surgery is therefore to a great extent the history of parathyroid *reoperation* and reports of failed operations continue to enhance our insight into the management of parathyroid surgery. Several of the early patients illustrated the varieties of parathyroid anatomy and pathology so crucial to successful parathyroid surgery. These patients also manifested many of the seriously incapacitating symptoms, only occasionally recognized or hardly even remembered today, that accompany chronic, untreated hyperparathyroidism. The disorders of calcium metabolism in these patients were associated with severe bone disease, renal stones and debilitating muscular weakness—that ended in death in renal failure. In recent years HPT, in a milder form, has been diagnosed with increasing frequency; it is characterized by weakness and psychiatric disorders as well as associated cardiovascular disease that significantly decreases survival. Serum calcium screening reveals the disease in at a milder stage, where the symptoms may be less obvious, and it has been suggested that these patients do not necessarily require surgery but can be observed. At the same time, training of specialized endocrine surgeons has advanced parathyroid surgery into an unusually successful procedure generally associated with low morbidity and few complications. However, increased diagnosis, liberal indications for surgery and more frequent operation by surgeons not specially trained in endocrine surgery have sometimes resulted in poor results.

Parathyroid reoperation is a serious undertaking which challenges the technical skills of the surgeon. It is associated with high complication rates and an outcome less certain than in primary surgery. Prior to reoperation it is essential that the diagnosis is made thoughtfully and that the indications for surgery are considered carefully . The various pathological and clinical forms of HPT must be appreciated, as these factors influence surgical strategy.

In this book we review recent aspects of the management of parathyroid surgery, with special emphasis on causes of failed operations, methods for preoperative glandular localization and the principles for reoperation. By presenting a comprehensive survey of the current knowledge about the parathyroid glands, we hope the book will be of value regarding both primary and reoperative parathyroid surgery. Accordingly, we include information about parathyroid pathophysiology and pathology, since recent knowledge may provide insight into the varieties of parathyroid disease. We also illustrate the principles of clinical diagnosis of primary and secondary HPT as well as specific features of hereditary disease and parathyroid malignancy. In discussing indications for primary and reoperative surgery we advocate a liberal attitude towards operation since this surgery can now be performed with great success and safety. However, when recommending liberal indications for surgery, all efforts should be undertaken to minimize failure. We believe important lessons in this respect may still be learned from descriptions of reoperative surgery.

Acknowledgment

We are indebted to Annika Åkerström for most efficient typing of the manuscripts.

CHAPTER 1

History of Parathyroid Operation and Reoperation

Henry Johansson

Our knowledge about the parathyroids now extends over slightly more than a century, but it is indeed intriguing for the scientist of today to realize that many of the important details of parathyroid anatomy, histology and even aspects on surgery were already known to the early discoverers in the field.

The parathyroid gland was first recognized in 1850 by Richard Owen, who was conservator and Professor of Comparative Anatomy at the Hunterian Museum of the Royal College of Surgeons, London. Owen made his discovery while undertaking an autopsy on an Indian rhinoceros, and his observation was reported to the Zoological Society of London, though the paper was not published until 1862, when it appeared in the *Transactions of the Society.*[1] In his paper Owen gives a clear description of a parathyroid gland as "a small compact yellow body attached to the thyroid at the point where the veins emerge". Apparently he had no prior knowledge of the presence of this organ, which "had a diameter and circumference no greater than a six penny piece". No microscopic examination of the gland was undertaken to confirm his finding, however, and Owen never mentioned the presence of these glands in other animals or in his later dissection studies. His observation passed unnoticed until 1905, when it was mentioned in an article in the *British Medical Journal.*

The credit for the discovery of the parathyroid glands is generally assigned the Uppsala anatomist Ivar Sandström (Fig. 1.1), who made a detailed anatomical and histological description of the gland in human and several animal species. His dissection studies were performed between 1877 and 1880, and included altogether 50 human autopsy cases. He named the new structures "glandulae parathyroideae". Sandström published his completed studies in a paper entitled "On a New Gland in Man and Several Animals". The original manuscript was first sent to Rudolf Virchow, the greatest pathologist of the time, but he declined its

Current Controversy in Parathyroid Operation and Reoperation, edited by Göran Åkerström.

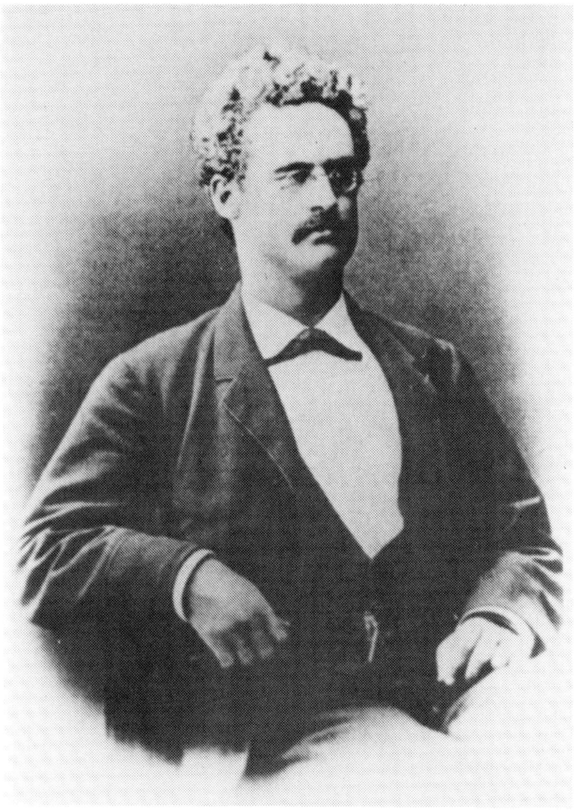

Fig. 1.1. Ivar Victor Sandström (1852-1889). Anatomy demonstrator at the University of Uppsala, Sweden.

publication in his archive because of the length of the paper, which comprised 30 pages. Therefore, Sandström published the manuscript in a Swedish journal, *Uppsala Läkareförenings Förhandlingar* in 1880.[2] His publication was in Swedish, and if two abstracts had not been published in a German yearbook of 1880, his work would probably have remained unrecognized for many years. Sandström's recognition and comprehensive description of these glands is often noted as the last anatomical discovery.

In Sandström's paper many of the anatomical and histological observations are of significance even for modern pathology and surgery. He presented a detailed gross description of the position, size, color, and the various forms of the glands. He mentioned that the parathyroid glands were most commonly found along the posterior capsule of the lateral lobe of the thyroid and "frequently they are both found along the inferior thyroid artery; one of them immediately above and the other one just below the place where the artery enters the thyroid gland" (Fig. 1.2). He also found that the parathyroids varied in both size and form, and he expressed this as follows: "Sometimes the glands are only 3 mm in their largest dimension, in other cases they reach a length of up to 15 mm. The most usual size is apparently about 6 mm. Their form is generally more or less compressed and plate-like, sometimes so much so that the thickness is hardly 2 mm, while the width and length are of the usual dimensions or even larger. The superior gland has not infrequently a rather elongated form". Sandström also noted a variable distribution between the parenchymal and fat cells, when examining histological sections of the glands by light microscopy. Using staining with osmic acid, he furthermore demonstrated that the parathyroid parenchymal cells often contained varying amounts of cytoplasmic fat droplets.

With reference to the possible physiological importance of the parathyroids, Sandström says in his paper, that "from reasons that are quite apparent I am not able to allow myself even to make a guess". However, he expressed speculations on their clinical relevance, and suggested that the glands could be of importance in pathological conditions, and he also said: "For the purpose of diagnosing a tumor of the parathyroid gland, I want to point out the proximity of the glands to the esophagus and the recurrent nerve, whereby in cases of pathological growth processes there may easily occur a compression of the former and a paralysis of the latter".

Sandström was disappointed with the reception of his discovery, and his disillusionment is reflected in a letter to his sister, where he writes: " I accepted an invitation from Stockholm to attend an international meeting of the Nature Scientists in order that I might do my part so that we Swedes should not succumb to our guests, which later on proved not to be the case at all. One should, of course, at a personal meeting of so many men who devote themselves to science, be inclined to expect less of a hurried reading of, more or less unimportant products of genius whose creators in any case would not forget to publish them if they are of any value, than rather a friendly exchange of thoughts and of trustful communication of personal experiences and impressions. Nothing of the kind was seen. Everyone seemed to be there with the intention of showing what *discoveries* he had made and at the same time give the astonished world the opportunity to have a look at the fortune discoverer, but for the discovery itself, for the revealed truth, the interest was little or none". These thoughts of Sandström's are the reflections of a man who was seriously devoted to science, and the spirit of his sentences indeed ought to be considered also by the scientists of the 20th century.

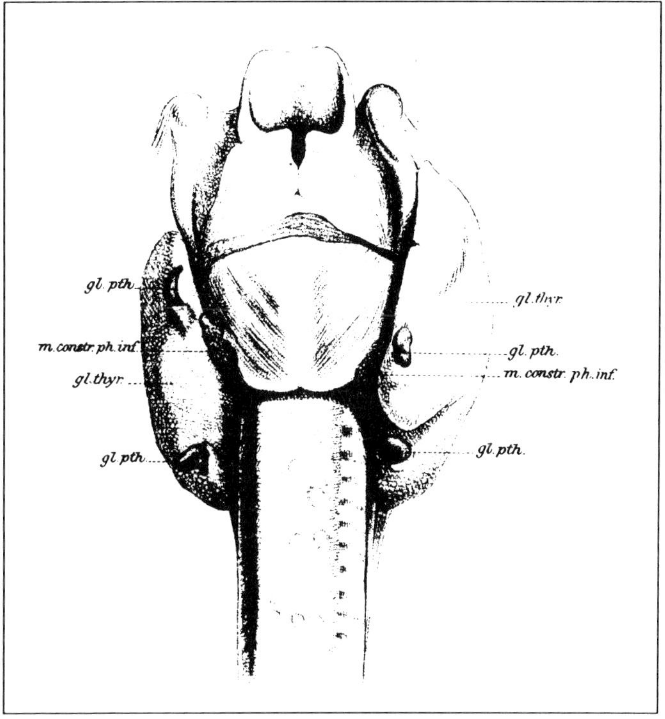

Fig. 1.2. Anatomical sketch of the parathyroid glands. Reprinted with permission from Sandström I.[2]

In 1891 Eugène Gley, Professor of Physiology in Paris, published the first report on a relationship between the parathyroid gland and tetany.[3] Shortly thereafter two Italians, Giulio Vassale and Francesco Generali, observed that tetany could be caused by parathyroidectomy. They suggested that tetany, which at that time was a common and harmful complication to thyroid surgery, was caused by intoxication, and that the parathyroids were the organs that were able to remove the toxin. This theory persisted for years, and it was not until 1924 that William MacCallum, who occupied a post as pathologist at Johns Hopkins Hospital, convincingly described how parathyroid tetany was directly related to calcium deficiency. At about the same time it was proved that tetany could be treated with parathyroid extract, and further research subsequently led to the successful isolation of parathyroid hormone (PTH) by James Collip in 1925.[4]

As early as 1891 von Recklinghausen described the typical parathyroid bone disease, and gave it the descriptive name "osteitis fibrosa cystica."[5] However, the association between this bone disorder and parathyroid disease was not established until 1904, when Max Askanazy described a patient with skeletal symptoms and the presence of a parathyroid tumor.[6] Subsequently the relationship between the parathyroid enlargement and the typical bone disease was further substantiated by the Viennese pathologist Jakob Erdheim who, in 1907 reported that patients dying of osteomalacic or fibrocystic bone disease frequently exhibited abnormally enlarged parathyroid glands.[7] From his studies on rats and also from observations in man, he concluded, however, that enlargement of the parathyroid glands was a compensatory phenomenon that occurred secondary to the bone disease. Not until 1915 was it suggested by Friedrich Schlagenhaufer that since often only one parathyroid gland was enlarged in this disease constellation, this should in fact be the primary lesion and the cause rather than the consequence of the bone disease.[8] On these grounds it appeared logical to treat patients who suffered from the bone disorder by excision of the abnormal parathyroid gland, rather than to give parathyroid extract, which indeed was the prevailing therapy at that time.

As a consequence of these reports the first surgical parathyroidectomy was subsequently performed by Felix Mandl of Vienna in 1925.[9] His patient Albert Jahne suffered from a severe, crippling parathyroid bone disease and had sustained a femur fracture. At first Mandl thought that the disease was due to parathyroid deficiency and performed parathyroid gland implantation. This, however, exacerbated the condition and he then explored Albert's neck, where he found and removed a parathyroid tumor, measuring 21 x 15 x 12 mm. The three remaining glands were identified and were considered normal. After this operation the patient's condition improved remarkably. Mandl's observation had for the first time unequivocally demonstrated that the bone disease was secondary to a lesion of the parathyroid gland, and the outcome of the operation substantiated Schlagenhaufer's idea that parathyroidectomy would be beneficial to patients with osteitis fibrosa.

However, in 1932 Mandl noted that the symptoms of Albert Jahne had recurred, and he had to reexplore the neck, which resulted in subtotal thyroid resection and excision of two normal parathyroid glands. The patient did not improve after this reoperation, however, and he died of uremia the same year. It is probable that the patient Albert Jahne was indeed suffering from multiglandular parathyroid disease—or he may even have had unrecognized parathyroid carcinoma.

Mandl's report of the first parathyroidectomy attracted considerable attention and aroused the interest among other surgeons about diseases of the parathyroid glands.

Another famous patient in the historical chapter on hyperparathyroidism (HPT) was Captain Charles Martel who was treated at the Mayo Clinic.[10] Like Albert Jahne this patient also has an interesting story, as he underwent a total of six operations, including total thyroidectomy and excision of two normal-sized parathyroid glands, until finally a mediastinal parathyroid tumor was successfully removed by Churchill and Cope in 1932.[11] At this the seventh operation a 30 x 30 mm encapsulated tumor was found medial to the superior vena cava. Because the normal parathyroid glands of this patient had been removed in conjunction with the previous operations, a remnant of the adenoma was transplanted in muscular tissue. In spite of this the patient developed tetany on the third postoperative day and required treatment with calcium and parathyroid hormone. He eventually recovered from the postoperative hypocalcemia but, like Mandl's first patient, Captain Martel too subsequently died of the renal complications he had acquired during the previous years, when the disease had defied all the efforts of the treating physicians.

During the decades to follow many surgeons recognized the reports of these early patients and subsequently entered the field of parathyroid surgery, which indeed was most highly regarded among surgeons. Primary HPT, however, continued for a long time to be a rare disorder, which was diagnosed virtually only in those who, like the early patients, suffered from severe bone disease. Around 1950 Albright and Reifenstein highlighted other aspects of the disease, when they suggested that the bone symptoms could be lacking in some patients with HPT, presenting with moderate hypercalcemia and symptoms of renal stones. As a consequence of their report HPT was subsequently diagnosed with increasing frequency, and more than 50% of the patients were actually found to suffer from a renal stone disorder. Albright and Reifenstein also reported on a patient with

HPT who had neither renal stones nor bone disease, and they anticipated that this might become a common mode of future presentation.

In Sweden, John Hellström, Professor of Surgery at the Karolinska Hospital in Stockholm, was the great pioneer of parathyroid surgery, and he ultimately presented no less than 138 patients, whom he personally had treated surgically for HPT.[12] His first operation was performed in 1930, but few patients were actually treated prior to 1950, and it was after this date that he had experienced a marked increase in parathyroid operations. In his studies Hellström confirmed the relationship between renal stones and HPT, which had initially been revealed by Fuller Albright in 1934.[13] Hellström also claimed that the only rational treatment for HPT was the surgical removal of all hyperfunctioning parathyroid tissue. He furthermore substantiated that surgical intervention in HPT is generally a simple and convenient procedure, particularly if a single adenoma is present in a normal location. However, he emphasized that the possible causes of inadequate and unsuccessful explorations are many, and thus almost 20% of his patients were reoperative cases, who had initially undergone surgery at other hospitals. In some of these cases, multiple parathyroid adenomas had been overlooked, while other patients had undergone inadequate resection of primary hyperplasia. However, the vast majority of failed primary explorations were the result of incomplete neck dissections, and Hellström strongly emphasized that parathyroid surgery should be carried out "in hospitals where the services of experienced surgeons and pathologists were available". Hellström's enthusiasm for parathyroid surgery was evident from his publications, and he summarized his experiences in an article which recounts detailed case reports on the type of improvement that may be obtained by parathyroid surgery. Altogether these patient histories illustrate a basic ideology in clinical research, implying that scientific endeavor should rely on clinical observations, and that meticulous review of the patient histories often affords important experience. In 1956 Hellström published a series of unsuccessful parathyroidectomies in HPT and emphasized some of the more common reasons for surgical failure.[14] These encompassed inability to retrieve glands in abnormal location and failure to recognize the presence of hyperplasia or multiple adenomas. Insufficient knowledge about the parathyroid anatomy and pathology was revealed as an important cause of unsuccessful surgery. Frozen section examination of excised specimens was considered as a crucial part of a parathyroid operation.[14]

At that time contemporary authors had already made important contributions in the context of parathyroid surgery. Albright[15] recognized parathyroid hyperplasia as a distinct histopathological entity, and Churchill and Cope[16] and Cope[17] described technical aspects of the operation and also emphasized the most efficient means to deal with mediastinal lesions. Norris[18] reported on multiple adenomas, Black and Haynes[19] substantiated the possible presence of intrathyroidal parathyroid tumors and Reifenstein[20] described the presence of ectopic adenomas posterior to the esophagus. Reoperative patients were reported by several authors, and although they provided important details on this surgery the patient series generally comprised only few cases. The parathyroid reoperation was invariably described as a difficult procedure which was associated with significant morbidity and even mortality.[21,22] It was substantiated that reoperation in HPT should first comprise a thorough reexploration of the neck, and a lateral approach via the vascular sheath was suggested to provide the safest access to the neck area after previous exploration.[21,23] This short review clearly illustrates that the pioneers of parathyroid surgery contributed information on parathyroid pathology and anatomy and that they gave suggestions on surgical strategy that are still most relevant today.

In Uppsala, the first parathyroid neck exploration was performed in 1941 on a woman but only one normal-sized parathyroid gland was found, and the patient was unimproved on discharge from the hospital. The first successful operation was, in fact, a reoperation undertaken in 1946 on a 37 year old woman with multiple spontaneous fractures, who one year earlier had undergone parathyroid surgery, which had failed to cure the disease. At the successful reoperation, a kidney-shaped, bean-sized adenoma was delivered from the mediastinum by sternotomy. However, the patient died of postoperative tetany, despite intravenous infusions of both calcium and parathyroid hormone.

In a personal experience considerable compilations of data concerning patients with primary HPT have been reported from Uppsala, and bear witness on the rapid development of parathyroid surgery, that took place from the mid-1960s and further on. Renal lithiasis often dominated the symptomatology, but non-specific symptoms, such as lassitude, muscular weakness and mental disturbances were found to play an increasingly prominent role.[24] A considerably more efficient diagnosis of parathyroid hyperplasia was also one of the developments during this period. Pernicious HPT, i.e. parathyroid disease presenting with hypercalcemic crisis, and the clinical management of this condition were described early from Uppsala, and it is particularly interesting to note that approximately half of the patients who presented with hypercalcemic crisis had previously been regarded as being asymptomatic. Parathyroid surgery was established as a very safe procedure with low morbidity. Mortality associated with parathyroid surgery was confined essentially only to those patients who presented with hypercalcemic crisis.

Subsequent studies on parathyroid histology described details of importance for distinguishing between the various entities of pathological parathyroid glands as well as between abnormal and normal glands. Careful anatomical studies of parathyroid glands were undertaken in Uppsala,[25] and provided a basis for a surgical strategy, which implied visualization of even normal-sized parathyroid glands, since this was found to constitute an important part of the histopathological evaluation. The experience gathered by the routine identification of normal parathyroid glands also resulted in successful and comparatively uncomplicated reoperative parathyroid surgery.

References

1. Owen R. On the anatomy of the Indian rhinoceros (*Rh. unicornis,* L). Trans Zool Soc Lond *iv* 1862; 31-58.
2. Sandström IV. On a new gland in man and several mammals—glandulae parathyroideae. Uppsala Läk Förenings Förh 1879-1880; 15: 441-71.
3. Gley E. Sur les functions du corps thyroide. Cr Séanc Soc Biol 1891; 43: 841-3.
4. Collip JB. Extraction of parathyroid hormone which will prevent or control parathyroid tetany and regulates level of blood calcium. J Biol Chem 1925; 63: 395-438.
5. von Recklinghausen FD. Die fibröse oder deformierende Ostitis, die Osteomalacie und die osteoplastische Karzinose in ihren gegenseitigen Beziehungen; in Festschrift für Rudolph Virchow Reimer, Berlin 1891: 1-89.
6. Askanazy M. Über Ostitis deformans ohne ostoides Gewebe. Arb Geb path anat Inst Tübingen 1903; 4: 398-422.
7. Erdheim J. Über die Dentinverkalkung im Nagezahn bei der Epithelkörperchen transplantation. Frankfurt Z Path 1911; 7: 295-342.
8. Schlaugenhaufer F. Zwei Fälle von Parathyreoideatumoren. Wien klin Wschr 1915; 28: 1362.
9. Mandl F. Therapeutischer Versuch bei Ostitis fibrosa generalisata mittels Extirpation eines Epithelkörperchentumors. Wien klin Wschr 1925; 50: 1343-4.
10. Bauer W, Federman DD. Hyperparathyroidism epitomized; the case of Captain Charles E. Martel. Metabolism 1962; 11: 21-9.
11. Cope O. The story of hyperparathyroidism at the Massachusetts General Hospital. New Engl J Med 1966; 21: 1174-82.

12. Hellström J. Primary hyperparathyroidism. Triangle 1962; 5: 171-8.
13. Albright F. Page out of history of hyperparathyroidism. J Clin Endocr Metab 1948; 8: 637-57.
14. Hellström J. The causes of unsuccessful or inadequate parathyroidectomy in hyperparathyroidism. Acta Chir Scandinav 1956; 112: 79-91.
15. Albright F, Bloomberg E, Castleman B et al. Hyperparathyroidism due to diffuse hyperplasia of all parathyroid glands rather than adenoma of one: Clinical studies on three such cases. Arch Intern Med 1934; 54: 315-29.
16. Churchill ED, Cope O. The surgical treatment of hyperparathyroidism: Based on 30 cases confirmed by operation. Ann Surg 1936; 104: 9-35.
17. Cope O. Surgery of hyperparathyroidism. The occurrence of parathyroids in the anterior mediastinum and the division of the operation into two stages. Ann Surg 1941; 114: 706-33.
18. Norris EH. Collective review; parathyroid adenoma; study of 322 cases. Internat Abstr Surg 1947; 84: 1-41.
19. Black BM, Haynes AL. Intrathyroid hyperfunctioning parathyroid adenomas: report of two cases. Proc Staff Meet Mayo Clin 1949; 24: 408-18.
20. Reifenstein EC Jr. Diseases of the parathyroid glands. Textbook of Endocrinology, Sec. Ed. 1955.
21. Clark O, Taylor S. Persistent and recurrent hyperparathyroidism. Brit J Surg 1972; 59: 555-8.
22. Beazley RM, Costa J, Ketcham AS. Reoperative parathyroid surgery. Am J Surg 1975; 130: 427-9.
23. Feind CR. Re-exploration for parathyroid adenoma. Am J Surg 1964; 108: 543-6.
24. Johansson H, Thorén L, Werner I. Hyperparathyroidism—Clinical experiences from 208 cases. Upsal J Med Sci 1972; 77: 41-6.
25. Åkerström G, Malmaeus J, Bergström R. Surgical anatomy of human parathyroid glands. Surgery 1984; 95: 14-21.

CHAPTER 2

PATHOPHYSIOLOGY OF HYPERPARATHYROIDISM

Per Hellman, Göran Åkerström, Claes Juhlin, Peter Ridefelt, Jonas Rastad

Calcium is the principal regulator of parathyroid hormone release. Recent findings suggest that this regulation is mediated by calcium receptors or receptors on the parathyroid cell surface. A membrane protein proposed to constitute such a receptor demonstrates reduced expression in hyperparathyroidism and seems causally related to the relative insensitivity of the secretion to external calcium in the pathological parathyroid cells. This protein consequently may be an important cause for the hypercalcemia of this disorder. Calcium sensing molecules seem to be involved in several cell types with prominent interactions in systemic calcium homeostasis. Interference with functions of such proteins comprises interesting means of future therapy in several disorders of mineral metabolism. Increased knowledge of these proteins and parathyroid pathophysiology in general will possibly clarify the presence of relevant mutations, secretory derangements and propensity for cell growth, whereby accurate classification of parathyroid diseases and improved treatment strategies might evolve.

Calcium is the most abundant cation in man, and its distribution within cells is essential for virtually all physiological functions. A precise hormonal system controlling Ca^{2+} fluxes has developed during evolution with a resulting tight maintenance of the physiologic serum Ca^{2+} concentration. The parathyroid glands play a key role in this homeostasis by their unique capacity to sense changes in the extracellular Ca^{2+} concentration and to respond rapidly with alterations in the parathyroid hormone (PTH) secretion. This 84 amino acid hormone increases the serum Ca^{2+} concentration by stimulating bone resorption and by enhancing Ca^{2+} reabsorption in the kidney tubule. Concomitantly it stimulates 1-α-hydroxylase activity of the proximal kidney tubule cells, which leads to increased formation of 1,25-dihydroxyvitamin D_3. This enzymatic activity is regulated not only by PTH, phosphate as well as calcitriol itself, but also by the extracellular Ca^{2+} concentration, indicationg presence of a

Current Controversy in Parathyroid Operation and Reoperation,
edited by Göran Åkerström.

Ca^{2+} sensing mechanism in the proximal tubular epithelium.[1-4] The active form of vitamin D enhances intestinal Ca^{2+} absorption and exerts a direct, functionally important feedback control on the parathyroid by its ability to interfere with PTH gene transcription and parathyroid cell proliferation.[5-7]

REGULATION OF PARATHYROID HORMONE RELEASE

The extracellular concentration of ionized Ca^{2+} is the principal regulator of PTH release.[8,9] The relationship between external Ca^{2+} and PTH release is inversely sigmoidal (Fig. 2.1A).[10,11] This dependency contrasts to the original concept of stimulus-secretion coupling prevailing in most secretory cells, where Ca^{2+} constitutes a universal stimulator of secretion. Analysis by sensitive immunoassays for the intact (1-84) PTH molecule has verified that the steepest part of the curve relating extracellular Ca^{2+} to secretion corresponds to the physiologic level of ionized plasma Ca^{2+}. Even small Ca^{2+} variations in this range thus exerts pronounced effects on PTH release.[12]

The principal intracellular messenger regulating PTH release is the concentration of cytoplasmic Ca^{2+} ($[Ca^{2+}]_i$), which exhibits a positive sigmoidal dependency on external Ca^{2+} (Fig. 2.1B).[13-15] The $[Ca^{2+}]_i$ response to stepwise increases in extracellular Ca^{2+} is biphasic, momentary, and unusually steep within the parathyroid cells. It consists of an initial transient peak followed by a sustained $[Ca^{2+}]_i$ elevation indicative of a receptormediated mechanism. As in many other cells, this receptor-activated response is regulated by metabolism of phosphoinositol phosphates in the plasma membrane. Inositol trisphosphate (IP_3) releases Ca^{2+} from intracellular stores located mainly within the endoplasmic reticulum, and creates the initial $[Ca^{2+}]_i$ transient typical of receptor activation.[16-18] It is possible that

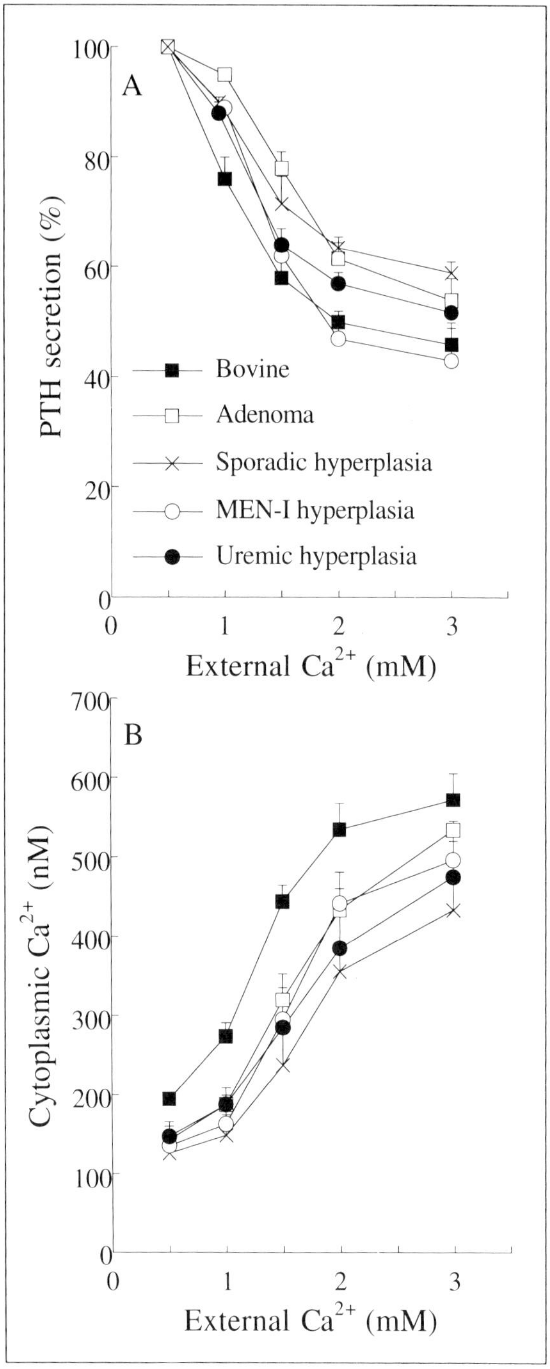

Fig. 2.1. Effects of extracellular ionized calcium on PTH release (A) and steady-state cytoplasmic calcium concentrations (B) of dispersed parathyroid cells from normal bovine glands, parathyroid adenomas (n=19), hyperplastic glands of sporadic primary HPT (n=6), familial HPT of MEN-1 (n=8), and hyperplastic glands of secondary HPT (n=20). PTH is expressed in percentages of the release at 0.5 mM Ca^{2+} and $[Ca^{2+}]_i$ is measured with quin-2 in a cuvette system.

phosphoinositol metabolites of parathyroid cells are responsible also for the Ca^{2+}-mediated Ca^{2+} gating through the plasma membrane. This gating constitutes a non-voltage dependent permeability and gives rise to the sustained increase in $[Ca^{2+}]_i$ upon a Ca^{2+} challenge. Protein kinase C (PKC) may also be involved in modulating the PTH release.[19-21] PKC is activated by diacylglycerol, which is another product of the phosphoinositol metabolism. Such activation at low extracellular Ca^{2+} concentrations inhibits the PTH release, while it stimulates the secretion at high external Ca^{2+}.[21] Discordant activations of PKC at low and IP_3 at high external Ca^{2+} levels substantiates that the precise role of PKC on the secretion remains to be elucidated. Cyclic AMP production of parathyroid cells has also been shown to be influenced by extracellular Ca^{2+} as well as by several other factors interfering with the PTH release. The secretory effect of cAMP is rather limited, however, and it mainly stimulates the release of stored PTH. This differs from the swift Ca^{2+} regulation of secretion, which preferentially involves newly synthesized hormone.[22] While the regulation of cAMP involves G proteins, it is unclear what role these proteins play in the mainstream of Ca^{2+} regulation of parathyroid $[Ca^{2+}]_i$ and PTH release.[23]

The parathyroid is exceptional among secretory cells, since Ca^{2+} inhibition of hormone release is related to cellular depolarization.[24,25] The Ca^{2+} influx associated with secretory inhibition occurs through non-voltage dependent channels activated by Ca^{2+}, and the resulting Ca^{2+} current seems to be the cause rather than a consequence of cellular depolarization.[26] Several other divalent cations as, e.g. Mg^{2+}, can also cause transient rises in $[Ca^{2+}]_i$ due to intracellular Ca^{2+} mobilization. Even the trivalent cation La^{3+}, which is restricted to the cell exterior and a potent Ca^{2+} antagonist may rise parathyroid $[Ca^{2+}]_i$ and inhibit the hormone release.[27-29] These findings comprise additional arguments for the presence of a surface cation-sensitive mechanism on the parathyroid cell, which exerts control of secretion and perhaps might be involved in replication.[28,30,31] Activation of this sensor seems to regulate phosphoinositol metabolism and PKC activity, while G protein involvement in the messenger cascade is questionable. Any coupling of such a sensor to parathyroid cAMP production remains to be elucidated. Moreover Ga^{3+} inhibits PTH release by an apparently different mechanism from the sensor coupled to $[Ca^{2+}]_i$ as the principal intracellular messenger.[32] Consequently there may be several cation-sensitive mechanisms involved in the regulation of PTH release. Indeed it has been postulated that, apart from the parathyroid, protein(s) with Ca^{2+} receptor function should be expressed also by other cell systems, including cells of the kidney tubule, placental cells, thyroid C-cells, possible osteoclasts and even alveolar pneumocytes type II, a.o.[33] The concept of cell surface Ca^{2+} sensors thus may be a more widely distributed function than previously anticipated.

In an attempt to identify functionally important surface structures specific to the parathyroid parenchyma, monoclonal antibodies were produced by immunizing mice with parathyroid adenoma cells.[34,35] The antibodies were all found to react with a surface-bound structure of human parathyroid epithelial cells, and with placental cytotrophoblasts as well as the brush border membrane of the proximal kidney tubule.[36] Two IgG2b antibodies, denoted G11 and B6, abolished Ca^{2+} regulation of $[Ca^{2+}]_i$ and hormone release of normal and pathological parathyroid cells.[35,37] In contrast, an IgG1 antibody denoted E11 lacked these effects and was subsequently found to recognize another domain of the same structure. The functionally active antibodies blocked both the Ca^{2+} induced $[Ca^{2+}]_i$ transient of intracellular Ca^{2+} mobilization as well as the steady-state elevation due to Ca^{2+} influx. These findings further supported expression of a Ca^{2+} sensor on parathyroid cells and indicated that the antibodies not only recognized but also interfered with the sensor rather than an associated Ca^{2+} channel.[35,37,38]

The human cytotrophoblast cells have shown virtually parathyroid-identical actions of extracellular Ca^{2+} on $[Ca^{2+}]_i$.[36] The steep sigmoidal relationship between external Ca^{2+} and $[Ca^{2+}]_i$, however, demonstrates a higher ED_{50} (set-point) than in the normal human parathyroid cells. This rise in set-point is consistent with the physiological elevation of the fetal plasma Ca^{2+} concentration due to active Ca^{2+} transfer from mother to fetus.[39] Moreover Ca^{2+} seems to regulate release of parathyroid hormone-related protein from the cytotrophoblast cells, which has been claimed to mediate the active materno-fetal Ca^{2+} transport. These findings suggest that the placental Ca^{2+} sensor protein exerts a key role in fetal Ca^{2+} homeostasis.[39] Studies on transformed cytotrophoblast cells also indicate that the Ca^{2+} sensor may interact in the regulation of cell proliferation.[40]

Cloning of the Ca^{2+} sensor recognized by the anti-parathyroid antibodies was possible by using the abundantly available human placental tissue. A 500 kDa glycoprotein was revealed, which exhibits a single membrane-spanning domain and structurally belongs to the LDL-receptor superfamily.[41,42] This placental protein subsequently was found to be identical to the antibody-reactive structure of the human parathyroid and kidney.[43] Particular homology was demonstrated between the Ca^{2+} sensor and the Heymann nephritis antigen.[42] This protein originally was isolated from rat kidney and comprises a large glycoprotein (gp330) claimed to be the autoantigen of experimental membranous glomerulonephritis.[44,45] Gp330 strongly binds Ca^{2+} and has been suggested to act as a Ca^{2+} receptor of the proximal kidney tubule.[46] The putative Ca^{2+}-binding motifs of the 500 kDa Ca^{2+} sensor and other members of the LDL-receptor superfamily probably comprise repetitive EGF-like modules. Each of these modules binds one Ca^{2+} ion in coagulation factors,[47-52] and they have been found to mediate Ca^{2+}-dependent protein/protein interaction.[53] The Ca^{2+} sensitivity of these proteins are in the range of the extracellular concentration of ionized Ca^{2+}, which constitutes the environment for Ca^{2+} actions on the sensor protein. Studies on kinetics of the parathyroid Ca^{2+} sensing mechanism indicates the presence of positive cooperativity for the interaction with Ca^{2+},[33] and several Ca^{2+} binding sites may comprise a requisite for this action. This allows efficient response to minimal alterations in ionized Ca^{2+}, which is required for adequate maintenance of the systemic Ca^{2+} homeostasis. A receptor-associated protein (RAP) is bound Ca^{2+}-dependently to the Heymann antigen.[54-56] This 44 kDa protein might be involved in translocating the large sensor protein to the cell surface, whereby it is interesting to note that the anti-parathyroid antibody-reactive structure is partially internalized in parathyroid carcinoma as well as in malignant tumors originating from both the kidney tubules and placental cytotrophoblasts.

Another protein with putative Ca^{2+} sensing function has recently been identified in the bovine parathyroid by expression cloning in oocytes.[57] This 120 kDa protein, is G-protein-coupled and expresses the characteristic seven transmembrane domains of peptide receptors, as well as putative Ca^{2+} binding sites. Transfection of this molecule to eukaryotic cells demonstrated linkage to regulation of $[Ca^{2+}]_i$.[58] Ca^{2+} sensitivity of this protein in the transfected cell system and oocytes is considerably higher than the concentration of ionized plasma Ca^{2+}. Message for this and related proteins is present also in the medulla of the kidney, CNS and the thyroid.[57] The protein shows significant homology to glutamate receptors mostly expressed in the CNS and with known association to voltage-dependent Ca^{2+} channels. Whether this protein is linked to the PTH release is at present not clear. The recently cloned calcitonin receptor comprise another seven transmembrane, G-protein-linked structure with Ca^{2+} receptor function.[59,60] Similar to the 120 kDa bovine sensor structure, Ca^{2+} sensitivity for this protein is several-fold higher than the ionized plasma Ca^{2+} concentration. Moreover it contrasts with the parathyroid Ca^{2+} sensor by its stimulatory action on secretion and its coupling to a voltage-sensitive Ca^{2+} permeability.

PATHOPHYSIOLOGY OF HYPERPARATHYROIDISM

Regulation of PTH release is disturbed in the pathological parathyroid tissue of patients with hyperparathyroidism (HPT) irrespective of the disorder being sporadic or familial, primary or secondary, benign or malignant, and uni- or multiglandular in character.[37,61-65] Moreover there exist quantitative rather than qualitative discrepancies in secretory regulation between these subgroups of patients. The derangement is characterized by relative insensitivities of $[Ca^{2+}]_i$ and PTH release to changes in external Ca^{2+}, whereby right-shifted dose-response relationships may be demonstrated in vitro (Fig. 2.1) and in vivo.[13,14,62] The set-points of PTH secretion and $[Ca^{2+}]_i$ correlate to each other and to the degree of hypercalcemia in both primary and uremic HPT.[13,62] Thus the derangement is less extensive in individuals with mild hypercalcemia, in whom chief cell hyperplasia of sporadic primary HPT is over-represented.[62,63] Since the extent of hypercalcemia largely correlates with total weight of the abnormal parathyroid tissue, the functional cellular abnormality tends to be more pronounced in the severely enlarged glands as indeed in the nodules of the hyperplastic parathyroid tissue.[63,65,66]

Immunohistochemistry with the monoclonal anti-parathyroid antibodies has revealed reduced expression of the 500 kDa Ca^{2+} sensor in the pathological parenchyma of parathyroid adenomas (Fig. 2.2) and primary as well as secondary hyperplasia.[67,68] This reduction is evidently not secondary to the hypercalcemia per se, since there is intense and overtly normal immunostaining in the rims of normal tissue

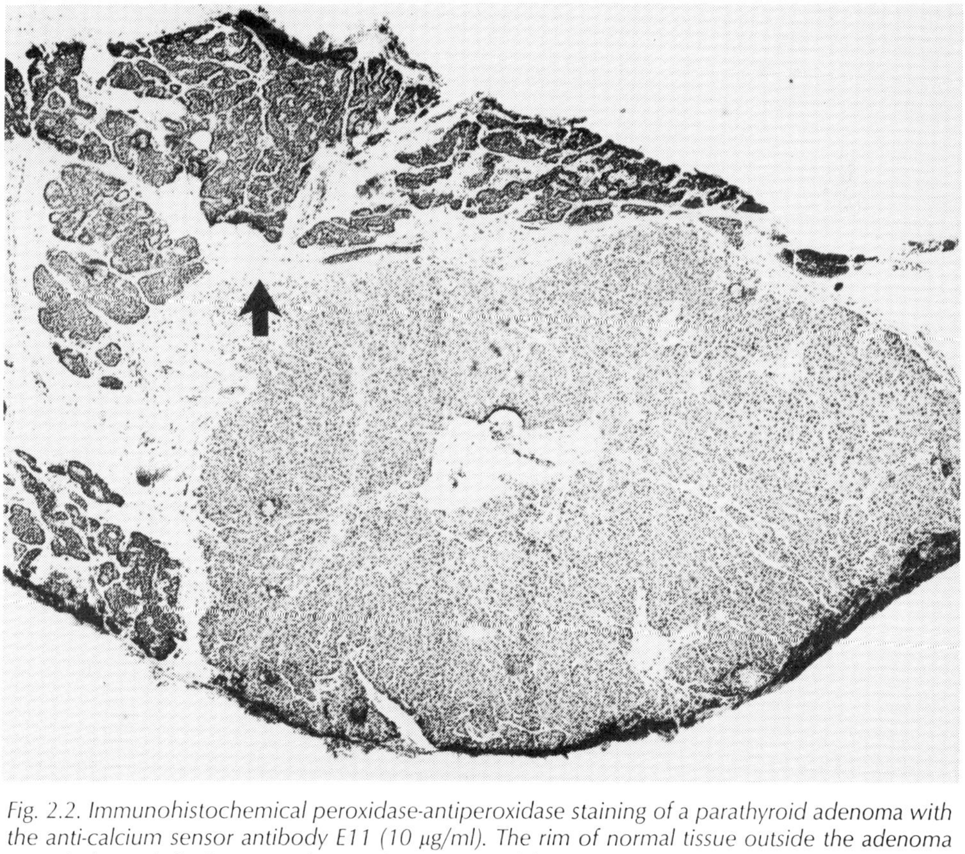

Fig. 2.2. Immunohistochemical peroxidase-antiperoxidase staining of a parathyroid adenoma with the anti-calcium sensor antibody E11 (10 μg/ml). The rim of normal tissue outside the adenoma capsule (arrow) displays more intense immunoreactivity.

outside adenoma capsules and in the normal-sized glands associated with single adenomas.[67,68] Down-regulation of the Ca^{2+} sensor in the hyperplastic parathyroid tissue often is particularly evident in well circumscribed nodules apparently representing clones of parathyroid cells with deviant histological features upon routine histological examination.[69] Both parathyroid adenoma and hyperplasia, however, frequently display additional parenchymal cell islands of reduced sensor expression, which may be indistinguishable from the surrounding parenchyma upon routine staining even with Oil-red O. The characteristic aberrance of parathyroid carcinoma largely comprises localization of the Ca^{2+} sensor immunoreactivity to the tumor cell cytoplasm.[68] Since the Ca^{2+} insensitivity of the PTH secretion has been related to defective Ca^{2+} sensor function within the different varieties of HPT, interference with this function might comprise an intriguing possibility for future pharmacological intervention in this disorder.

Another derangement of the pathological parathyroid cells of HPT may comprise elevated PKC activity leading to hypersecretion of PTH.[19,37] This elevation is presumed to cause right-shifts in the dependence of $[Ca^{2+}]_i$ on extracellular Ca^{2+} mainly through partial uncoupling of the Ca^{2+} sensor from the signaling machinery of the parathyroid cells.[19] Recent studies have suggested that this uncoupling may be due to PKC-mediated effects directly on the sensor.[21] In addition to Ca^{2+} sensor and PKC abnormalities in HPT, reduced inhibition of PTH mRNA expression could be due to nonfunctioning calcitriol receptors in parathyroid adenomas.[70] Calcitriol thus has been found to inhibit hormone release by interfering with PTH gene transcription and to normalize its right-shifted dependence on external Ca^{2+} in HPT. Furthermore there is evidence for a decreased number of calcitriol receptors in the enlarged glands of patients with uremic HPT, which may contribute to the hypersecretion of PTH and comprise an important rationale for calcitriol therapy in this disorder.[71] Evidence for inhibition of PTH mRNA expression and secretion by all-trans- and 9-cis-retinoic acid through nuclear receptors has recently been presented,[72] but the role of vitamin A metabolites in HPT currently is unclear.

It is not presently known to what extent the putative Ca^{2+} sensors exert the functionally crucial regulation of secretion from the normal and diseased parathyroid parenchyma. Both the 120 kDa, 7 transmembrane protein and the 500 kDa, antibody-reactive structure appear to be involved in this regulation, and these proteins may even be structurally and functionally coupled to each other. The constantly reduced expression of the 500 kDa sensor in all varieties of HPT, its prominent interaction in the secretion and $[Ca^{2+}]_i$ regulated by Ca^{2+} and other cations, and its ability to bind Ca^{2+} in the physiologic concentration range support an essential role in the normal and pathologic Ca^{2+} homeostasis.[35,38,67-69]

PARATHYROID CELL GROWTH

HPT invariably is associated with an increased proliferation of the parathyroid cells, which seems to differ considerably between patients as well as within and between the glands of each individual. Little, however, currently is known about relevant factors regulating parathyroid cell replication. The cell turnover normally is very low, and the cells can be triggered to leave the quiescent G_0 stage and enter the G_1 phase by hypocalcemia and calcitriol deficiency.[73-75] These findings may be clinically relevant as reduced 1,25-dihydroxyvitamin D_3 levels characteristically is found even in subclinical disturbances of renal function. Indeed this circumstance also includes many of the overtly healthy elderly, who seem to display an unusual propensity for the development of primary HPT especially in climates associated with limited sun exposure. Although relative calcitriol deficiency may cause parathyroid cell proliferation and reduced inhibition of PTH secretion by decreased genomic control,[6,75] it remains to be established that therapeutic rather than prophylactic replenishment may reverse not only the increased proliferation but actually participate in reducing an established elevation in parathyroid cell mass.

Bovine parathyroid cells in monolayer culture demonstrate gradually increasing set-points for $[Ca^{2+}]_i$ and PTH release, which seem to develop in parallel to the enhanced proliferation.[75] This functional dedifferentiation has not been noted when culturing normal or abnormal human parathyroid cells, which indeed tend to replicate considerably slower than the cells of adult cattle. Moreover calcitriol has been found to inhibit the replication without altering the functional dedifferentiation.[75] Hitherto unidentified factors in the circulation may interact in the coupling of function to proliferation within the parathyroid, since culture in serum-free medium abolishes the hypertrophy, hyperplasia and decreased Ca^{2+} sensitivity of parathyroid cells.[76] In this context it is interesting to note that the increased parathyroid cell replication of multiple endocrine neoplasia type 1 (MEN-1) has been associated with the presence of a circulating mitogenic agent resembling basic fibroblastic growth factor.[77]

Several studies have indicated that the hypersecretion of PTH in HPT is related more to functional dedifferentiation of the parathyroid cells than to tumor size. Indeed it has been suggested that a primary mutation increasing the secretory set-point might initiate and stimulate the proliferation, and that this stimulation declines when plasma Ca^{2+} settles at the genomically determined level.[78] Such a line of reasoning remains to be substantiated, but generally fits with the observation on the relationship between the secretory set-point, serum Ca^{2+} and tumor weight in HPT, the highly variable parathyroid gland enlargement between the patients, and the clinical impression that the hypercalcemia tends to aggravate stepwise in HPT. The increased cell mass nevertheless may determine the portion of PTH secretion not suppressible by Ca^{2+},[79] whereby the hypercalcemia might relate to a complex mixture of increases in cell number and rates of hormone secretion per cell. This supposition is hampered by the fact that studies on quantitative PTH release are difficult to perform on the scarcely available normal human parathyroid cells, and that dynamic shifts in secretory set-point seem to occur in vivo during longer alterations in the serum calcium value.[80] While awaiting rapid tests on the extent of functional parathyroid cell derangements, e.g. by intraoperative anti-parathyroid antibody stainings, parathyroid gland size (at least intraindividually) may comprise a practically useful manner of tissue selection. This line of reasoning is strengthened by the possibly lower rate of cell proliferation in small versus more massively enlarged glands. Parathyroid autografts during total parathyroidectomy as well as remnants of tissue during subtotal resection thus should encompass preferentially the smallest parathyroid gland of each individual. Moreover apparently nodulated glands should be avoided in this respect in order to minimize the incidence of recurrence.[66]

The MEN-1 gene has been mapped to chromosome 11q13. In agreement with the two hit theory of hereditary neoplasia the constitutional mutation is unmasked by loss of the wild type allele, which suggests that tumorgenesis relates to inactivation of a suppressor gene at the MEN-1 locus.[81] Similar allelic losses have been found also in subsets of sporadic parathyroid adenomas.[82,83] Mainly large parathyroid adenomas have displayed rearrangement of the PTH gene on chromosome 11p15 and overexpression of the proto-oncogene PRAD1 on 11q13.[84,85] The PRAD1 gene product constitutes the cell cycle-regulating protein cyclin D1, which may be important in the G1-S phase transition that commits cells to divide.[86] Despite the genomic location of PRAD 1 on 11q13 and its role in sporadic parathyroid neoplasia, it is apparently not any major predisposing gene in MEN-1. Secondary mutations in the 11q13 area involving this gene, however, may hypothetically contribute to the characteristically asymmetric parathyroid tumor development of MEN-1. Rare patients with MEN-1 indeed present only a singularly enlarged parathyroid gland associated with parathyroids of overtly normal size.[87,88] Mere excision of such a gland has been accompanied by lower rates of recurrence than in individuals with multiglandular enlargement subjected to more radical procedures of parathyroid operation. This discrepancy suggests the presence of important variations in the propensity for growth of the parathyroid parenchyma in MEN-1, which apparently varies between individuals, between the glands of each individual, as well as within the singular glands themselves.

Current knowledge strongly indicates that the MEN-1 lesion and a major proportion of sporadic parathyroid adenomas are monoclonal tumors. This is consistent with findings upon analysis of X chromosome inactivation.[89] In the multiglandular parathyroid involvement of sporadic and MEN-1-associated primary HPT there is considerable variation in expression of the 500 kDa Ca^{2+} sensor protein. This phenotypic variation is particularly striking between individual chief cell nodules,[68,69] and further substantiates that such homogeneously appearing nodules may represent individual cell clones. The pathological glands of sporadic parathyroid hyperplasia have displayed no monoclonal pattern upon analysis of restriction length polymorphisms.[89] This circumstance, however, cannot be considered to exclude the presence of multiple monoclonal lesions, which indeed has been suggested by recent analysis of X-chromosome inactivation.[90] Similarly the characteristically multiglandular and asymmetric parathyroid enlargement in uremic HPT may represent both monoclonal and polyclonal components together with complex admixtures of vitamin D deficiency and vitamin D resistance. Indeed the larger nodules from patients with hypercalcemia of uremic HPT have displayed clonal allelic losses involving the MEN-1 gene on chromosome 11.[91] This and hitherto unrecognized secondary alterations may contribute to the appearance of very complex and heterogeneous characteristics upon analysis of the pathological parathyroid tissue, and underline the limitations in our current knowledge on mechanisms contributing to the parathyroid cell derangements in HPT.

Parathyroid carcinomas have demonstrated allelic losses of the retinoblastoma gene, which contrasts with the findings in parathyroid adenomas.[92] Moreover increased expression of mRNA for the protooncgenes c-myc and c-fos has been associated with parathyroid cell proliferation,[93] while neither ras nor p53 gene mutations have been implicated in parathyroid tumours.[94] It also is evident that scarce information is available on the actions of growth factors on the human parathyroid tissue. Insulin-like growth factor 1 and its receptor thus seems to be expressed by the parathyroid tissue, and epidermal growth factor may interact in parathyroid cell proliferation.[95,96]

FAMILIAL HYPOCALCIURIC HYPERCALCEMIA

Familial hypocalciuric hypercalcemia (FHH) is an autosomal dominant trait with virtually complete penetrance.[97] The disorder is characterized by increased levels of serum Ca^{2+}, low urinary Ca^{2+} concentrations, often slight hypermagnesemia, but generally normal or only minimally elevated serum PTH concentrations, and normal-sized parathyroid glands.[98,99] The carriers exhibit subtle or no symptoms or signs of complications to the disease. They should not undergo parathyroid surgery and comprise a well recognized cause of failed parathyroid exploration. Biochemical studies in vivo indicate slightly reduced Ca^{2+} sensitivity of the PTH secretion due possibly to a set-point error.[79] The inappropriate tubular Ca^{2+} reabsorption persists after total parathyroidectomy and consequently is independent of PTH and has been related to deficient handling of Hg^{2+} and Ca^{2+} within the medullary thick ascending loop of Henle's.[100] The homozygous form of FHH manifests itself in severe neonatal hypercalcemia immediately after birth.[101] These patients have a striking right-shift in the Ca^{2+} regulated PTH release, largely hyperplastic glands, and benefit from parathyroid surgery. It has been proposed that the derangements of FHH may involve a Ca^{2+} sensor protein.[97,102] By linkage analysis using highly polymorphic DNA probes, the gene for FHH was mapped to chromosome 3q21-24 in four families,[103] i.e. the location of the recently cloned 120 kDa Ca^{2+} binding protein.[58] One FHH family has displayed a mutation in the extracellular domain of this protein, which was accompanied by loss of its $[Ca^{2+}]_i$ regulatory property upon transfection studies and indicates a role for this protein in FHH pathogenesis.[57,58] However other FHH families display linkage with chromosome 19 as well as "non-3, non-19" aberrations supporting that different genes could be responsible for development of this disease.

References

1. Colston KW, Evans IMA, Galante L et al. Regulation of vitamin D metabolism: factors influencing the rate of formation of 1,25-dihydroxycholecalciferol by kidney homogenates. Biochem J 1973; 134: 817-20.
2. Bikle DD, Murphy EW, Rasmussen H. The ionic control of 1,25-dihydroxyvitamin D_3 synthesis in isolated chick renal mitochondria. The role of calcium as influenced by inorganic phosphate and hydrogen ion. J Clin Invest 1975; 55: 299-304.
3. Henry HL, Norman AW. Regulation of 25-hydroxyvitamin D_3-1-hydroxylase in isolated renal mithocondria. Arch Biochem Biophys 1976; 172: 582-9.
4. Matsumoto T, Ikeda K, Morita K et al. Blood Ca^{2+} modulates responsiveness of renal 25(OH)D_3-1-alfa-hydroxylase to PTH in rats. Am J Physiol 1987; 253:E503-7.
5. Habener JF, Rosenblatt M, Potts Jr JT Parathyroid hormone: biochemical aspects of biosynthesis, secretion, action and metabolism. Physiol Rev 1984; 64: 985-1053.
6. Cantley LK, Russel J, Lettieri D et al. 1,25-dihydroxyvitamin D_3 suppresses parathyroid hormone secretion from bovine parathyroid cells in tissue culture. Endocrinology 1985; 117: 2114-9.
7. Farrow SM, Hawa NS, Karmali R et al. Binding of the receptor for 1,25-dihydroxyvitamin D_3 to the 5'-flanking region of the bovine parathyroid hormone gene. J Endocrinol 1990; 126: 355-9.
8. Sherwood LM, Potts Jr JT, Care AD et al. Evaluation by radioimmunoassay of factors controlling the secretion of parathyroid hormone. Nature 1966; 209: 52-5.
9. Brown E. PTH secretion in vivo and in vitro. Regulation by calcium and other secretagogues. Miner Electrolyte Metab 1982; 8: 130-50.
10. Brown EM. Four-parameter model of the sigmoidal relationship between parathyroid hormone release and extracellular calcium concentration in normal and abnormal parathyroid tissue. J Clin Endocrinol Metab 1983; 56: 572-81.
11. Shoback D, Thatcher J, Leombruno R et al. Effects of extracellular Ca^{++} and Mg^{++} on cytosolic Ca^{++} in dispersed bovine parathyroid cells. Endocrinology 1983; 113: 424-6.
12. Ljunghall S, Larsson K, Lindh E et al. Disturbance of basal and stimulated serum levels of intact parathyroid hormone in primary hyperparathyroidism. Surgery 1991; 110: 47-53.
13. Larsson R, Wallfelt C, Abrahamsson H et al. Defective regulation of the cytosolic Ca^{2+} activity in parathyroid cells from patients with hyperparathyroidism. Biosci Rep 1984; 4: 909-15.
14. LeBoff MS, Shoback D, Brown EM et al. Regulation of parathyroid hormone release and cytosolic calcium by extracellular calcium in dispersed and cultured bovine and pathological human parathyroid cells. J Clin Invest 1985; 75: 49-57.
15. Johansson H, Larsson R, Nygren P et al. Cytoplasmic Ca^{2+} concentration of single normal human and bovine parathyroid cells measured by dual wavelength microfluorometry. Biosci Rep 1987; 7: 705-12.
16. Brown EM, Enyedi P, LeBoff M et al. High extracellular Ca^{2+} and Mg^{2+} stimulate accumulation of inositol phosphates in bovine parathyroid cells. FEBS Lett 1987; 218: 113-7.
17. Shoback D, Membreno L, McGhee J. High calcium and other divalent cations increase

inositol triphosphate in bovine parathyroid cells. Endocrinology 1988; 123: 283-9.
18. Kifor O, Brown EM. Relationship between diacylglycerol levels and extracellular Ca^{2+} in dispersed bovine parathyroid cells. Endocrinology 1988; 123: 2723-7.
19. Ridefelt P, Nygren P, Hellman P et al. Regulation of parathyroid hormone release in normal and pathological parathyroid cells exposed to modulators of protein kinase C. Acta Endocrinol 1992; 126: 505-9.
20. Racke FK, Nemeth EF. Cytosolic calcium homeostasis in bovine parathyroid cells and its modulation by protein kinase C. J Physiol 1993; 468: 141-62.
21. Racke FK, Nemeth EF. Protein kinase C modulates hormone secretion regulated by extracellular polycations in bovine parathyroid cells. J Physiol 1993; 468: 163-76.
22. Morrissey JJ, Cohn DV. Regulation of secretion of parathormone and secretory protein-I from separate intracellular pools by calcium, dibutyryl cAMP and (1)-isoproterenol. J Cell Biol 1979; 82: 93-102.
23. Ridefelt P, Hellman P, Rastad J et al. Fluoride interactions with stimulus-secretion coupling of normal and pathological parathyroid cells. Acta Physiol Scand 1992; 145: 275-85.
24. Bruce BR, Anderson Jr NC. Hyperpolarization in mouse parathyroid cells by low calcium. Am J Physiol 1979; 236:nC15-21.
25. Lopez-Barneo J, Armstrong CM. Depolarizing response of rat parathyroid cells to divalent cations. J Gen Physiol 1983; 82: 269-94.
26. Wallfelt C, Larsson R, Johansson H et al. Stimulus-secretion coupling of parathyroid hormone release: Studies of ^{45}Ca and ^{86}Rb fluxes. Acta Physiol Scand 1985; 124: 239-45.
27. Wallace J, Scarpa A. Regulation of parathyroid hormone secretion in vitro by divalent cations and cellular metabolism. J Biol Chem 1982; 257: 10613-9.
28. Gylfe E, Johansson H, Larsson R et al. Activation of Ca^{2+} influx into parathyroid cells by external cation binding. In: Cohn DV, Martin TJ, Meunier PJ, eds. Calcium Regulation and Bone Metabolism: Basic and Clinical Aspects. Amsterdam: Elsevier. 1987: 33-8.
29. Johansson H, Larsson R, Wallfelt C et al. Calcium-agonistic action of Mn^{2+} in the parathyroid cell. Mol Cell Endocrinol 1988; 59: 77-82.
30. Gylfe E, Larsson R, Johansson H et al. Calcium-activated calcium permeability in parathyroid cells. FEBS Lett 1986; 205: 132-5.
31. Nemeth E, Scarpa A. Rapid mobilization of cellular Ca^{2+} in bovine parathyroid cells evoked by extracellular divalent cations. J Biol Chem 1987; 262: 5188-96.
32. Ridefelt P, Hellman P, Ljunggren Ö et al. Ga^{3+} inhibits parathyroid hormone release without interacting with the Ca^{2+} receptor of the parathyroid cell. Biochim Biophys Res Commun 1992; 186: 556-61.
33. Brown E. Extracellular Ca^{2+} sensing, regulation of parathyroid cell function, and role of Ca^{2+} and other ions as extracellular (first) messengers. Physiol Rev 1991; 71: 371-411.
34. Juhlin C, Holmdahl R, Johansson H et al. Monoclonal antibodies with exclusive reactivity against parathyroid cells and tubule cells of the kidney. Proc Natl Acad Sci, USA 1987; 84: 2990-4.
35. Juhlin C, Johansson H, Holmdahl R et al. Monoclonal anti-parathyroid antibodies interfering with a Ca^{2+}-sensor of human parathyroid cells. Biochem Biophys Res Commun 1987; 143: 570-4.
36. Juhlin C, Lundgren S, Johansson H, et al. 500-kilodalton calcium sensor regulating cytoplasmic Ca^{2+} in cytotrophoblast cells of human placenta. J Biol Chem 1990; 265: 8275-9.
37. Nygren P, Gylfe E, Larsson R et al. Modulation of the Ca^{2+}-sensing function of parathyroid cells in vitro and in hyperparathyroidism. Biochim Biophys Acta 1988; 968: 253-60.
38. Johansson H, Larsson R, Juhlin C et al. Interaction of monoclonal antiparathyroid antibody with Ca^{2+} agonistic actions of Mn^{2+} in normal human parathyroid cells. Cell Calcium 1989; 10: 11-5.
39. Hellman P, Ridefelt P, Juhlin C et al. Parathyroid-like regulation of parathyroid hormone-related protein release and cytoplasmic calcium in cytotrophoblast cells of

human placenta. Arch Biochem Biophys 1992; 293: 174-80.

40. Hellman P, Hellman B, Juhlin C et al. Regulation of proliferation in JEG-3 cells by a 500-kDa Ca^{2+} sensor and parathyroid hormone-related protein. Arch Biochem Biophys 1993; 307: 379-85.
41. Lundgren S, Hjälm G, Hellman P et al. A protein involved in calcium sensing of the human parathyroid, and placental cytotrphoblast belongs to the LDL-receptor protein superfamily. Exp Cell Res 1994; 212:344-350.
42. Raychowdhury R, Niles JL, McCluskey RT et al. Autoimmune target in Heymann nephritis is a glycoprotein with homology to the LDL receptor. Science 1989; 244: 1163-5.
43. Lundgren S, Hellman P, Juhlin C et al. Messenger RNA and protein expression and sequence analysis of a 500 kDa glycoprotein with calcium sensing properties. J Bone Miner Res 1994;9(suppl):S342 (Abstr.)
44. Heymann W, Hackel DB, Harwood S et al. Production of nephrotic syndrome in rats by Freund's adjuvants and rat kidney suspension. Proc Soc Exp Biol Med 1959; 100: 660-4.
45. Edgington TS, Glasscock RJ, Dixon FJ. Autologous immune-complex pathogenesis of experimental allergic glomerulonephritis. Science 1967; 155: 1432-4.
46. Christensen EI, Gliemann J, Moestrup SK. Renal tubule gp330 is a calcium binding receptor for endocytic uptake of protein. J Histochem Cytochem 1992; 40: 1481-90.
47. Öhlin AK, Linse S, Stenflo J. Calcium binding to the epidermal growth factor homology region of bovine protein C. J Biol Chem 1988; 263: 7411-7.
48. Öhlin AK, Landes G, Bourdan P et al. β-hydroxyaspartic acid in the first epidermal growth factor-like domain of protein C. Its role in Ca^{2+} binding and biological activity. J Biol Chem 1988; 263: 19240-19248.
49. Huang LH, Ke X-H, Sweeny W et al. Calcium binding and putative activity of the epidermal growth factor domain of blood coagulation factor IX. Biochem Biophys Res Commun 1989; 160: 133-9.
50. Persson E, Selander M, Linse S et al. Calcium binding to the isolated β-hydroxyaspartic acid-containing epidermal growth factor-like domain of bovine factor X. J Biol Chem 1989; 264: 16897-904.
51. Handford PA, Baron M, Mayhew M et al. The first EGF-like domain from human factor IX contains a high-affinity calcium binding site. EMBO J 1990; 9: 475-80.
52. Selander-Sunnerhagen M, Ullner M, Persson C et al. How an epidermal growth factor (EGF)-like domain binds calcium. High resolution NMR structure of the calcium form of the NH2-terminal EGF-like domain in coagulation factor X. J Biol Chem 1992; 267: 19642-9.
53. Rebay I, Fleming RJ, Felion RG et al. Specific EGF repeats of Notch mediate interactions with Delta and Serrate: Implications for Notch as a multifunctional receptor. Cell 1991; 67: 687-99.
54. Furukawa T, Ozawa M, Huang R-P, Muramatsu T. A heparin binding protein whose expression increases during differentiation of embryonal carcinoma cells to parietal endoderm cells: cDNA cloning and sequence analysis. J Biochem 1990; 108: 297-302.
55. Pietromonaco S, Kerjaschki D, Binder S et al. Molecular cloning of a cDNA encoding a major pathogenic domain of the Heymann nephritis antigen gp330. Proc Natl Acad Sci, USA 1990; 87: 1811-5.
56. Strickland DK, Ashcom JD, Williams S et al. Primary structure of α_2-macroglobulin receptor-associated protein. J Biol Chem 1991; 266: 13364-9.
57. Brown EM, Gamba G, Riccardi D et al. Cloning and characterization of an extracellular Ca^{2+}-sensing receptor from bovine parathyroid. Nature 1993; 366: 575-80.
58. Pollak MR, Brown EM, Wu Chou Y-H et al. Mutations in the human Ca^{2+}-sensing receptor gene cause familial hypocalciuric hypercalcemia and neonatal severe hyperparathyroidism. Cell 1993; 75: 1297-303.
59. Lin HY, Harris TL, Flannry MS et al. Expression cloning of an adenylate cyclase-coupled calcitonin receptor. Science 1991; 254: 1022-4.
60. Stroop SD, Thompson DL, Kuestner RE et al. A recombinant human calcitonin recep-

tor functions as an extracellular calcium sensor. J Biol Chem 1993; 268: 19927-30.
61. Brown EM, Gardner DG, Brennan MF et al. Calcium-regulated parathyroid hormone release in primary hyperparathyroidism: Studies in vitro with dispersed parathyroid cells. Am J Med 1979; 66: 923-31.
62. Wallfelt C, Gylfe E, Larsson R et al. Relationship between external and cytoplasmic calcium concentrations, parathyroid hormone release and weight of parathyroid glands in human hyperparathyroidism. J Endocrinol 1988; 116: 457-64.
63. Wallfelt C, Ljunghall S, Bergström R et al. Clinical characteristics and surgical treatment of sporadic primary hyperparathyroidism with emphasis on chief cell hyperplasia. Surgery 1990; 107: 13-9.
64. Brown EM, Brennan MF, Hurwitz S et al. Dispersed cells prepared from human parathyroid glands: Distinct calcium sensitivity of adenomas vs. primary hyperplasia. J Clin Endocrinol Metab 1978; 46: 267-75.
65. Benson L, Rastad J, Ljunghall S et al. Parathyroid hormone release in vitro in hyperparathyroidism associated with multiple endocrine neoplasia type 1. Acta Endocrinol 1987; 114: 12-6.
66. Wallfelt C, Larsson R, Gylfe E et al. Secretory disturbance in hyperplastic parathyroid nodules of uremic hyperparathyroidism: Implications for parathyroid autotransplantation. World J Surg 1988; 12: 431-6.
67. Juhlin C, Klareskog L, Nygren P et al. Hyperparathyroidism is associated with reduced expression of a parathyroid calcium receptor mechanism defined by monoclonal antiparathyroid antibodies. Endocrinology 1988; 122: 2999-3001.
68. Juhlin C, Rastad J, Klareskog L et al. Parathyroid histology and cytology with monoclonal antibodies recognizing a calcium sensor of parathyroid cells. Am J Pathol 1989; 135: 321-8.
69. Bjerneroth G, Juhlin C, Grimelius L et al. Improvement in histological diagnosis of primary hyperparathyroidism with a monoclonal antiparathyroid antibody. Endocr Pathol 1992; 3: 83-92.
70. Karmali R, Farrow S, Hewison M et al. Effects of 1,25-dihydroxyvitamin D_3 and cortisol on bovine and human parathyroid cells. J Endocrinol 1989; 123: 137-41.
71. Brown AJ, Dusso A, Lopez-Hilker S et al. 1,25-$(OH)_2D_3$ receptors are decreased in parathyroid glands from chronically uremic dogs. Kidney Int 1989; 35: 19-23.
72. MacDonald PN, Ritter C, Brown AJ et al. Retinoic acid suppresses parathyroid hormone (PTH) secretion and preproPTH mRNA levels in bovine parathyroid cell culture. J Clin Invest 1994; 93: 725-30.
73. Brandi ML, Fitzpatrick LA, Coon HG et al. Bovine parathyroid cells: Cultures maintained for more than 140 population doublings. Proc Natl Acad Sci USA 1986; 83: 1709-13.
74. Sakaguchi K, Santora A, Zimering M et al. Functional epithelial cell line cloned from rat parathyroid glands. Proc Natl Acad Sci, USA 1987; 84: 3269-73.
75. Nygren P, Larsson R, Johansson H et al. 1,25$(OH)_2D_3$ inhibits hormone secretion and proliferation but not functional dedifferentiation of cultured bovine parathyroid cells. Calcif Tissue Int 1988; 43: 213-8.
76. Nygren P, Larsson R, Johansson H et al. Inhibition of cell growth retains the differentiated function of bovine parathyroid cells in monolayer culture. Bone Miner 1988; 4: 123-32.
77. Brandi M-L, Aurbach GD, Fitzpatrick LA et al. Parathyroid mitogenic activity in plasma from patients with familial multiple endocrine neoplasia type 1. N Engl J Med 1986; 314: 1287-93.
78. Parfitt AM, Willgoss D, Jacobi J et al. Cell kinetics in parathyroid adenomas: evidence for decline in rates of cell birth and tumour growth, assuming clonal origin. Clin Endocrinol 1991; 35: 151-7.
79. Khosla S, Ebeling PR, Firek AF et al. Calcium infusion suggests a "set-point" abnormality of parathyroid gland function in familial benign hypercalcemia and more complex disturbances in primary hyperparathyroidism. J Clin Endocrinol Metab 1993; 76: 715-20.
80. Graf W, Rastad J, Åkerström G et al. Dynamics of parathyroid hormone release

and serum calcium regulation after surgery for primary hyperparathyroidism. World J Surg 1992; 16: 625-31.
81. Byström C, Larsson C, Blomberg C et al. Localization of the gene for multiple endocrine neoplasia type 1 to a small region within chromosome 11q13 by deletion mapping in tumors. Proc Natl Acad Sci, USA 1990; 87: 1968-72.
82. Thakker RV, Bouloux P, Wooding C et al. Association of parathyroid tumors in multiple endocrine neoplasia type 1 with loss of alleles on chromosome 11. N Engl J Med 1989; 321: 218-24.
83. Friedman E, de Marco L, Gejman PV et al. Allelic loss from chromosome 11 in parathyroid tumors. Cancer Res 1992; 52: 6804-9.
84. Arnold A, Kim HG, Gaz RD et al. Molecular cloning and chromosomal mapping of DNA rearranged with the parathyroid hormone gene in parathyroid adenoma. J Clin Invest 1989; 83: 2034-40.
85. Rosenberg CL, Kim HG, Shows TB et al. Rearrangement and overexpression of D11S287E, a candidate oncogene on chromosome 11q13 in benign parathyroid tumors. Oncogene 1991; 6: 449-53.
86. Motokura T, Bloom T, Kim HG et al. A novel cyclin encoded by a bcl1-linked candidate oncogene. Nature 1991; 350: 512-5.
87. Hellman P, Skogseid B, Juhlin C et al. Findings and long-term results of parathyroid surgery in multiple endocrine neoplasia type 1. World J Surg 1992; 16: 718-23.
88. Kraimps JL, Duh QY, Demeure M et al. Hyperparathyroidism in multiple endocrine neoplasia syndrome. Surgery 1992; 112: 1080-6.
89. Arnold A, Staunton CE, Kim HG et al. Monoclonality and abnormal parathyroid hormone genes in parathyroid adenomas. N Engl J Med 1988; 318: 658-62.
90. Arnold A, Brown M, Urena P et al. X-inactivation analysis of clonality in primary and secondary parathyroid hyperplasia. J Bone Miner Res 1992; 7 (suppl 1): S153 (Abstr).
91. Falchetti A, Bale AE, Amorosi A et al. Progression of uremic hyperparathyroidism involves allelic loss on chromosome 11. J Clin Endocrinol Metab 1993; 76: 139-44.
92. Cryns V, Thor A, Xu HJ et al. Loss of the retinoblastoma tumor-supressor gene in parathyroid carcinoma. N Engl J Med 1994; 330: 757-61.
93. Kremer R, Bolivar I, Goltzman D et al. Influence of calcium and 1,25-dihydroxycholecalciferol on proliferation and proto-oncogene expression in primary cultures of bovine parathyroid cells. Endocrinology 1989; 125: 935-41.
94. Friedman E, Bale AE, Marx SJ et al. Genetic abnormalities in sporadic parathyroid adenomas. J Clin Endocrinol Metab 1990; 71: 293-7.
95. Tanaka R, Tsushima T, Kawakami M et al. Insulin-like growth factor-1 receptors and insulin-like growth factor-binding protein in human parathyroid tumors. World J Surg, in press.
96. Duh Q-Y, Gum ET, Sancho JJ et al. Epidermal growth factor receptors in parathyroid tumors. J Surg Res 1986; 40: 569-73.
97. Marx SJ. Familial hypocalciuric hypercalcemia. In: Favus MJ, ed. Primer on Metabolic Bone Diseases and Disorders of Mineral Metabolism. Richmond, VA: William Byrd Press. 1990: 113-5.
98. Marx SJ, Attie MF, Levine MA et al. The hypocalciuric or benign variant of familial hypercalcemia: clinical and biochemical features in fifteen kindreds. Medicine 1981; 60: 397-412.
99. Law Jr WM, Heath III H. Familial benign hypercalcemia (hypocalciuric hypercalcemia). Clinical and pathogenetic studies in 21 families. Ann Intern Med 1985; 102: 511-9.
100. Attie MF, Grill Jr JR, Stock JL et al. Urinary calcium excretion in familial hypocalciuric hypercalcemia: persistence of relative hypocalciuria after induction of hypoparathyroidism. J Clin Invest 1983; 72: 667-76.
101. Marx SJ, Attie MF, Spiegel AM et al. An association between neonatal severe primary hyperparathyroidism and familial hypocalciuric hypercalcemia in three kindreds. N Engl J Med 1982; 306: 257-64.
102. Marx SJ, Spiegel AM, Brown EM et al.

Familial hypocalciuric hypercalcemia. In: deLuca HF, Anast CS. Pediatric Diseases related to Calcium. New York, N.Y: Elsevier North Holland Inc. 1980: 413-26.

103. Chou Y-HW, Brown EM, Levi T et al. The gene responsible for familial hypocalciuric hypercalcemia maps to chromosome 3q in four unrelated families. Nature Genet 1992; 1: 295-300.

CHAPTER 3

PARATHYROID PATHOLOGY

Göran Åkerström, Lars Grimelius

The details of parathyroid pathology have continued to intrigue surgeons and pathologists involved in the treatment of hyperparathyroidism, and inadequately defined diagnostic criteria have generated considerable argument concerning the surgical management of the different varieties of the disease.

During the early years of parathyroid surgery adenoma was the predominant pathological entity, and if more than one enlarged gland was identified in a patient with primary hyperparathyroidism (HPT) it was thought generally to represent multiple adenoma. The exception was water clear cell hyperplasia, which was described in 1934 by Albright et al, who considered that this entity resulted from some form of external glandular stimulation.[1] Parathyroid chief cell hyperplasia was recognized by Cope et al in 1958, and was believed to have similar genesis, also because the histopathological features appeared much the same as in patients with HPT secondary to uremia.[2] However, many of the patients with primary parathyroid chief cell hyperplasia in the early series displayed either a family history or were affected by endocrinopathies later known to be part of a multiple endocrine neoplasia type 1 (MEN-1) syndrome.[2] The distinction between adenoma and hyperplasia has even nowadays continued to present difficulties, and many surgeons have been particularly indecisive about the value of an intraoperative histopathological examination. The surgical strategy thus commonly has been based on the gross features of the glands, as they are revealed at operation, and the principal histological entities have often been classified as uniglandular or multiglandular disease, rather than adenoma and hyperplasia. Better precision in diagnosis and treatment will, however, be obtained if the histopathological criteria for these different lesions are appreciated.

NORMAL PARATHYROID GLANDS

MACROSCOPIC FEATURES

Normal parathyroid glands characteristically exhibit a light yellowish to brownish color, which serves to distinguish them from surrounding

Current Controversy in Parathyroid Operation and Reoperation,
edited by Göran Åkerström.

fat or a neighboring thyroid.[3] The color may be more reddish-brown in glands with a lower content of stromal fat cells. The glands are soft in consistency, but still slightly more solid and thereby generally well delineated from the surrounding fat tissue. Most glands are oval or bean shaped, but may occasionally be round or considerably elongated, and sometimes also multilobated or flattened out into thin leaf-like structures[3] (Fig. 3.1). Owing to the variable shape of the glands their diameters vary, but a normal gland often measures approximately 5 x 4 x 2 mm. The weight of a gland is a more appropriate estimate of its size, and therefore constitutes a more valuable diagnostic parameter. The weights of normal glands are known to vary considerably, both within and between individuals, and have been reported to range from only a few mg to maximally 70 mg.[4,5] Autopsy studies have revealed an average of 30-40 mg for the weights of normal glands, with slightly higher values for inferior than superior ones.[4,5] As glandular weight includes also stromal fat cells, the histopathological evaluation should be more appropriate if the amount of functioning parenchyma, i.e. the parenchymal cell weights of the glands are considered.[4,5] Such estimates may be roughly calculated from the glandular weight

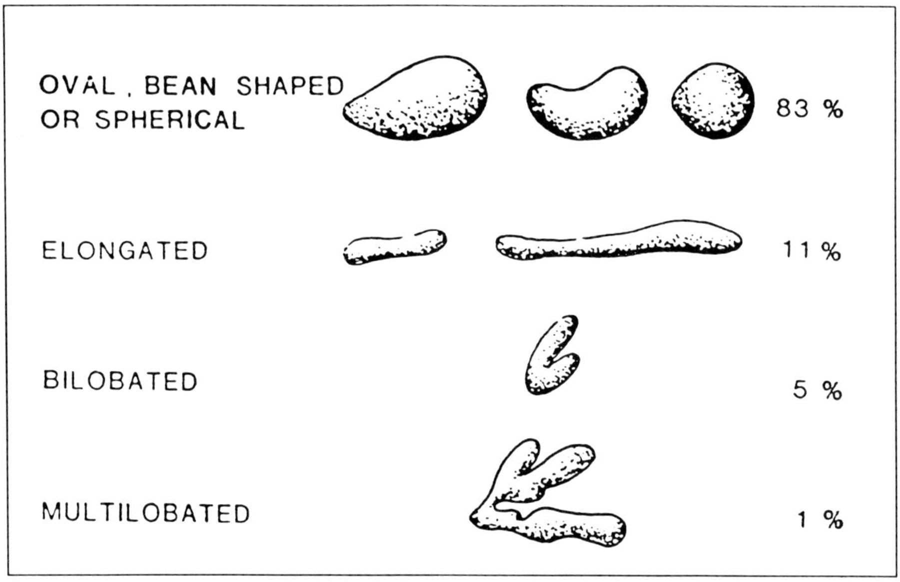

Fig. 3.1. Different shapes of parathyroid glands and their frequencies. Reprinted with permission from Åkerström et al.[3]

Table 3.1. Individual total gland and parenchymal cell weights (mg) of normal human parathyroid glands[5]

		Single Gland	Largest Gland	All Glands
Glandular weight	Mean	31	41	122
	Upper limit[a]	59	72	208
Parenchymal weight	Mean	22	28	87
	Upper limit[a]	39	49	144

[a] Upper 95% limit of the frequency distribution.

and microscopic evaluation of the distribution of parenchymal versus fat cells in representative light microscopy sections of the gland. The average parenchymal cell weight of a normal gland has been estimated in autopsy studies to be 22 mg, and the maximal weight to be 39 mg.[5] The total parathyroid glandular weight, i.e. the sum weight of all parathyroid glands in one person averages 122 mg, while the corresponding total parenchymal cell weight has been estimated to be 87 mg[5] (Table 3.1). The maximal total glandular weight amounts normally to 208 mg, and the corresponding maximal parenchymal weight to 144 mg.[5] Even if these weights generally have little influence on the histopathological evaluation of parathyroid glands, merely a rough appreciation of the limits may often aid in determining the nature of an equivocal lesion.

Histology

A normal parathyroid gland consists of parenchymal cells, sparse stroma, and intermingled fat cells (Fig. 3.2). Pathologists often have paid attention to the amount of fat cells, and have generally interpreted a low fat cell content as a sign of hyperplasia. However, the fat content also depends on age and constitutional factors, so that prior to adolescence the glands usually contain a minimal amount of fat cells, but after 30 years of age the fat occupies up to 30% of the glandular volume.[5,6] The number of fat cells will also generally be considerably increased in obese individuals, while the parathyroids of lean or cachectic persons may be almost devoid of fat cells.[5] The evaluation of the content of fat cells in histological sections is furthermore often difficult because of uneven distribution within the glands, with a tendency to concentration of fat cells to one or a few areas, often in the vicinity of a glandular pole.[6,7]

The parenchymal cells of normal parathyroid glands are mainly of the chief cell type.[6] Oxyphil and transitional oxyphil cells occur very sparsely in younger individuals, but their proportion increases to about 5% at the age of 80 years.[6,8] These cells also tend to increase in number in patients with subclinical renal impairment and will generally become numerous in renal failure of longer duration.[8,9] When the oxyphil cells are prevalent they often have a tendency to assemble into more or less circumscribed nodules, which may be an early indication of parathyroid abnormality.[8,9] The parenchymal cells of normal parathyroid glands are often arranged into trabecular or irregular strands separated by dispersed individual fat cells or groups of such cells.[6] Almost all chief cells of these glands characteristically contain numerous cytoplasmic fat droplets, with a size slightly smaller than the cell nucleus. This cytoplasmic fat may be visualized with the "Oil red O" method, and is considered to reflect the endocrine activity of the glands.[10]

PRIMARY HYPERPARATHYROIDISM

Primary HPT may be caused by adenoma, hyperplasia or rarely occurring parathyroid carcinoma. Essentially due to lack of generally accepted histopathological criteria, the reported incidence of adenoma versus hyperplasia in primary HPT has varied considerably, and this has caused uncertainty about the adequacy of the histopathological diagnosis.[11] When more distinct criteria have been applied, however, approximately 80-90% of the patients with primary HPT have harbored adenoma,

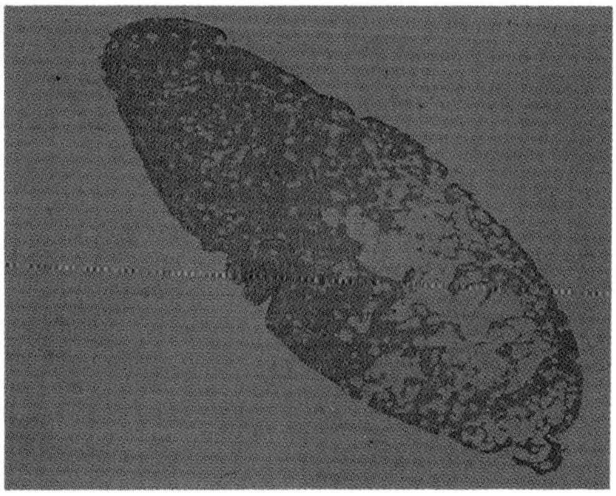

Fig. 3.2. A normal-sized parathyroid gland with uneven distribution of fat cells

and the remaining have had hyperplasia, almost invariably of the chief cell type.[12-14] Water clear cell hyperplasia has remained an unusual entity, and has during the recent decades become even more rare.[12,15] Parathyroid carcinoma should affect less than 1% of the patients with primary HPT.[12] (See chapter 10).

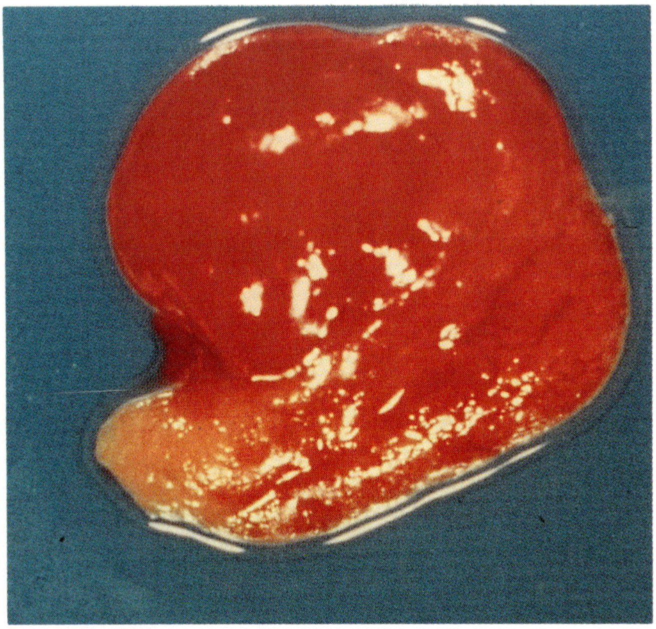

Fig. 3.3. A tiny parathyroid adenoma with a light brownish-colored glandular part, representing the normal glandular remnant. Reprinted with permission from Åkerström et al.[124]

Adenoma

The size of parathyroid adenomas has varied considerably, with weights ranging from less than 100 mg to more than 100 g, although weights of around 300-1000 mg have been the most common in our experience. The size of the adenoma tends to correlate to some extent with the degree of hypercalcemia and also roughly with the parathyroid hormone (PTH) values of the patients.[16-18] An adenoma is characteristically reddish-brown and displays a somewhat firmer consistency than a normal parathyroid gland, but is still more homogenous and soft than thyroid tissue or lymph nodes. Sometimes a tiny brown-yellowish cap may be grossly visible on the surface of the adenoma, and may represent the remnant of normal parathyroid tissue from which the adenoma has evolved (Figs. 3.3 and 3.4). Selection of tissue for frozen section diagnosis should aim to include this remnant, and may be facilitated if the surgeon marks the remnant or the vascular stalk

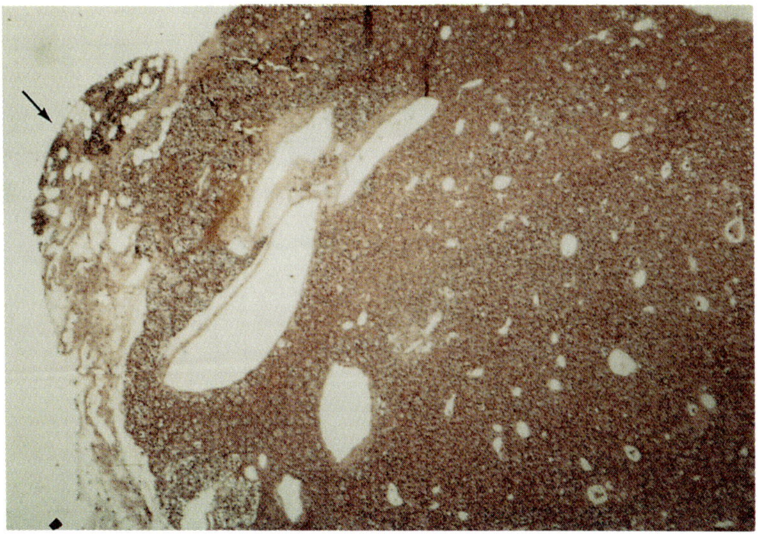

Fig. 3.4. Parathyroid adenoma with a rim of normal fat cell rich glandular tissue in the periphery (arrow). Reprinted with permission from Åkerström et al.[124]

of the gland, since the adenoma vessels often attach where the normal remnant is situated.[18] The shape of parathyroid adenomas is often kidney-like, oval or rounded, but may sometimes be flattened or elongated and occasionally even lobulated or multinodular.[12] It is surrounded by a thin fibrous capsule, which generally permits easy dissection from the adjacent tissue.

The histological architecture is variable, some adenomas consist of solid cell masses, while others are trabecular or nodular or usually exhibit a mixture of different patterns. In some adenomas a multinodular growth pattern indicates the presence of separate clones of cells with distinct arrangement, which indeed may mimic nodular chief cell hyperplasia.[19-21] Occasional adenomas display a predominantly follicular structure, and may thus be difficult to distinguish from thyroid tissue, as even colloid content may be present within the follicles[21] (Fig. 3.5). Rare adenomas contain amyloid deposits, which if extensive may raise suspicion of medullary thyroid carcinoma.[22] Fat cells are generally virtually absent in adenomas, and only rare lesions exhibit more numerous fat cells.[20,21] In approximately 50% of the adenomas a remnant of histologically normal, fat cell-rich, "atrophic" glandular tissue may be histologically visible outside the adenoma capsule, and cells in this remnant will appear uniform in size and invariably smaller than the adenoma cells[20,21,23,24] (Fig. 3.4). Visualization of this remnant is valuable as it constitutes one of the classical *"adenoma criteria"*, being suggestive of adenomatous rather than hyperplastic disease. Chief cells predominate in the majority of parathyroid adenomas, but a mixture of oxyphil or transitional oxyphil cells is common, and these cells may be diffusely scattered or may infrequently form circumscribed nodules. Adenomatous chief cells are generally larger than the chief cells of normal glands, and tend to display increased and more variable nuclear size.[25,26] Occasional adenomas exhibit pronounced nuclear pleomorphism, including giant and multiple nuclei, and this constitutes another of the so called "adenoma criteria", which may be of help in distinguishing the adenoma from a hyperplastic gland.[27-30] The chief cells of parathyroid adenomas characteristically contain reduced content of cytoplasmic fat, and only in a minority of adenomas larger amounts of such fat are

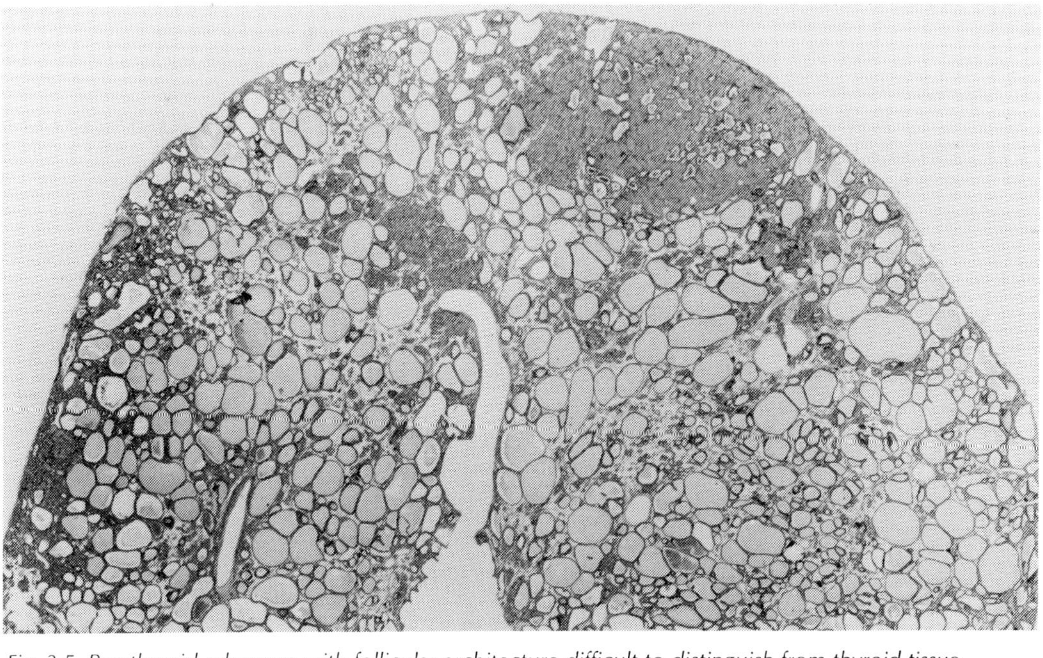

Fig. 3.5. Parathyroid adenoma with follicular architecture difficult to distinguish from thyroid tissue.

seen in the chief cells, either focally or diffusely spread.[10,18,31,32]

Double adenomas may occur in 1-2% of patients with primary HPT; some authors have described higher figures and even triple adenomas, but many of these cases probably represent pronounced asymetrical involvement in nodular chief cell hyperplasia.[23,29,33-38] The majority of multiple adenomas seem to occur asynchronously, and may then be the cause of recurrent HPT in patients previously operated on with excision of solitary adenomas.[14]

Occasional adenomas are composed almost exclusively of oxyphil cells, and although some of these tumors are non-functioning, at least 3-8% of all adenomas associated with primary HPT have been classified as *oxyphil cell adenoma.*[39-42]

Rare so called *lipoadenomas* contain an abundance of adipous and/or myxoid stroma, with only scattered nests or cords of parenchyma. Grossly these lesions will exhibit a more yellowish-tan color, and they can evidently attain a considerable size. Some lipoadenomas are associated with clinically detectable HPT, and others are apparently non-functioning.[43-47]

Normal glands associated with adenoma

The normal parathyroid glands associated with adenoma characteristically exhibit similar histologic features as the parathyroids of euparathyroid individuals. Many of these glands have lower parenchymal weight and contain more numerous fat cells than the completely normal glands.[48,49] They also generally exhibit an abundance of cytoplasmic fat reflecting a lower endocrine activity, and electronmicroscopic investigation of such glands have revealed signs of secretory inactivity.[10,18,31,50] Occasionally, however, these glands may contain nodules of chief or oxyphil cells, indicating abnormality within multiple glands.[14]

Parathyroid Hyperplasia

Parathyroid hyperplasia has long been considered to result from some yet unidentified stimulation, affecting all parathyroid glands of an individual.[1] This should most likely cause diffuse hyperplasia with uniformly enlarged glands, which however, is unusual in patients with primary HPT, who more frequently display markedly uneven glandular enlargement. Two pathological entities of parathyroid hyperplasia are encountered, the more common chief cell hyperplasia and the rare water clear cell hyperplasia.

Chief Cell Hyperplasia

The glands of chief cell hyperplasia are usually affected very assymetrically, and greatly enlarged glands often coexist with normal sized ones.[13,14,16,19-21,24,30,33,51-55] There are generally some but vague relations between the extent of glandular enlargement and the level of hypercalcemia and raised PTH values in the patients with chief cell hyperplasia.[16,56] Individuals with more severe hypercalcemia or more extensively enlarged glands due to nodular chief cell hyperplasia should be expected to suffer from a MEN-1 syndrome.[13] In cases without the MEN-1 association the proportional incidence of chief cell hyperplasia has been inversely related to the degree of hypercalcemia, and thus most commonly revealed in individuals with only moderately raised serum calcium values.[13,16,56] Occasionally the glandular enlargement is only slight and the presence of micronodular hyperplasia is merely recognized microscopically, but this probably largely represents subclinical rather than clinical disease.[8,57,58] At gross examination the larger glands in chief cell hyperplasia will generally appear indistinguishable from adenomas.

The cellular arrangement in chief cell hyperplasia varies between and within the glands.[21,31,33,51-56] Diffusely hyperplastic areas with solid cell masses may be seen (Fig. 3.6), although a nodular and more variable pattern is considerably more common (Fig. 3.7). Hyperplastic nodules may lack encapsulation, and are then evident by variation in cell type or cellular architecture, but individual nodules may also be limited by a compressed stroma, creating the appearance of fibrous encapsulation. Trabecular, acinar

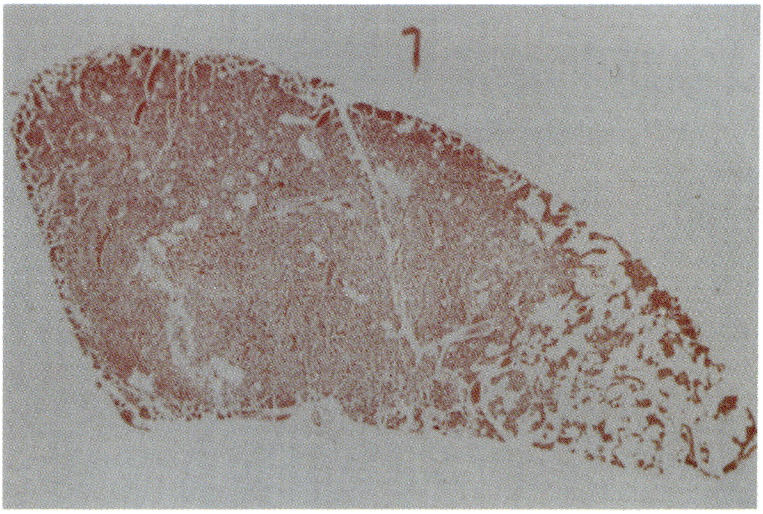

Fig. 3.6. Enlarged, diffusely hyperplastic parathyroid gland with fat cells still remaining at the glandular pole.

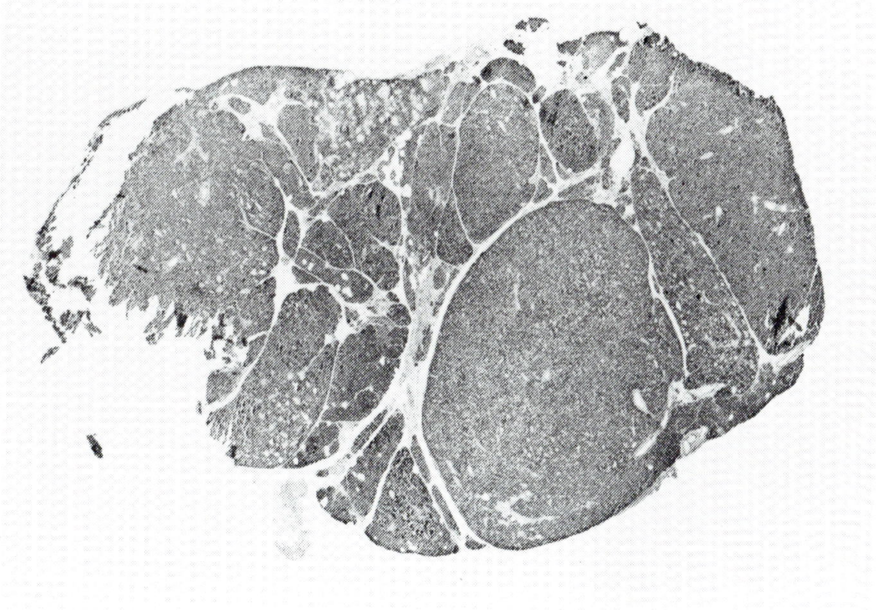

Fig. 3.7. Parathyroid gland exhibiting nodular chief cell hyperplasia.

as well as follicular components may be recognized in these nodules. Occasionally a hyperplastic gland is dominated by a single nodule, which may mimic or actually represent an adenoma occurring in a background of micronodular hyperplasia.[23,59] The micronodular hyperplasia may also focally involve only part of a gland, and the remaining, unaffected glandular part may appear with normal amount and distribution of fat cells. More commonly the involvement of individual glands is irregular but more or less universal. In between nodules may be encountered areas of diffuse hyperplasia, or compressed normal, fat cell-rich tissue, which may resemble the rim of normal parathyroid tissue considered as a criterion for adenoma[12,20,21,24,54,60-62]

(Fig. 3.8). The chief cells of hyperplastic glands are generally increased in size and exhibit larger nuclei than the chief cells of normal parathyroid glands, and slight variation in nuclear size, as well as occasional mitotic figures may be encountered.[60,63] Chief cells generally predominate, but oxyphil and transitional oxyphil cells are often present, sometimes in abundance, and large clear cells may be seen focally. Chief cells of the nodules often contain little or almost no cytoplasmic lipid.[10,18,31]

In rare cases of diffuse *lipohyperplasia* an abundance of stromal fat cells may occur, and the glands may appear almost completely composed of fat cells.[64] There may also be conspicuous nodules of parenchymal cells occurring in this fat rich tissue, and we have encountered this condition in association with clinical HPT.

Water Clear Cell Hyperplasia

Water clear cell hyperplasia differs from the more common chief cell hyperplasia by having a male rather than female predominance, and by being accompanied generally by more severe clinical symptoms and more pronounced hypercalcemia.[15,21,33,51,53,65] The glands of water clear cell hyperplasia are usually markedly and asymmetrically enlarged. Moreover, the glands tend to be irregular in shape and exhibit characteristic indentations and pseudopod-like extensions as well as characteristic dark brown to chocolate brown color. The water clear cells predominate in these glands and fat, chief cells and oxyphil cells are more or less absent. The growth pattern may be solid, acinar and trabecular or a mixture of these patterns. The water clear cells are polygonal in shape, with a distinct cell membrane and a huge cytoplasm which looks empty in lower magnification. Ultrastructurally the cytoplasm appears filled with vacuoles. Cytoplasmic lipid is not found in these cells.[18] The cell nuclei are usually relatively small and uniform in size, tend to be located peripherally in the cell cytoplasm, and exhibit dense chromatin patterns. Only some of the cells are multinucleated. Cystic degeneration can occur in these glands.[33]

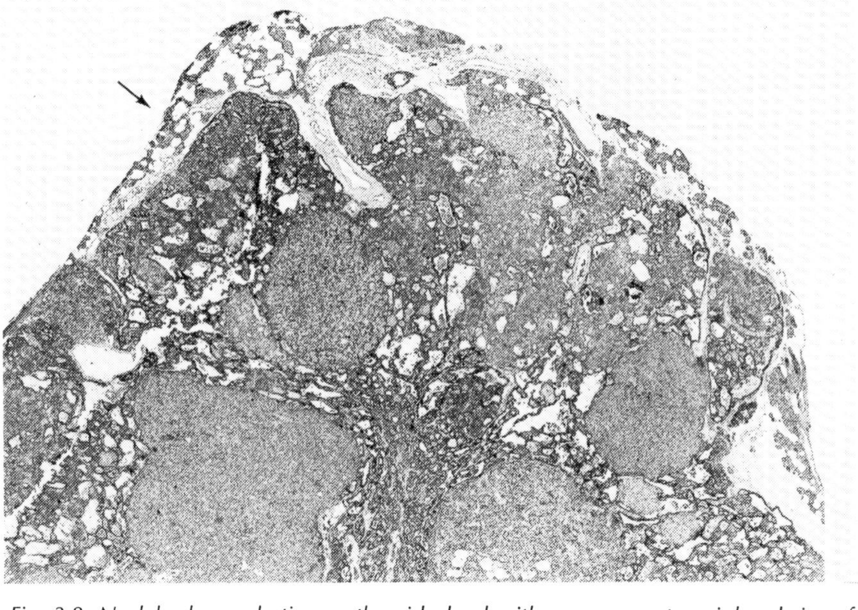

Fig. 3.8. Nodular hyperplastic parathyroid gland with an apparent peripheral rim of normal tissue (arrow).

CYSTIC PARATHYROID LESIONS

Degenerative changes which may occur in adenomas and more rarely in individual hyperplastic glands may result in cystic parathyroid lesions.[33-35,66-71] Such cystic lesions are rare, however, and only infrequently encountered in patients with clinically detected HPT.[34,35,66-71] Cysts of branchial cleft origin may assume a considerable size and mimic a growing thyroid nodule or a mediastinal mass.[70,71] These cysts are generally non-functioning, and rarely associated with clinical parathyroid disease. The diagnosis of cystic lesions may be obtained by fine needle aspiration of typically water-like fluid containing high concentration of PTH.[71]

SECONDARY HPT

Secondary parathyroid hyperplasia occurs as a common and possibly inevitable result of chronic renal insufficiency. It has long been considered as an adaptive response to a commonly prevailing hypocalcemia, secondary to phosphate retention in renal failure.[72] However, signs of parathyroid stimulation may be revealed early in renal disease, often prior to any notable changes in serum calcium and phosphate.[73,74] The development and progression of secondary HPT have therefore more recently been related principally to reduced synthesis of $1,25(OH)_2D_3$, leading to inappropriate feed-back control of the parathyroids, with inadequate suppression of both hormone secretion and proliferation.[74-76] The decreased $1,25(OH)_2D_3$ levels and hyperphosphatemia at later stages of the renal disease also contribute to a relative skeletal resistance to the peripheral actions of PTH, which together with reduced intestinal calcium absorption may indeed cause a negative calcium balance and a state of chronic hypocalcemia.[77] Although secondary HPT occurs by far most commonly in association with renal disorders, it may also be observed in other conditions leading to hypocalcemia and/or vitamin D deficiency, such as malabsorption.[78]

High incidence of micronodular chief cell hyperplasia has been demonstrated by autopsy in an elderly population, and related to decreased levels of $1,25(OH)_2D_3$, which in these age groups is common, even in the absence of significant renal impairment.[8] The histopathological changes may occur as single or multiple apparently clonal lesions in otherwise completely normal glands (Fig. 3.9). Contrasting to this is the finding in individuals with slight renal impairment, where the parathyroid glands appear to increase more or less uniformly in size, due mainly to diffuse parathyroid hyperplasia.[9,79] In more severe and prolonged renal insufficiency the parathyroid

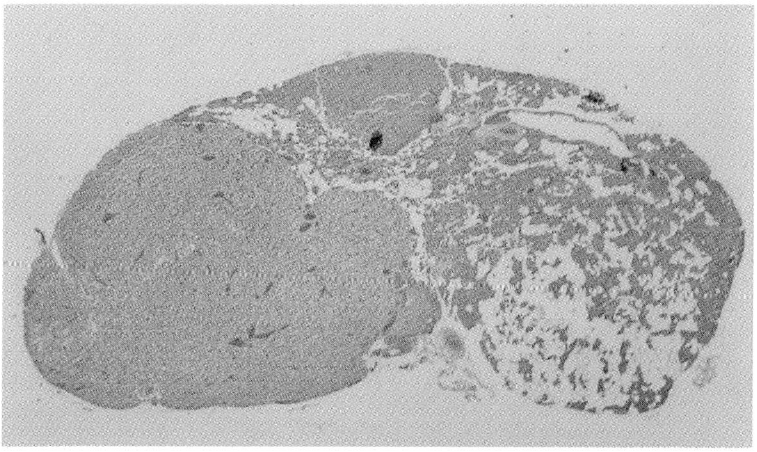

Fig. 3.9. Minimally enlarged parathyroid gland with focal areas of nodular hyperplasia. Reprinted with permission from Åkerström et al.[124]

glands tend to exhibit increasingly abnormal morphological features, with more considerably raised weights and also pronounced nodularity, comprising both chief and/or oxyphil cells[9,79,80] (Fig. 3.10). Chief cells tend to predominate in these secondary hyperplastic glands, but oxyphil and transitional oxyphil cells are often numerous, and their number increases with the degree of renal impairment.[9,79-81] The fat cells are generally sparse, but may be more frequent in individuals with slighter glandular enlargement, and in obese individuals. The cytoplasmic fat content of the chief cells is often markedly reduced or absent.

During further progression of the parathyroid disease in renal failure, one or a few nodules, which have acquired more pronounced growth potential, will frequently become predominant[9,82] (Fig. 3.11). These larger nodules tend to exhibit pronounced insensitivity for regulation by calcium, with resulting more or less unregulated hormone release and development of hypercalcemia.[82] This condition has been named "tertiary" HPT, which should imply that a more or less autonomous tumor originates as a consequence of the chronic glandular stimulation in secondary parathyroid hyperplasia.[83] The "tertiary" HPT has been related to the presence of markedly asymmetrical glandular enlargement, and development of conspicuously large nodules, with sometimes distinct adenoma-like features.[82-88] There may even be functional suppression of the tissue outside the expanding nodules, and normal-sized glands may be encountered together with the enlarged ones. However, hyperplastic changes will invariably be present and generally also obvious enlargement of some of the associated glands, apparently substantiating that the condition results from clonal, variably expanding lesions in the setting of polyclonal hyperplasia.[82-88]

The chief cells usually predominate also in the glands of the tertiary nodular parathyroid hyperplasia, but there is often a pronounced admixture of oxyphil cells forming nodules. The cellular architecture generally varies considerably between individual nodules, which may display solid, trabecular, follicular, as well as acinar patterns.[85] Pronounced variability in PTH immunoreactivity occurs within these lesions, with apparent hormone suppression in the normal-looking or diffusely hyperplastic tissue.[85] Fat cells are usually sparse

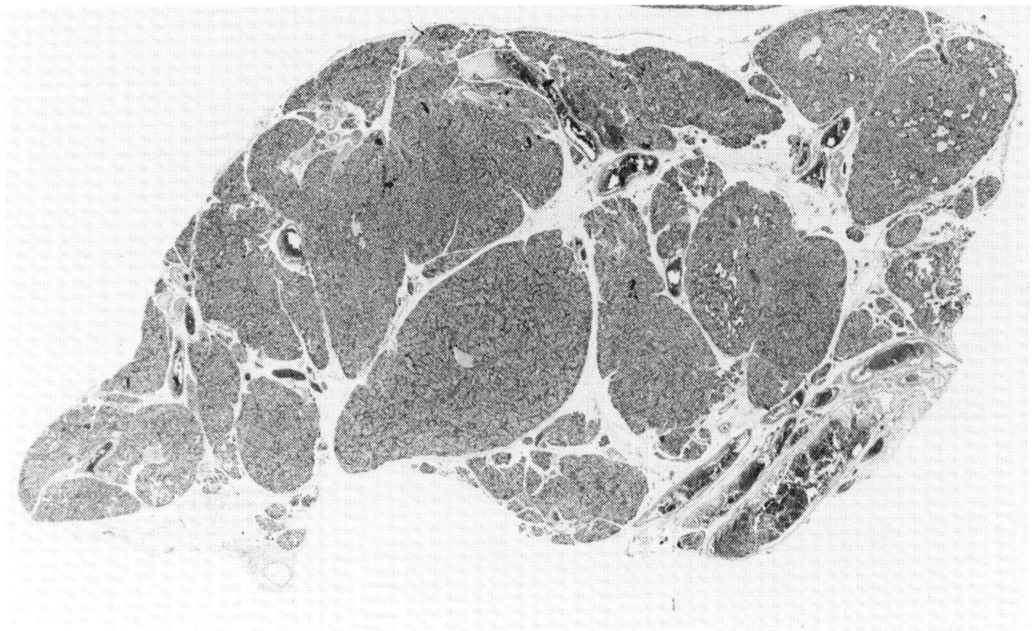

Fig. 3.10. Parathyroid gland exhibiting nodular chief cell hyperplasia in a patient with uremia. Reprinted with permission from Åkerström et al.[125]

or absent, but may be more prevalent in the compressed parathyroid tissue occurring between the nodules, or in smaller glands. The cytoplasmic fat content is generally markedly reduced in chief cells of the nodules, but may be more abundant in the normal-looking tissue. Degenerative changes are common, especially in the larger glands, displaying more or less focal areas of fibrosis and sometimes also calcifications.

It is generally concluded that the pathological changes of "tertiary" HPT secondary to chronic renal failure invariably involves parathyroid hyperplasia. In contrast, the patients with HPT secondary to a malabsorption syndrome and vitamin D deficiency very rarely exhibit clinical parathyroid disease, but if they do they will frequently be found to harbor adenoma.[78]

PARATHYROID HISTOPATHOLOGY

A principal obstacle in parathyroid histopathological diagnosis as well as in parathyroid surgery has been the difficulties associated with the discrimination between parathyroid adenoma and chief cell hyperplasia.[21,24,54,89] This evolves partly from unreliable diagnostic criteria, but also from lack of knowledge about the genesis and pathophysiology behind the different lesions. It has in fact been suggested that adenoma and hyperplasia should not always represent distinct entities, but instead that adenomatous disease could develop from nodular hyperplasia, if a nodule in one gland becomes dominant enough to functionally suppress the other glands.[24,54,89] This hypothesis is to some extent supported by histological similarity between large hyperplastic nodules and adenomas, and also by the observation that chief cell hyperplasia is more common in patients with mild hypercalcemia, but should probably be valid only for minorities of adenoma.[8,13,16]

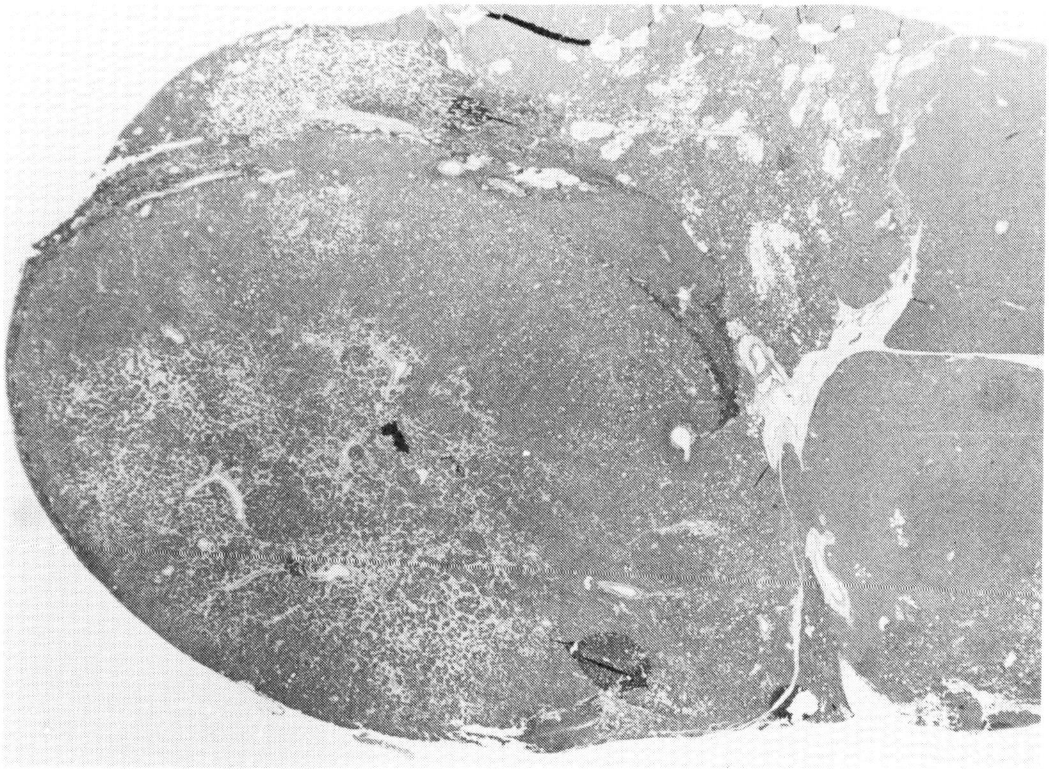

Fig. 3.11. Conspicuously enlarged nodule in a parathyroid gland from a patient with uremia and "tertiary" HPT.

DNA QUANTITATION IN PARATHYROID LESIONS

Several authors have reported measurement of nuclear DNA content, in attempts to distinguish between the various parathyroid lesions.[90-101] Although variable results have been reported in such studies, the majority opinion indicates that parathyroid adenomas differ from normal parathyroid glands by greater prevalence of tetraploid nuclei.[90-92,101] However, tetraploid nuclei have been revealed also in normal-sized glands associated with adenoma, indicating possibly a multiglandular abnormality in some of these cases.[92,93] Concerning hyperplastic glands the results have been even more variable, but tetraploidy may evidently be present in many of these lesions, and thus the method should provide no reliable discrimination between adenoma and hyperplasia.[101] Nor can DNA measurements be used during operation to determine whether border-line enlarged glands are normal.[90] Aneuploid cell populations have been demonstrated in up to 10% of parathyroid adenomas, but occur with considerably higher frequency in parathyroid carcinoma, being revealed in up to 60% of the primary and a majority of metastatic lesions.[94,95,97,98,100] The presence of aneuploidy thus supports, but is not necessary for a carcinoma diagnosis, and the overlap between the two entities prohibits reliable discrimination.[94,96,98,99] However, the presence of aneuploidy in parathyroid carcinoma indicates a more aggressive tumor, and has been associated with presence of metastases, early recurrence and death from malignancy.[96,98]

MONOCLONALITY OF PARATHYROID LESIONS

The majority of parathyroid adenomas are solitary and histopathologically solid, apparently clonal tumors. In some adenomas the pattern may be more heterogenous, consisting of multiple nodules, which may sometimes even be separated by more or less distinct encapsulation. In micronodular chief cell hyperplasia the histological pattern likewise creates the impression of multiple, variably expanding clones of cells. When molecular techniques were utilized to determine the clonality of parathyroid lesions, this initially revealed heterogeneity regarding glycose-6-phosphate dehydrogenase isoenzymes, suggesting that many adenomas were multicellular in origin.[102-104] However, subsequent investigations utilizing X chromosome inactivation analysis, have clearly demonstrated monoclonal patterns in the majority of parathyroid adenomas but this was not revealed in hyperplastic glands.[105] Genetic rearrangement within the PTH gene in a minority of adenomas further supports the clonality of these lesions.[106] More recently allelic deletions of chromosome 11 were demonstrated in a majority of MEN-1 associated parathyroid tumors, inferring that the inherited defect conveys susceptibility to develop neoplasia in all cells of the target tissue, and that a final genetic hit results in development of a monoclonal tumor.[104,107-111] Similar allelic deletions of chromosome 11 were revealed in up to 30% of sporadic parathyroid adenoma, further substantiating that a majority of adenoma represented monoclonal lesions.[111,112] The chromosome 11 allelic deletion was in fact demonstrated also in occasional larger glands of patients with "tertiary" HPT, indicating that monoclonal lesions could develop also in this setting.[113] A recent report, evaluating more thoroughly the clonality in hyperplastic lesions by the X chromosome inactivation analysis, revealed that also 27% of primary hyperplastic glands, as well as the majority of secondary hyperplastic glands, showed patterns consistent with monoclonality.[114] Thus, available data seem to substantiate an impression, suggested both from histopathology and clinical experience, namely that monoclonal, neoplastic tumors may emerge in a background of polyclonal hyperplasia, in familial as well as non-familial primary parathyroid hyperplasia, and in the "tertiary" hyperplasia of uremia.

INTRAOPERATIVE HISTOPATHOLOGY

The majority of patients with HPT will ultimately be revealed to have adenomatous disease, and in such cases the histopathological diagnosis, as well as the required surgical procedure are generally obvious merely from the gross findings at operation. Emphasizing the difficulties sometimes experienced in parathyroid histology and in order to avoid unexpected errors at surgery, the diagnosis should, however, always be confirmed histopathologically by intraoperative frozen section examination. Because of the irregular distribution of abnormality in hyperplasia appropriate visualization of four parathyroid glands during surgery is crucial for the histopathological evaluation.[115] Moreover, the surgeon has to be familiar with the size limits of normal parathyroid glands, as well as the characteristic gross features of pathological glands, in order to be able to correctly select specimens for excision and histopathological examination. It is also important that the surgeon informs the pathologist about the size of the glands detected in the operative field, and no glands should be excised or biopsied until the exploration is completed on both sides. An adequate diagnosis of hyperplasia or multiglandular parathyroid disease generally requires that two or more glands are obviously diseased, and also that the microscopic analysis will encompass intact glands or considerable parts of the glands. Tiny glandular biopsies are often difficult to interpret, due to the irregular distribution of the histopathological changes, and may be used mainly to determine whether an equivocal lesion really represents a parathyroid gland. In cases where gross findings indicate adenoma and the associated glands appear normal, it is usually sufficient to excise the adenoma and leave the other glands intact even if focal nodular changes can be expected in a proportion of the associated normal-sized glands.[116] The histopathological evaluation is generally most difficult in the patients with multiple glandular enlargement, especially when they exhibit only slight hypercalcemia, as this is associated generally with only minimal increases in glandular size. The intraoperative examination should thus include precise weight measurements and light microscopic analysis of frozen sections stained with hematoxylin and eosin, and it should be especially important to recognize the occasional normal parathyroid gland, which has become enlarged because of an unusually high fat cell content, but still exhibits a parenchymal weight within normal limits.

The presence of nodular accumulations of chief or oxyphil cells indicate abnormality, but such changes may occur also in the glands of euparathyroid, elderly individuals.[8,115] Staining of the frozen section specimens with "Oil red O" will allow visualization of cytoplasmic fat in the parathyroid chief cells and is particularly useful in supporting a diagnosis of a normal parathyroid gland.[10,18,31,117-119] This investigation is not without obstacles, but still generally constitutes a significant improvement in the diagnostic interpretation.[10,18,31,117-119]

MONOCLONAL ANTIPARATHYROID ANTIBODIES

It has recently been suggested that the parathyroid cell is equipped with a specialized calcium sensing receptor mechanism, by which extracellular calcium regulates the PTH release.[120] Monoclonal antiparathyroid antibodies, which seem to react with this calcium sensor mechanism have revealed heterogenous, but universally reduced expression in pathological parathyroid tissue, in contrast to intense staining of cell membrane structures in normal parathyroid cells.[120-123] Although functional aspects of this sensor mechanism still need to be clarified, the antibodies seem to efficiently distinguish between normal and abnormal parathyroid tissue, by appropriately revealing parathyroid cells with a functional abnormality.[120-123]

Moreover, the variable staining patterns within abnormal glands seem to substantiate the presence of clones of cells with variable phenotype and functional derangement.[122] Streaks of normal-looking chief cells may be efficiently visualized by the antibodies in normal tissue remnants associated with adenoma, and also in the normal-looking tissue appearing in between nodules in chief cell hyperplasia.[123] Although the staining pattern with these antibodies largely corresponds to that obtained with the "Oil red O" staining, the distribution within normal cells appears more sharply and efficiently defined with the antiparathyroid antibodies.[123] However, the swiftness in performance of the "Oil red O" stainings makes it possible to apply them to intraoperative evaluation and in this respect the antibody stainings require improvement. The antiparathyroid antibodies should provide important means for histological recognition of parathyroid cells, which may be of particular value in parathyroid adenomas with a follicular arrangement, and may also be used to identify parathyroid cells in needle biopsy specimens.[115,122,123]

REEVALUATION OF HISTOPATHOLOGY FACING A PARATHYROID REOPERATION

It is essential to carefully reexamine previous histopathological specimens in patients scheduled for parathyroid reoperation. Unfortunately operative notes and histopathology reports from primary operations often provide insufficient data on location and size of excised or remaining glands. Frequently the weights have not been determined and normal-sized glands may have been sequentially excised with the incorrect impression that they represented hyperplastic lesions. Reoperation in such cases may have to remove a parathyroid adenoma, representing the only remaining parathyroid in that particular patient. If weights of excised glands have not been recorded it is possible to obtain a rough estimate of the glandular size by measuring perpendicular diameters in available tissue sections.

REFERENCES

1. Albright F, Bloomberg E, Castleman B et al. Hyperparathyroidism due to diffuse hyperplasia of all parathyroid glands rather than adenoma of one. Arch Intern Med 1934; 54: 315-29.
2. Cope O, Keynes WM, Roth SI et al. Primary chief-cell hyperplasia of the parathyroid glands—A new entity in the surgery of hyperparathyroidism. Ann Surg 1958; 148: 375-88.
3. Åkerström G, Malmaeus J, Bergström R. Surgical anatomy of human parathyroid glands. Surgery 1984; 95: 14-21.
4. Gilmour JR, Martin WJ. The weight of the parathyroid glands. J Pathol 1937; 44: 431-62.
5. Åkerström G, Grimelius L, Johansson H et al. The parenchymal cell mass in normal human parathyroid glands. Acta Pathol Microbiol Immunol Scand (A) 1981; 89: 367-75.
6. Gilmour JR. The normal histology of the parathyroid glands. J Pathol 1939; 48: 187-222.
7. Grimelius L, Åkerström G, Johansson et al. Estimation of the parenchymal cell content of human parathyroid glands using the image analyzing computer technique. Am J Pathol 1978; 93: 793-800.
8. Åkerström G, Rudberg C, Grimelius L et al. Histologic parathyroid abnormalities in an autopsy series. Hum Pathol 1986; 17: 520-7.
9. Åkerström G, Malmaeus J, Grimelius L et al. Histological changes in parathyroid glands in subclinical and clinical renal disease. Scand J Urol Nephrol 1984; 18: 74-84.
10. Ljungberg O, Tibblin S. Peroperative fat staining of frozen sections in primary hyperparathyroidism. Am J Pathol 1979; 95: 633-41.
11. Edis AJ. Surgical anatomy and technique of neck exploration for primary hyperparathyroidism. Surg Clin North Am 1977; 57: 495-504.
12. van Heerden JA, Beahrs OH, Woolner LB. The pathology and surgical management of primary hyperparathyroidism. Surg Clin North Am 1977; 57: 557-63.

13. Åkerström G, Bergström R, Grimelius L et al. Relation between changes in clinical and histological features of primary hyperparathyroidism. World J Surg 1986; 10: 696-702.
14. Rudberg C, Åkerström G, Palmér M et al. Late results of operation for primary hyperparathyroidism in 441 patients. Surgery 1986; 99: 643-51.
15. Palmér M, Ljunghall S, Åkerström G et al. Patients with primary hyperparathyroidism operated on over a 24-year period: temporal trends of clinical and laboratory findings. J Chronic Dis 1987; 40: 121-30.
16. Wallfelt C, Ljunghall S, Bergström R et al. Clinical characteristics and surgical treatment of sporadic primary hyperparathyroidism with emphasis on chief cell hyperplasia. Surgery 1990; 107: 13-19.
17. Rutledge R, Stiegel M, Thomas CG et al. The relation of serum calcium and immunoparathormone levels to parathyroid size and weight in primary hyperparathyroidism. Surgery 1985; 98: 1107-12.
18. Bondeson A-G, Bondeson L, Ljungberg O et al. Fat staining in parathyroid disease—diagnostic value and impact on surgical strategy: Clinicopathologic analysis of 191 cases. Hum Pathol 1985; 16: 1255-63.
19. Williams ED. Pathology of the parathyroid glands. Clin Endocrinol Metab 1974; 3: 285-303.
20. Roth SI. Recent advances in parathyroid gland pathology. Am J Med 1971; 50: 612-22.
21. Grimelius L, Åkerström G, Johansson H et al. Anatomy and histopathology of human parathyroid glands. Pathol Annu 1981; 16: (II): 1-24.
22. Leedham PW, Pollock DJ. Intrafollicular amyloid in primary hyperparathyroidism. J Clin Pathol 1970; 23: 811-18.
23. Straus FH, Paloyan E. The pathology of hyperparathyroidism. Surg Clin North Am 1969; 49: 27-42.
24. Black WC, Utley JR. The differential diagnosis of parathyroid adenoma and chief cell hyperplasia. Am J Clin Pathol 1968; 49: 761-75.
25. Lloyd HM, Jacobi JM, Cooke RA. Nuclear diameter in parathyroid adenomas. J Clin Pathol 1979; 32: 1278-81.
26. Rudberg C, Grimelius L, Johansson H et al. Alteration in density, morphology and parathyroid hormone release of dispersed parathyroid cells from patients with hyperparathyroidism. Acta Path Microbiol Immunol Scand (A) 1986; 94: 253-61.
27. Roth SI. Pathology of the parathyroids in hyperparathyroidism. Discussion of recent advances in the anatomy and pathology of the parathyroid glands. Arch Pathol 1962; 73: 495-510.
28. Castleman B, Mallory TB. The pathology of the parathyroid gland in hyperparathyroidism—a study of 25 cases. Am J Pathol 1935; 11:1-72.
29. Norris EH. The parathyroid adenoma—a study of 322 cases. Surgery 1947; 84: 1-41.
30. Woolner LB, Keating FR Jr, Black BM. Tumors and hyperplasia of the parathyroid glands-a review of the pathological findings in 140 cases of primary hyperparathyroidism. Cancer 1952; 5: 1069-88.
31. Roth SI, Gallagher MJ. The rapid identification of "normal" parathyroid glands by the presence of intracellular fat. Am J Pathol 1976; 84: 521-28.
32. King DT, Hirose FM. Chief cell intracytoplasmic fat used to evaluate parathyroid disease by frozen section. Arch Pathol Lab Med 1979; 103: 609-12.
33. Ackerman's Surgical Pathology, Chapter 9, Parathyroid glands, 6th Ed. St. Louis: CV Mosby 1981: 379-99.
34. Wang CA. Surgery of the parathyroid gland. Adv Surg 1966; 5: 109.
35. Hoehn JG, Bearhs OH, Woolner LB. Unusual surgical lesions of the parathyroid gland. Am J Surg 1969; 118: 770-8.
36. Harness JK, Ramsburg SR, Nishiyama RH et al. Multiple adenomas of the parathyroids: do they exist? Arch Surg 1979; 114: 468-74.
37. Attie JN, Bock G, Auguste L-J. Multiple parathyroid adenomas: Report of thirty-three cases. Surgery 1990; 108: 1014-20.
38. Utley JR, Black WC. Hyperparathyroidism-a clinicopathologic evaluation. Am J Surg 1967; 113: 788-95.

39. Poole GV, Albertsson DA, Marshall RB et al. Oxyphil cell adenoma and hyperparathyroidism. Surgery 1982; 92: 799-805.
40. Ordonez NG, Ibanez ML, Mackay B et al. Functioning oxyphil cell adenomas of parathyroid glands: immunoperoxidase evidence of hormonal activity in oxyphil cells. Am J Clin Pathol 1982; 78: 681-89.
41. Bedetti CD, Dekker A, Watson CG. Functioning oxyphil cell adenoma of the parathyroid gland: a clinicopathologic study of ten patients with hyperparathyroidism. Hum Pathol 1984; 15: 1121-26.
42. Wolpert HR, Vickery AL, Wang C-A. Functioning oxyphil cell adenomas of the parathyroid gland. A study of 15 cases. Am J Surg Pathol 1989; 13: 500-4.
43. Abul-Haj SK, Conklin H, Hewitt WC: Functioning lipoadenoma of the parathyroid gland: Report of a unique case. N Engl J Med 1962; 266: 121-3.
44. Ober WB, Kaiser GA. Hamartoma of the parathyroid. Cancer 1958; 11: 601-6.
45. Daroca PJ Jr, Landau RL, Reed RJ et al. Functioning lipoadenoma of the parathyroid gland. Arch Pathol Lab Med 1977; 101: 28-30.
46. Legolvan DP, Moore BP, Nishiyama RH. Parathyroid hamartoma. Report of two cases and review of the litterature. Am J Clin Pathol 1977; 67: 31-5.
47. Weiland LH, Garrison RC, ReMine WH et al. Lipoadenoma of the parathyroid gland. Am J Surg Pathol 1978; 2: 3-7.
48. Ejerblad S, Grimelius L, Johansson H et al. Studies on the nonadenomatous glands in patients with a solitary parathyroid adenoma. Ups J Med Sci 1979; 81: 31-6.
49. Åkerström G, Grimelius L, Johansson H et al. Parenchymal cell mass determination in parathyroid glands and its application in a material of hyperparathyroidism. World J Surg 1981; 5: 555-63.
50. Roth SI, Munger BL. The cytology of the adenomatous, atrophic, and hyperplastic parathyroid glands of man: A light- and electron-microscopic study. Virchows Arch. (Pathol Anat) 1962; 335: 389-410.
51. Adams PH, Chalmers TM, Peters N et al. Primary chief cell hyperplasisa of the parathyroid glands. Ann Intern Med 1965; 63: 454-67.
52. Block MA, Greenawald K, Horn RC Jr et al. Involvement of multiple parathyroids in hyperparathyroidism. Surgical aspects. Am J Surg 1967; 114: 530-7.
53. Castleman B, Schantz A, Roth SI. Parathyroid hyperplasia in primary hyperparathyroidism. A review of 85 cases. Cancer 1976; 38: 1668-75.
54. Black WC, Haff RC. The surgical pathology of parathyroid chief cell hyperplasia. Amer J Clin Path 1970; 53: 565-79.
55. Bruining HA, van Houten H, Juttman JR et al. Results of operative treatment of 615 patients with primary hyperparathyroidism. World J Surg 1981; 5: 85-90.
56. Tominaga Y, Grimelius L, Rudberg C et al. Histological and clinical features of non-familial primary parathyroid hyperplasia. Pathol Res Pract 1992; 188: 115-22.
57. Block MA, Frame B, Jackson CE et al. Primary diffuse microscopical hyperplasia of the parathyroid glands. Surgical importance. Arch Surg 1976; 111: 348-54.
58. Badder EM, Graham WP, Harrison TS. Functional insignificance of microscopic parathyroid hyperplasia. Surg Gyn Obstet 1977; 145: 863-8.
59. Golden A, Canary JJ, Kerwin DM. Concurrence of hyperplasia and neoplasia of the parathyroid glands. Am J Med 1965; 38: 562-78.
60. Kay S. The abnormal parathyroid. Progress in human pathology. Hum Pathol 1976; 7: 127-38.
61. Schantz A. The microscopical pathology of primary parathyroid hyperplasia. Ann Clin Lab Sci 1979; 9: 314-8.
62. Lawrence DA. A histological comparison of adenomatous and hyperplastic parathyroid glands. J Clin Pathol 1978; 31: 626-32.
63. Banerjee SS, Faragher B, Hasleton PS. Nuclear diameter in parathyroid disease. J Clin Pathol 1983; 36: 143-8.
64. Strauss FH, Kaplan E, Nishiyama RH et al. Five cases of parathyroid lipohyperplasia. Surgery 1983; 94: 901-5.
65. Tisell LE, Hedman J, Hansson G. Clinical characteristics and surgical results in hyperparathyroidism caused by water-clear cell hyperplasia. World J Surg 1981; 5:565-71.

66. Arnaud CD, Walker JA, Ewer RW. Primary hyperparathyroidism associated with a cystic lesions in the neck: probable parathyroid cysts. J Clin Endocr 1961; 21: 833-8.
67. Shields TW, Staley CJ. Functioning parathyroid cysts. Arch Surg 1961; 82: 937-42.
68. Haid SP, Method HL, Beal JM. Parathyroid cysts. Report of two cases and review of the litterature. Arch Surg 1967; 94: 421-6.
69. Buchanan G, Gregory MM. Giant functioning cervicomediastinal parathyroid cysts. Ann Otol Rhinol Laryngol 1979; 88: 545-9.
70. Linos DA, Schoretsanitis G, Carrunis E. Parathyroid cysts of the neck and mediastinum. Case report. Acta Chir Scand 1989; 155: 211-16.
71. Prinz RA, Peters JR, Kane JM et al. Needle aspiration of non-functioning parathyroid cysts. Am Surg 1990; 56: 420-22.
72. Slatopolsky E, Caglar S, Pennell JP et al. On the pathogenesis of hyperparathyroidism in chronic experimental renal insufficiency in the dog. Clin Invest 1971; 50: 492-9.
73. Bonjour JP. 1,25-Dihydroxy vitamin D and phosphate homeostasis in early chronic renal failure: the "trade off hypothesis" revisited. In Davison AM, ed. Nephrology Vol II Bailliere Tindall, London 1988:1059.
74. Reichel H, Deibert B, Schmidt-Gayk H et al. Calcium metabolism in early chronic renal failure: Implications for the pathogenesis of hyperparathyroidism. Nephrol Dial Transplant 1991; 6: 162-9.
75. Russel J, Lettieri D, Sherwood LM. Suppression by 1,25$(OH)_2D_3$ of transcription of the parathyroid hormone gene. Endocrinology 1986; 119: 2864-6.
76. Pitts TO, Piraino BH, Mitro R et al. Hyperparathyroidism and 1,25-dihydroxyvitamin D deficiency in mild, moderate, and severe renal failure. J Clin Endocrinol Metab 1988; 67: 876-81.
77. Massry SG, Coburn JW, Lee DB et al. Skeletal resistance to parathyroid hormone in renal failure. Studies in 105 human subjects. Ann Intern Med 1973; 78: 357-64.
78. Smith JF. Parathyroid adenomas associated with the malabsorption syndrome and chronic renal disease. J Clin Pathol 1970; 23: 362-9.
79. Malmaeus J, Grimelius L, Johansson H et al. Parathyroid pathology in hyperparathyroidism secondary to chronic renal failure. Scand J Urol Nephrol 1984; 18: 157-66.
80. Hasleton PS, Ali HH. The parathyroid in chronic renal failure–a light and electron microscopical study. J Pathol 1980; 132: 307-23.
81. Christie AC. The parathyroid oxyphil cells. J Clin Pathol 1967; 20: 591-602.
82. Wallfelt C, Larsson R, Gylfe E et al. Secretory disturbances in hyperplastic parathyroid nodules of uremic hyperparathyroidism. Implication for parathyroid autotransplantation. World J Surg 1988; 1: 431-8.
83. St Goar WT. Case records of the Massachusetts General Hospital. Case 29. N Engl J Med 1963; 268: 943-53.
84. Krause MW, Hedinger CE. Pathologic study of parathyroid glands in tertiary hyperparathyroidism. Hum Pathol 1985; 16: 772-84.
85. Harach HR, Jasani B. Parathyroid hyperplasia in tertiary hyperparathyroidism: a pathological and immunohistochemical reappraisal. Histopathology 1992; 21: 513-19.
86. Davies DR, Dent CE, Watson L. Tertiary hyperparathyroidism. Br Med J 1968; iii: 395-9.
87. Black WC, Slatopolsky E, Elkan I et al. Parathyroid morphology in suppressible and nonsuppressible renal hyperparathyroidism. Lab Invest 1970; 23: 497-509.
88. Anderson TJ, Boyle IT. Autonomous nodular hyperplasia of the parathyroid glands. J Pathol 1971; 105: 211-14.
89. Reiss E, Canterbury JM. Primary hyperparathyroidism: differentiation of adenoma and hyperplasia and localization of hyperfunctioning glands. New Engl J Med 1969; 280: 1381-85.
90. Mallette LE. DNA quantitation in the study of parathyroid lesions. A review. Am J Clin Pathol 1992; 98: 305-11.
91. Bengtsson A, Grimelius L, Johansson H et al. Nuclear DNA-content of parathyroid cells in adenomas, hyperplastic and normal glands. Acta Pathol Microbiol Scand Sect A 1977; 85: 455-60.
92. Irvin GL, Bagwell CB. Identification of

histologically undetectable parathyroid hyperplasia by flow cytometry. Am J Surg 1979; 138: 567-71.
93. Rosen IB, Musclow E. DNA histogram of parathyroid tissue in determining extent of parathyroidectomy. Surgery 1985; 98: 1024-30.
94. Bowlby LS, DeBault LE, Abraham SR. Flow cytometric DNA analysis of parathyroid glands, relationship between nuclear DNA and pathologic classifications. Am J Pathol 1987; 128: 338-44.
95. Irvin GL, Taupier MA, Block NL et al. DNA patterns in parathyroid disease predict postoperative parathyroid hormone secretion. Surgery 1988; 104: 1115-20.
96. Levin KE, Chew KL, Ljung B-M et al. Deoxyribonucleic acid cytometry helps identify parathyroid carcinomas. J Clin Endocrinol Metab 1988; 67: 779-84.
97. Joensuu H, Klemi P. DNA aneuploidy in adenomas of endocrine organs. Am J Pathol 1988; 132: 145-51.
98. Obara T, Fujimoto Y, Kanaji Y et al. Flow cytometric DNA analysis of parathyroid tumors. Implication of aneuploidy for pathologic and biologic classification. Cancer 1990; 66: 1555-62.
99. Shenton BK, Ellis H, Johnston IDA et al. DNA analysis and parathyroid pathology. World J Surg 1990; 14: 296-302.
100. Harlow S, Roth SI, Bauer K et al. Flow cytometric DNA analysis of normal and pathologic parathyroid glands. Mod Pathol 1991; 4: 310-5.
101. Bonjer HJ, Bruining HA, Birkenhager JC et al. Single and multigland disease in primary hyperparathyroidism: Clinical follow-up, histopathology, and flow cytometric DNA analysis. World J Surg 1992; 16: 737-44.
102. Fialkow PJ, Jackson CE, Block MA et al. Multicellular origin of parathyroid "adenomas". N Engl J Med 1977; 297: 696-8.
103. Jackson CE, Cerny JC, Block MA et al. Probable clonal origin of aldosteronomas versus multicellular origin of parathyroid "adenomas". Surgery 1982; 92: 875-9.
104. Bäckdahl M, Howe JR, Lairmore TC et al. The molecular biology of parathyroid disease. World J Surg 1991; 15: 756-62.
105. Arnold A, Staunton CE, Hyung GK et al. Monoclonality and abnormal parathyroid hormone genes in parathyroid adenomas. N Engl J Med 1988; 318: 658-62.
106. Arnold A, Hyung GK, Gaz RD et al. Molecular cloning and chromosomal mapping of DNA rearranged with the parathyroid hormone gene in a parathyroid adenoma. J Clin Invest 1989; 83: 2034-40.
107. Larsson C, Skogseid B, Öberg K et al. Multiple endocrine neoplasia type I gene maps to chromosome 11 and is lost in insulinoma. Nature 1988; 332: 85-87.
108. Friedman E, Sakaguchi K, Bale AE et al. Clonality of parathyroid tumors in familial multiple endocrine neoplasia type I. N Engl J Med 1989; 321: 213-18.
109. Thakker RV, Bouloux P, Wooding C et al. Association of parathyroid tumors in multiple endocrine neoplasia type 1 with loss of alleles on chromosome 11. N Engl J Med 1989; 321: 218-24.
110. Radford DM, Ashley SW, Wells SA et al. Loss of heterozygosity of markers on chromosome 11 in tumors from patients with multiple endocrine neoplasia syndrome type 1. Cancer Res 1990; 50: 6529-33.
111. Byström C, Larsson C, Blomberg C et al. Localization of the MEN 1 gene to a small region within chromosome 11q13 by deletion mapping in tumors. Proc Natl Acad Sci USA 1990; 87: 1968-72.
112. Friedman E, De Marco L, Gejman PV et al. Allelic loss from chromosome 11 in parathyroid tumors. Cancer Res 1992; 52: 6804-9.
113. Falchetti A, Bale AE, Amorosi A et al. Progression of uremic hyperparathyroidism involves allelic loss on chromosome 11. J Clin Endocrinol Metab 1993; 76: 139-44.
114. Arnold A, Brown M, Urena P et al. X-inactivation analysis of clonality in primary and secondary parathyroid hyperplasia. J Bone Min Res 1992; 7 (suppl 1): S153.
115. Grimelius L, Åkerström G, Bondeson L et al. The role of the pathologist in diagnosis and surgical decision making in hyperparathyroidism. World J Surg 1991; 15: 698-705.
116. Cusumano RJ, Mahadevia P, Silver CE. Intraoperative histologic evaluation in ex-

ploration of the parathyroid glands. Surg Gynecol Obstet 1989; 169: 506-10.

117. Monchik JM, Farrugia R, Teplitz C et al. Parathyroid surgery: The role of chief cell intracellular fat staining with osmium carmine in the intraoperative management of patients with primary hyperparathyroidism. Surgery 1983; 94: 877-86.

118. Dekker AL, Watson CG, Barnes EL. The pathologic assessment of primary hyperparathyroidism and its impact on the therapy. A prospective evaluation of 50 cases with Oil-red-O stain. Ann Surg 1979; 190: 671-5.

119. Cinti S, Sbarbati A, Zancanaro C et al. Morphometric evaluation of intracytoplasmic lipid in normal and pathological glands. J Pathol 1990; 160: 31-4.

120. Juhlin C, Holmdahl R, Johansson H et al. Monoclonal antibodies with exclusive reactivity against parathyroid cells and tubule cells of the kidney. Proc Natl Acad Sci USA 1987; 84: 2990-4.

121. Juhlin C, Klareskog L, Nygren P et al. Hyperparathyroidism is associated with reduced expression of a parathyroid calcium receptor mechanism defined by monoclonal antiparathyroid antibodies. Endocrinology 1988; 122: 2999-3001.

122. Juhlin C, Rastad J, Klareskog L et al. Parathyroid histology and cytology with monoclonal antibodies recognizing a calcium sensor of parathyroid cells. Am J Pathol 1989; 135: 321-8.

123. Bjerneroth G, Juhlin C, Grimelius L et al. Improvement in histological diagnosis of primary hyperparathyroidism with a monoclonal antiparathyroid antibody. Endocr Pathol 1992; 3: 83-92.

124. Åkerström G, Ljunghall S. Medical and radiological evaluation and operative treatment of primary hyperparathyroidism. Curr Opinion Gen Surg 1993; 130-138.

125. Grimeluis L, Åkerström G, Johansson H, Juklin C, Rastad J. The parathyroid glands. In Functional Endocrine Pathology, vol 2. Eds. Kovaes K; Asa SL. Blackwell Scientific Publications 1991; 375-95.

CHAPTER 4

Anatomy and Strategy of Parathyroid Operation

Göran Åkerström

Appreciation of variation in anatomy is crucial for the outcome of parathyroid surgery and the majority of glands retrieved by reoperation will be found to occupy normal locations or common ectopic sites which should have been explored at the initial operation.

Few surgical diseases have such variable anatomy as hyperparathyroidism (HPT), and rarely is knowledge about variation in this respect as critical for the surgical procedure. Recognition of the embryological development and the details of normal and ectopic location of parathyroid glands is thus more or less essential for a successful outcome of parathyroid explorations. This is required since an unequivocal histopathological diagnosis in HPT often has to be based on visualization of both the enlarged and obviously diseased parathyroid glands, as well as those of apparent normal size. This can only be achieved routinely if the neck dissection is cautiously and diligently performed without any great distortion of the normal anatomy in the area. The dissection should therefore preferably utilize the normal cleavage planes between the more or less distinct fasciae layers of the neck, and the glands should be searched for with a systematic, carefully considered strategy. In association with reoperative parathyroid surgery it is even more crucial to appreciate these details of the neck anatomy, since previous surgery has frequently resulted in extensive fibrotic adhesions, and the parathyroid glands will more frequently be hidden in ectopic locations, where they may be exceedingly difficult to find.

EMBRYOLOGY

The *superior parathyroid glands* originate within the fourth branchial pouch and descend together with the developing lateral lobes of the thyroid to become located, most commonly, in contact with the thyroid capsule, at the posterior edge of the middle or cranial parts of the thyroid[1-5]

Current Controversy in Parathyroid Operation and Reoperation, edited by Göran Åkerström. © 1994 R.G. Landes Company.

(Fig. 4.1). Lobules of fat, which are generally found surrounding superior parathyroid glands in this location, have been thought to represent involuted thymic remnants. Such remnants may thus originate from the fourth branchial pouch, but have failed to develop into mature thymic tissue.[6] The superior parathyroid glands normally have a comparatively short cervical descent, and are therefore fairly constant in their adult location[3-5] (Fig. 4.1). If the superior glands descend further they tend to move posteriorly and somewhat laterally, and may be found in more or less ectopic positions lateral or posterior to the esophagus or in the posterior superior mediastinum. Rare cases of ectopic parathyroids in the middle mediastinum, i.e. located between the aorta, the pulmonary artery or the right main bronchus, are consequently thought to represent embryologically superior glands.[7] The same origin has been claimed for likewise rare ectopic glands found in the lateral triangle of the neck, i.e. lateral to the jugular vein and the carotid artery.[8,9] It has been suggested that these glands develop because the parathyroid primordium is divided or pushed laterally by the passage of the carotid artery trunk during the embryological development, and such lateral glands may indeed often be supernumerary.[8,9]

The *inferior parathyroid glands* and the adult thymus both develop from the third branchial pouch[1-5] (Fig. 4.1). These parathyroids have a longer descent, as they develop together, with or separated from the thymus, to become located most commonly around the inferior thyroid pole or in the vestigial fibrous tissue connecting the thyroid with the cervical thymic horns, being generally referred to as the thyreothymic ligament.[1-3] Due to their long embryological descent the inferior parathyroid glands are more likely to attain an inconsistent location, and they may be found anywhere along the embryological pathway, extending from high up in the neck down into the anterior mediastinum[3-5] (Fig. 4.2). During this descent the inferior glands have a tendency to move anteriorly. Failure of the inferior parathyroids, and then often also the thymus, to descend normally may occasionally leave the glands together with thymic tissue high in the neck, within or attached medially to the carotid sheath at the level of the carotid artery bifurcation.[10,11] Abnormally descended inferior glands may also be encountered within or associated with the vascular sheath down to the level of the lower thyroid pole.[11] Sometimes the thyreothymic ligament and the cervical thymus have not been properly attached to the thyroid, but deviates laterally from it, and may then contain an inferior gland in its tip or point towards such a gland in an aberrant lateral location. An in-

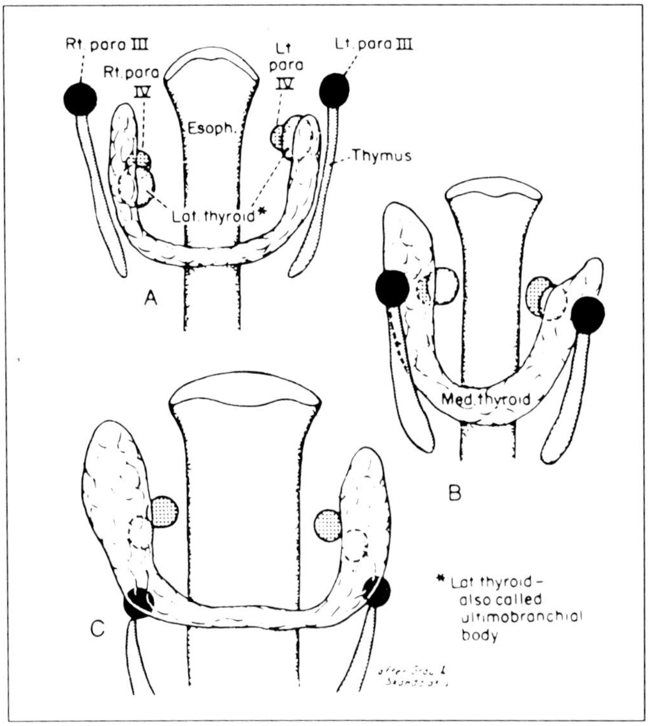

Fig. 4.1 (A and B). Schematic presentation of the embryologic shifts in locations of the thyroid, parafollicular and parathyroid tissues. (C) Approximate adult position. Reprinted with permission from H Gray et al[3] and Skandalaleis et al.[59]

ferior gland may also be entrapped within the descending thymus, and pulled into the anterior mediastinum.[11] Embryologic relationships between the thymus and the developing primordium of the heart may enable the glands to be carried even further down and take a position in proximity with the ascending aorta or the pericardium.[11] Such glands are generally located in the thymus, but may occasionally also be found in the perithymic tissue on the mediastinal pleural or pericardial surfaces.[11] Inferior parathyroid glands may also become incorporated into the developing thyroid gland, and occupy an intrathyroidal position, within the middle or lower parts of the thyroid.[11,12] This contrasts to the superior parathyroid glands, which although they have a particularly intimate connection with the lateral thyroid lobes during embryological development more seldomly achieve an intrathyroidal position.[11,12]

NORMAL PARATHYROID GLAND ANATOMY

Number of Parathyroid Glands

Virtually every individual seems to have at least four parathyroid glands.[13-15] Autopsy studies have reported the presence of less than four glands in occasional individuals, but the low total parathyroid glandular weights in most of these cases indicate that not all glands have been identified.[13,14] At least 13% of all normal persons have one or even several supernumerary glands, and as many as 11-12 glands have been encountered sporadically.[14] Half of these supernumerary glands occur as proper glands, implying that they are of more or less normal size and located well away from the other glands.[14] Such proper supernumerary glands seem to be slightly more common in individuals where the other parathyroids are bi- or multilobar.[14] Sequestration from the glandular primordium during embryogenesis may also give rise to either bi- or multilobar glands or completely divided ones, as well as to the presence of rudimentary glands, which often tend to lie close to the normal parathyroids or within the thymus.[14] Scattered nests of minute parathyroid tissue, have in fact been reported as a fairly common finding if the thymus has been subjected to serial sectioning, and may represent an embryological remnant, since Gilmour reported supernumerary parathyroids in 21% of all embryos.[16] A condition where such clusters of parathyroid cells

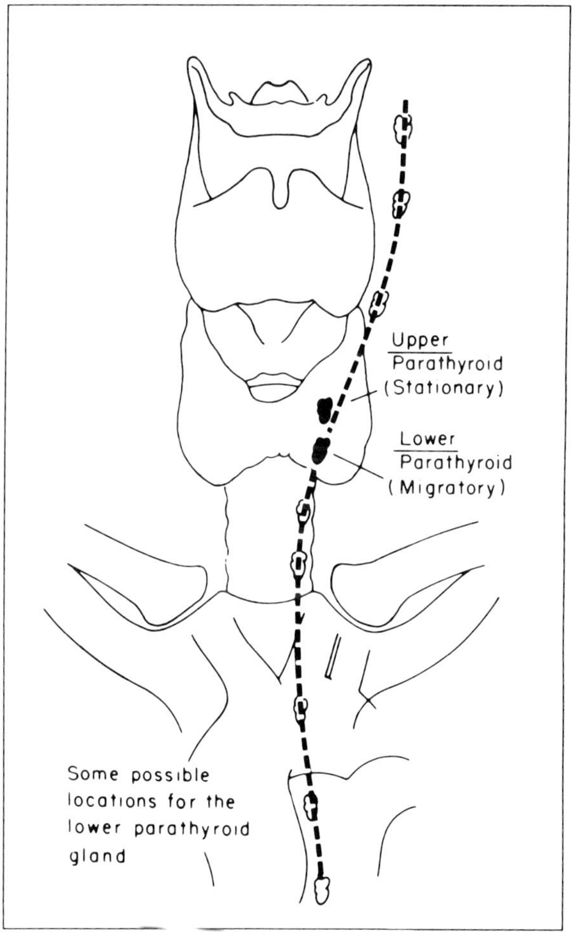

Fig. 4.2. Descent of the lower parathyroid. The upper parathyroid occupies a relatively constant position in relation to the middle or upper third of the lateral thyroid lobe, but the lower parathyroid normally migrates in embryonic life and may end up anywhere along the course of the dotted line. When this gland is in the chest, it is nearly always in the anterior mediastinum. Reprinted with permission from Kaplan EL et al.[5]

have been found diffusely scattered within the adipose tissue of the neck or the mediastinum has been denoted parathyromatosis, and is generally considered due to spillage and implantation of parathyroid cells during operation, but may occur in the absence of previous parathyroid surgery.[17-20] When such nests consist of normal parathyroid cells they should generally have no functional implication, but they may indeed become enlarged in hyperplasia, and be the cause of clinically overt parathyroid disease.[17-20] Implantated cells resulting from violation of the capsule of a diseased parathyroid gland during surgery on the other hand have a marked tendency to attach and may grow as free grafts and cause recurrent HPT.[18-22]

LOCATION OF PARATHYROID GLANDS

Consistent with their short embryological descent the location of the **superior parathyroid glands** is fairly constant in adult life.[11,13-15] These glands are most commonly found within or close to the posterior aspects of the thyroid capsule in an area of about 2 cm^2 centered 1 cm rostral of the intersection between the recurrent laryngeal nerve and the inferior thyroid artery (Fig. 4.3a). As approximately 80% of superior glands will be found in this location, the depicted area serves as the important predictable anatomical landmark, where the superior glands should be initially and most thoroughly searched for.[11,14] Within this area the thyroid is enveloped between two sheaths of the pretracheal fascia, which extends and joins more laterally to form the anterior and posterior layers of the carotid sheath.[11,14,15] The superior glands behind the upper thyroid pole are characteristically located between these two fasciae layers, and external to the thyroid capsula. When the outer fascia layer is cut open a parathyroid gland is often easily identified by its firm consistency and brown-reddish color, and by its tendency to move freely within a surrounding lobulated fat pad, being enveloped by the same

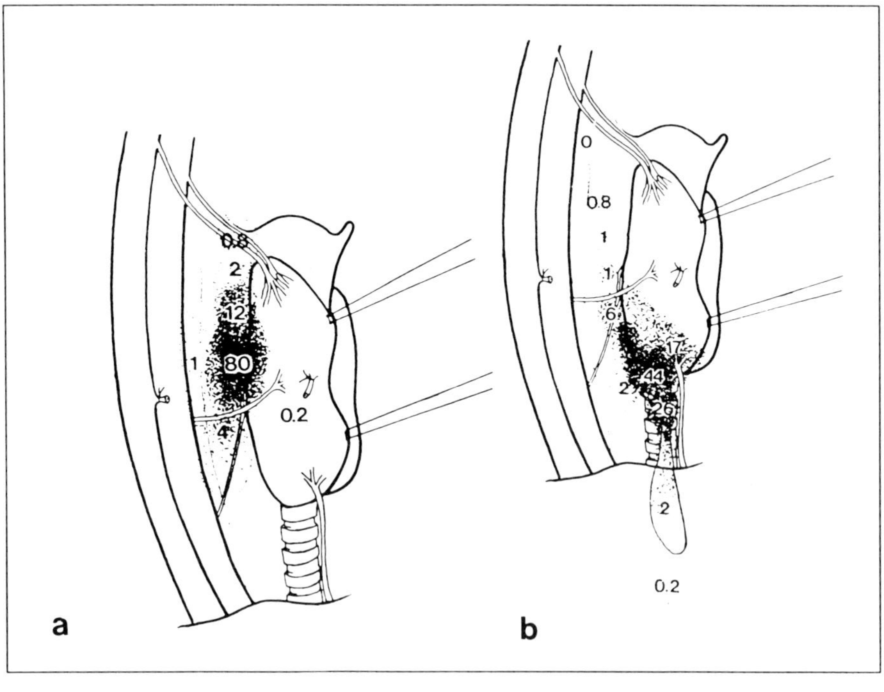

Fig. 4.3. Locations of superior (a) and inferior (b) parathyroid glands. The more common locations are indicated by the darker shading. The numbers represent the percentages of glands found at the different locations. Reprinted with permission from Åkerström G et al.[14]

fasciae layers. When the fascia and fat pad is incised the gland thus frequently tends to literally pop out from the surrounding fat. Occasionally a superior gland is located directly on the posterior border of the thyroid lobe, and it may also be situated higher up on the ventrolateral thyroid surface, and occasionally also medially. In either case is it often more or less fixed to the thyroid surface as it tends to lie between the layers of the surgical thyroid capsule. Only rarely are the superior glands located in the vascular pedicle at the top or above the thyroid pole, or medial to the thyroid in this area. The superior glands can also lie more caudally, along the posterior or the lateral thyroid surfaces, and may then be obscured by branches from the inferior thyroid artery or by the recurrent nerve or the nerve/artery intersection. Such a gland may also be covered by a common dorsal protrusion of the thyroid gland in this area, the so called thyroid tubercle of Zuckerkandl. The superior glands may be engulfed within the clefts of a goiterous thyroid, but rarely do they occur deeper within the thyroid tissue itself.

When the superior glands occupy an ectopic location, they have from embryological reasons a tendency to lie more posteriorly in the neck, in the para-or retropharyngeal and retroesophageal spaces. The lower they are in location, the more posterior generally is their position.

Due to their comparatively longer embryological descent, the **inferior parathyroid glands** are more widely distributed than the superior ones[11,13-15] (Fig. 4.3b). The inferior glands are most commonly situated around the lower thyroid pole, around its caudal, lateroposterior or ventral surfaces. Frequently is may be present in the proximity with or within the thyreothymic ligament or the upper parts of the cervical thymus. Inferior glands may also be found slightly cranially, lateral to the thyroid, up to the recurrent laryngeal nerve/inferior thyroid artery intersection, and occasionally even above this point. Some inferior glands located on the lateral or ventral aspects of the lower thyroid lobe, may be closely adherent or actually engulfed within the layers of the surgical thyroid capsule, but they generally remain outside the thyroid and the inner layers of this capsule. Glands in this position are thus generally possible to dissect with retained their vascular supply. Occasionally inferior parathyroid glands may appear deeply hidden within nodular thyroid tissue. Although these glands are generally located on the thyroid surface rather than within the gland, their mobilization will more easily result in compromising their blood supply. Occasional inferior parathyroid glands are truly intrathyroidal, but may then be deeply buried in the middle or the lower parts of the thyroid. Inferior glands located further down in the mediastinum, may be found in around 2% of normal individuals, and the majority of these glands will be located within the thymus. More rarely, mediastinal glands may be found in the parathymic tissue or even below the thymus, and may then be attached to the pleura or the pericardium. Incomplete descent may sometimes leave an inferior gland high up in the neck, and it is then often located together with undescended thymic tissue, which also has failed to descend properly during the embryological development.[10] This aberration should be suspected if no thymic tissue is found below the thyroid lobe. The undescended parathyroid gland, often named parathymus, tends to lie between the pharynx and the vascular sheath or even within this sheath at the level of the carotid artery bifurcation. In another developmental aberration the thymus may occupy an ordinary position below the thyroid but deviates laterally and may contain an inferior parathyroid gland.

Although the position of individual parathyroid glands may vary considerably, there is still often a *remarkable symmetry*, of location of four glandsin 60% in normal individuals.[14] The superior pair of parathyroid glands tend to be symmetrically located on contralateral sides of the neck in around 80%, and for inferior glands such symmetry may be noted in 70%. In approximately

50% of normal individuals the superior glands are located above, and the inferior glands below the intersection between the recurrent laryngeal nerve and the inferior thyroid artery. Less commonly are the pairs of superior and inferior glands on one side either below or above the nerve/artery intersection, and it may then be difficult to judge with certainty which glands really constitute the true superior or inferior ones. The most commonly recognized asymmetrical alignment of glands is when an inferior gland is situated lower down in the thymus (Fig. 4.4). Another asymmetrical positioning of glands may be present when two glands on one side are located above or below the nerve/artery intersection[14] (Fig. 4.4).

In cases with *supernumerary glands* a fifth gland is most frequently found in the thyreothymic ligament or within the thymus (Fig. 4.5). In rare instances with a higher number of parathyroid glands these may be distributed as a string of pearls stretching from behind the thyroid down to the thymus, evidently representing the extended line of embryological descent[14] (Fig. 4.6).

VASCULAR SUPPLY

Knowledge of the parathyroid blood supply originates from dissection and injection studies from the beginning of this century, but has recently been amplified in a study by Nobori et al.[23-27] According to this study the parathyroid glands receive their main arterial blood supply from end arteries, which together with the main venous effluent gain access to the gland via a more or less distinct hilus. The arterial supply to the superior glands is claimed to originate most often from the inferior thyroid artery, but in approximately 40% of cases the feeding artery may come from a more or less prominent anastomosing ramification between the superior and inferior thyroid arteries, which runs along the posterior margin of the thyroid lobe[25-27] (Fig. 4.7). Since the principal blood supply to the superior parathyroid may originate in this posterior branch of the superior thyroid artery it may be best to try to

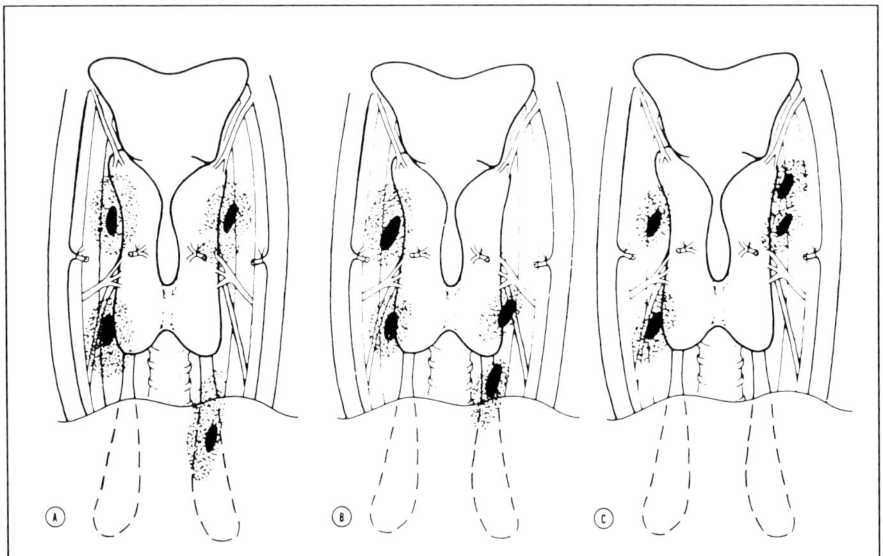

Fig. 4.4. Positions of asymmetrically located parathyroids in an autopsy series. A. Three glands located in the vicinity of the thyroid gland, and the fourth gland from either side located well below in the thymus (13%). B,C. On one side the superior gland is above and the inferior is below the nerve artery intersection, on the other side two glands are located below (B, 5%). or above (C, 2%) the intersection. Reprinted with permission from Åkerström G et al.[14]

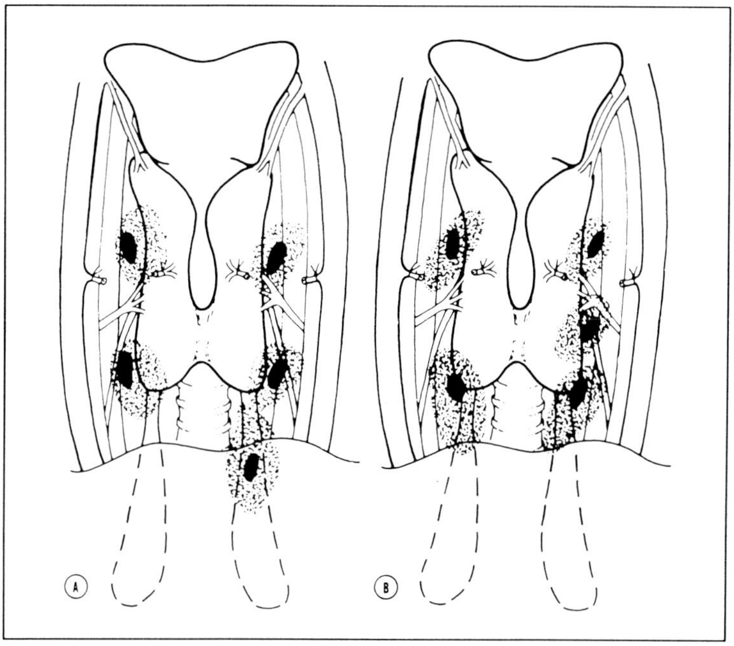

Fig. 4.5. Positions of proper supernumerary glands in an autopsy series. A. In approximately two thirds of the cases the supernumerary gland was found below the thyroid in association with the thyrothymic ligament or the thymus on either side. B. In one third the supernumerary gland was found in the vicinity of the thyroid between two other glands. Reprinted with permission from Åkerström G et al.[14]

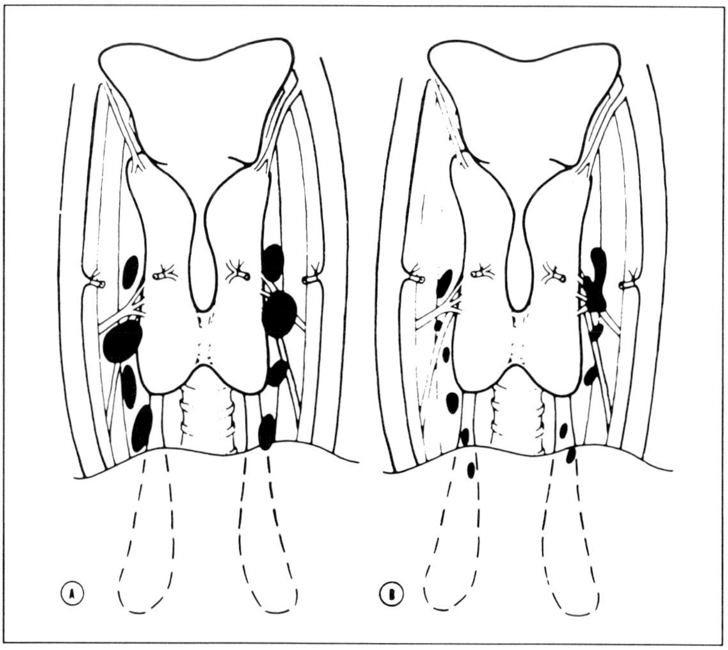

Fig. 4.6A. Distribution of eight parathyroid glands in a case with renal function impairment before death. At autopsy the parathyroid glands were enlarged (33 to 92 mg). B. Distribution of 11 parathyroid glands in an autopsy case. Reprinted with permission from Åkerström G et al.[14]

preserve this particular branch during thyroid and parathyroid surgery.[27] Occasionally the artery to a superior parathyroid gland can be of surprising length, possibly aiding in a posterior and caudal dislocation of such a gland.[27] The inferior glands are almost invariably supplied by arterial branches from the inferior thyroid artery, or from similar anastomosing ramifications. When an inferior gland is located below the lower thyroid lobe the parathyroid artery may occasionally be of conspicuous size and length and may arise close to the origin of the inferior thyroid artery. This may give the impression of a an additional artery appearing behind the carotid sheath just caudal to the main inferior artery trunk, and such an arterial branch may lead to a parathyroid gland in the upper mediastinum. When inferior glands are located in lower parts of the cervical thymus they may be supplied by thymic arteries, and when situated in the mediastinal thymus the arterial supply generally originates from direct branches of the internal mammary artery. Generally one parathyroid artery enters the hilus of the parathyroid gland, but there may occasionally be several additional feeding branches, and the surrounding fat or connective tissue around the parathyroids may also provide collateral vessels with direct entry into the capsule[26,27] (Fig. 4.8). Likewise, parathyroids located in close contact with the thyroid may obtain similar additional, small arteries directly from the lateral surface of this gland. Although the anastomosing ramifications as well as these small additional arteries are believed to provide sufficient blood supply, this is doubtful and it is strongly recommended that ligation of the inferior thyroid artery during neck surgery should always be performed distal to the origin of the individual parathyroid end arteries.[11,25]

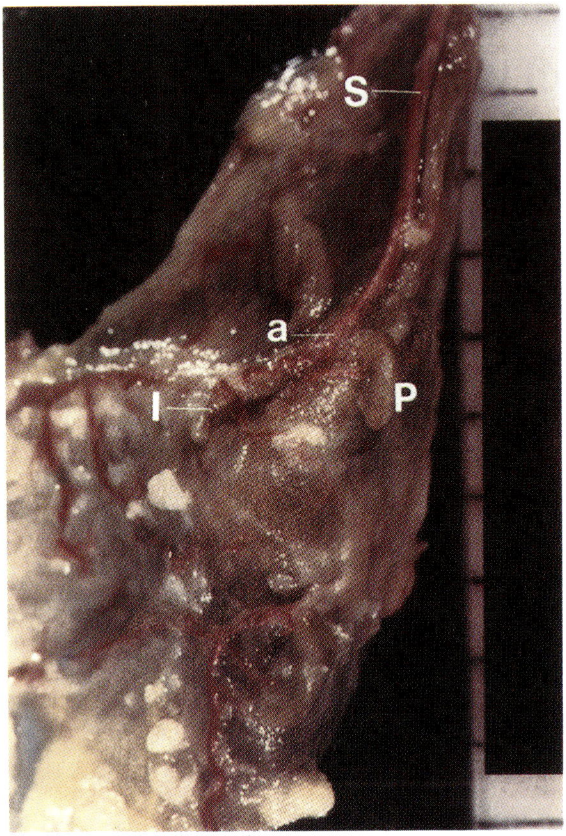

Fig. 4.7. Posterior aspect of the right thyroid lobe shows an anastomosing branch (a) between the posterior branch of the superior thyroid artery (S) and the inferior thyroid artery (I), from which an artery to the upper parathyroid gland (P) arises. Distal cut end of inferior thyroid artery (I) is shown. Reprinted with permission from Nobori MN et al.[27]

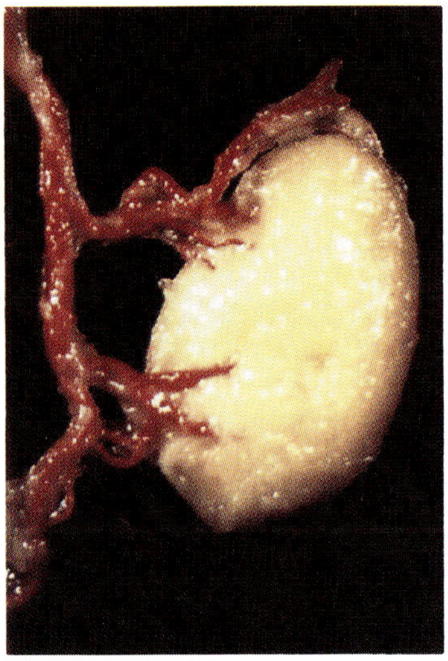

Fig. 4.8. An upper parathyroid gland with six parathyroid arteries. Reprinted with permission from Nobori MN et al.[27]

FASCIAL LAYERS

A neck exploration may be facilitated if the appropriate cleavage planes between the different fasciae layers of the neck are utilized during the operative approach.[11] This should result in minimal distortion of the anatomy and cause less chance tof obscuring the characteristic consistency and color of the parathyroid glands. The thyroid is thus covered by the superficial cervical fascia, but it is under that also enveloped in the pretracheal fascia, which is distinct around the superior thyroid lobe but more friable at the middle and lower parts of this gland. The pretracheal fasica engulfs the superior thyroid lobe in two layers, which join laterally to form the vascular sheath,[11] while more caudally the dorsal fascia covers a compartment containing the recurrent laryngeal nerve. Early in the exploration it is essential to separate the superficial cervical fascial layers from the vascular sheath in order to mobilize the thyroid. Transection of this fascia is performed close to the thyroid at its upper part. In the lower neck this transection is adjacent to the vascular sheath in order to ensure that the central neck structures, including the recurrent laryngeal nerve can be safely pushed towards the midline by blunt dissection. When the thyroid has been efficiently mobilized by this maneuver, the ventral layer of the pretracheal fascia still has to be detached from the surgical thyroid capsule along the superior/posterior thyroid border in order to expose the superior parathyroid gland. Likewise the more friable part of this fascia around the inferior thyroid pole is transected, whereby free-dissection of the thyreothymic ligament and the cervical thymus may be undertaken. For exposure of the recurrent laryngeal nerve a thin dorsal layer of the pretracheal fascia is cut longitudinally along the direction of the nerve.

NECK EXPLORATION IN HPT

It needs to be repeatedly emphasized that by far the best opportunity to successfully treat a patient with HPT is at the time of the initial neck exploration, since repeat parathyroid surgery may be a considerably more cumbersome procedure often associated with less certain outcome.[28]

Optimal access to the operative field at any parathyroid operation is provided by maximal neck extension and support to elevate the shoulders. The neck is opened by a generous collar incision, being placed no higher than two finger-breadths above the sternal notch, whereafter a platysma/skin flap is dissected and the strap muscles are separated from the upper part of the thyroid cartilage to the sternum.

On the side to be explored first the fascial layers are divided adjacent to the thyroid in order to initially expose the most common locations of both the superior and inferior glands. These pertinent sites are the lateral and posterior aspects of the superior thyroid lobe and the tip of the thymus, respectively[29] (Fig. 4.9). The deeper fascial layers or the recurrent laryngeal nerve need not be explored at this stage, since too much and incautious dissection will easily obscure the initially often very characteristic features of the parathyroids. Instead the surgeon should *carefully inspect* the dissected areas in order to recognize the typical brownish color and characteristic consistency of these glands.

If not already identified by this early inspection the *superior parathyroid gland*, which has the most constant position, is first searched for more thoroughly at the posterior edge of the upper thyroid pole. Transection of the fascial attachments to the thyroid may frequently reveal the gland floating or extruding from the surrounding fat in this area. If still not identified the dissection continues around the ventral and latero–posterior thyroid surfaces, where the gland may be concealed in a cleft of the thyroid or obscured by a prominent thyroid tubercle. By medial rotation of the thyroid its medial aspects will come into view. In further dissections the superficial branches of the inferior thyroid artery may have to be divided, whereby the recurrent laryngeal nerve and the nerve/artery intersection can be completely visualized. The superior gland may occasionally be deeply

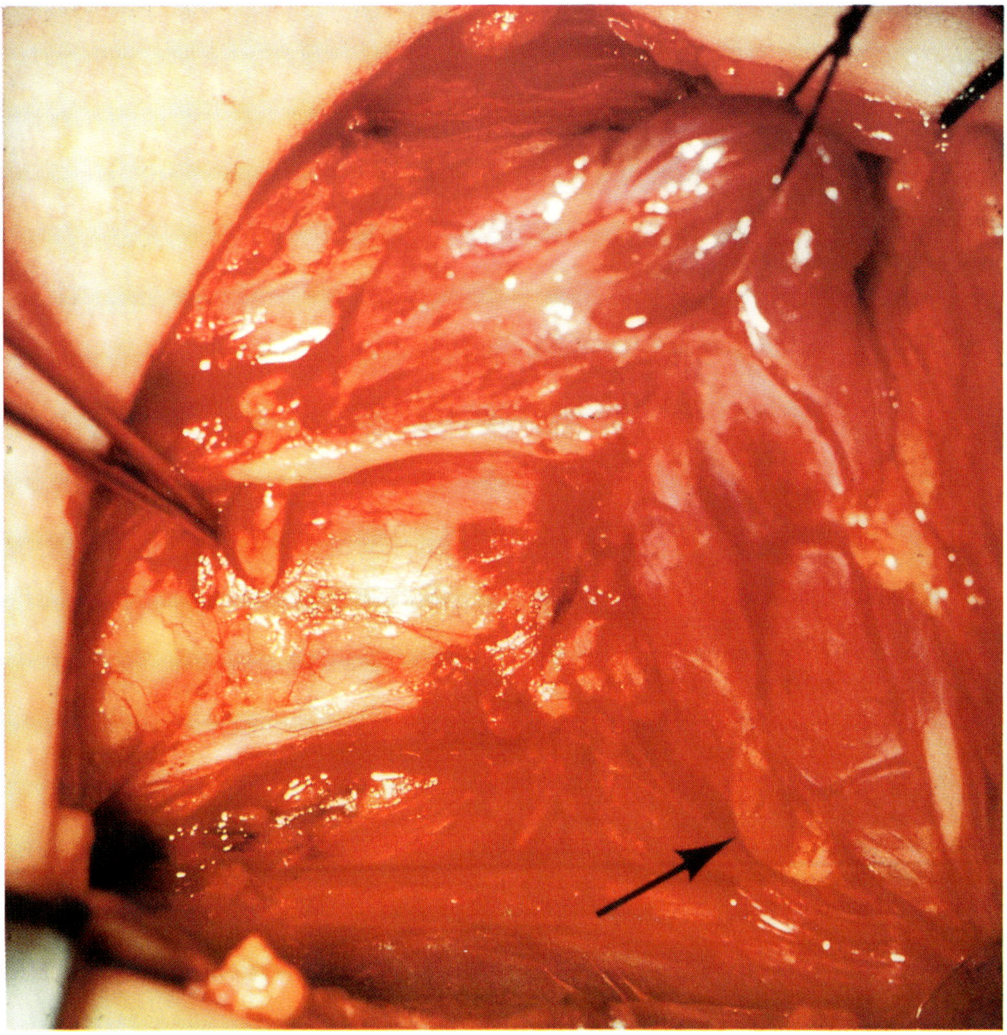

Fig. 4.9. Typical location and gross features of normal parathyroid glands. Reprinted with permission from Åkerström G et al.[29]

hidden in this area, under the nerve, the nerve/artery intersection or sometimes even within the ligament of Berry. If unrewarding at this time-point the search should also be directed towards the common ectopic positions for the superior gland, in the tracheoesophageal groove or lateral to or behind the esophagus in the middle or lower neck or towards the superior, posterior mediastinum.

Thompson has emphasized that expeditious exposure of such glands may be obtained early by division of the pretracheal fascia from the level of the inferior thyroid artery to the upper thyroid pole, whereafter a finger is allowed to explore the sites lateral to and behind the esophagus as well as towards the superior mediastinum, where a superior gland adenoma frequently hides[11,30] (Fig. 4.10).

Search for the *inferior parathyroid gland* commences around the inferior, low lateral and ventral aspects of the lower thyroid pole and includes the thyreothymic ligament and upper parts of the thymus. In this search the thymus is carefully dissected from surrounding fat, inspected on all sides and its fascia is cut open over any suspicious lesion. If an inferior gland is not readily identified the dissection will have

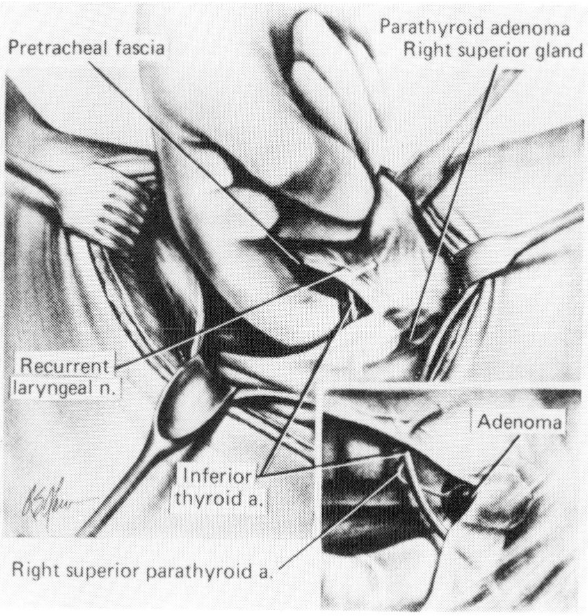

Fig. 4.10. The exposure and digital maneuver used to locate many superior gland adenomas, the pretracheal fascia has been excised allowing the finger to slide along the prevertebral fascia in an avascular plane beneath both the recurrent laryngeal nerve and the inferior thyroid artery. Reprinted with permission from Thompson NW.[11]

to proceed in the cephalad direction along the lateral and posterior border of the thyroid, between the branches of the inferior thyroid artery and also laterally, along the line of embryological descent, anterior and medial to the carotid sheath up to and above the hyoid bone. The thyroid lobe is also carefully palpated and any nodularity on its surface or within its parenchyma is free-dissected and excised. If the thyroid is totally normal it is unlikely that it contains a parathyroid adenoma, but if enlarged or nodular, an incision or partial resection of the lower thyroid pole may be indicated. These measures are preferred in our opinion rather than hemithyroidectomy which may seriously complicate following reoperative surgery. An alternative and attractive approach is to utilize intraoperative ultrasound in order to visualize an enlarged intrathyroidal inferior gland at this stage of the exploration. Finally as much as possible of the thymus is pulled up from the anterior mediastinum by blunt dissection and ligation of venous effluents, and the carotid sheath is also opened all the way down to the clavicle.

Some general aspects are important to consider in these dissections. One of them is that it is generally advisable to postpone any glandular excision until the exploration is complete on both sides. This requirement may be easier to fulfill if it is emphasized that close to 80% of all parathyroid glands also in patients with HPT will occur with a symmetrical, anatomically more or less typical distribution. It is therefore often more awarding to carefully explore the normal locations of the parathyroid glands before turning to the more abnormal ones. However, due to an occasional variable and overlapping location it may sometimes be difficult to determine whether a recognized gland is a superior or inferior one. Dissection of the recurrent laryngeal nerve as well as the inferior thyroid artery and the intersection between these two may then help, and this is in fact often required in difficult explorations. In this context may the inferior cornu of the hyoid cartilage serve as a landmark for the laryngeal entrance of the recurrent laryngeal nerve.[31] Superior glands tend to be located posterior to the nerve and superior to the artery while inferior ones are generally ventral to the nerve and inferior to the artery unless they have been arrested in descent.

ABNORMAL ANATOMY IN HPT

Studies of the parathyroid anatomy in patients undergoing surgery for HPT have reported a variable distribution of glands in normal versus ectopic location. This may not necessarily reflect true variations, but could be due to selection bias associated with patient referral, as well as to different opinions about what really represents the ectopic location of these glands. Variation in thyroid anatomy and particularly the presence of a nodular goiter would also influence such judgment. Thompson et al have emphasized that enlarged superior parathyroid glands may more frequently achieve an aberrant location.[11,30] These authors have found up to 30-40% of superior gland adenomas to be displaced into a paraesophageal, retropharyngeal or retroesophageal position, which contrasts with the 1-4% incidence of normal superior parathyroid glands in this location.[11,30] The authors infered that the superior gland in conjunction with enlargement may have a tendency to migrate in a plane between the pretracheal sheath and the prevertebral fascia to achieve a common position along the esophagus, caudal and posterior to the inferior thyroid artery. From here they may descend further caudally into the posterior mediastinum or medially into the tracheoesophageal groove, where they tend to be posterior or lateral to the recurrent laryngeal nerve. In our experience such ectopic location is slightly less frequent, and it may in fact be particularly valid for the more severely enlarged superior glands. Unusual superior gland adenomas are located higher up around the superior thyroid pole or on the medial surface of the thyroid lobe. Rarely are the superior parathyroid glands intrathyroidal, but more commonly they may be deeply hidden within the thyroid tissue, especially if the patient has nodular goiter, which in fact has been reported to occur in up to 30-40% of the parathyroid operations.[32] Inferior glands seem to lack a similar tendency to be displaced in association with enlargement, but are still more variably distributed than the superior ones.[11,30,32] Like normal glands the enlarged inferior ones are most commonly found around the inferior thyroid pole, in the thyreothymic ligament or within the cervical thymus. Fewer than 2% of adenomas in inferior glands appear in the mediastinum out of reach from the cervical incision.[11,30] The incidence of intrathyroidal inferior glands has varied, possibly because of difficulties to distinguishing the glands that are entrapped within the surgical thyroid capsule or engulfed within nodular thyroid tissue. True intrathyroidal glands seem to occur in no more than 1% or less.[11,12,30] Undescended inferior glands are strictly uncommon, as are ectopic parathyroids concealed within the sheath of the carotid artery.[10,11,30,32] Even more uncommon are locations in the lateral triangle of the neck, glands buried in the esophageal wall, as well as those intimately related to the aortic arch or the great vessels in the superior mediastinum.[9,11,30,32,33] Very rare glands are also those deep in the middle mediastinum or at the aortopulmonary window.[7] Glands inside the pericardium, within the vagal nerve, or in the mucosa of the pyriform sinus represent great curiosities.[34-36]

Several authors have substantiated that the incidence of clinically significant *supernumerary parathyroid glands* may be increased in patients with parathyroid hyperplasia.[11,14,27,37-42] The incidence may be even more significant in patients with HPT secondary to uremia, where more or less every third patient may be exhibiting such additional glands (Table 4.1).[27] This substantiates the need to carefully explore possible sites of supernumerary glands when treating patients with any type of multiglandular parathyroid involvement. Since in such patients even the rudimentary parathyroids may be stimulated to grow to clinically significant lesions, it should be important to include cervical thymectomy and possibly also excision of fat pads around the proper parathyroids as part of the operative procedure.[11,14] This is now frequently suggested as routine in operations for multiple endocrine neoplasia type 1 (MEN-1) associated HPT and the secondary parathyroid hyperplasia of dialysis patients.[11,14,41,42]

The *principle aims of the neck exploration in HPT* are to establish the most likely cause of the disease as well as to perform adequate excision of pathological glands. Parathyroid adenomas are known to cause the disease in 85-90% of patients with primary HPT, while 10-15% can be expected to harbor hyperplasia or multiple parathyroid adenoma, i.e. multiglandular disease, and probably less than 0.5% will have parathyroid carcinoma. Safe establishment

Table 4.1. Incidence of supernumerary parathyroid glands reported in the literature

Authors* (yr)	Incidence	Comment
Autopsy study of embryos		
Norris (1937)	2/130 (2%)	2 cases had 5 glands
Gilmour (1937)	3/14 (21.4%)	1 case had 5 glands; 2 had 6 glands
Boyd (1950)	5/35 (14.3)	5 or 6 glands were present
Autopsy study of adults		
Gilmour (1938)	27/427 (6.5%)	2 cases had 6 glands
Alveryd (1968)	13/354 (3.7%)	All 13 cases had 5 glands
Wang (1975)	4/160 (2.5%)	3 cases had 5 glands; 1 had 6 glands
Åkerström (1984)	63/504 (13%)	39 cases had rudimentary or split glands; 24 had proper supernumerary glands; 18 cases had 5 glands, 3 had 6, 1 had 7, 1 had 8, and 1 had 11 glands
Nobori (1987)	70/754 (9.3%)	65 cases had 5 glands, 3 had 6, and 2 had 7 glands
Surgical study of primary hyperparathyroidism excluding cases of hyperplasia		
Palmer (1978)	3/365 (0.8%)	
Wang (1979)	6/762 (0.8%)	5 cases had 5 glands; 1 had 6 glands
Surgical study of primary hyperparathyroidism caused by parathyroid hyperplasia		
Reddick (1977)	3/40 (7.5%)	
Edis (1979)	5/55 (13%)	
Thompson (1982)	1/42 (2.4%)	
Surgical study of secondary hyperparathyroidism		
Wells (1977)	5/13 (38%)	
Meakins (1984)	3/12 (25%)	
Edis (1987)	3/20 (15%)	
Yamamoto (1991)	6/30 (20%)	5 cases had 5 glands; 1 had 7 glands

*Literature references for supernumerary parathyroid glands are available from Nobori et al[27] on request.

of a correct diagnosis often requires that both sides of the neck have been explored and the size and gross features of four glands have been assessed. Pathophysiological derangement is often suspected by the glandular inspection, as it relates grossly to the size of the glands, and consequently a diagnosis of adenoma should not be considered securely established unless three normal-sized associated glands have been visualized together with an enlarged one (Fig. 4.9). *Routine biopsy or excision of normal-sized glands* should be avoided as the identity of a normal gland is usually evident from size, consistency and color. Biopsies are needed only when there is doubt whether a recognized lesion involves a parathyroid, and partial glandular biopsies generally do not allow establishment of a correct histological diagnosis (see chapter 3).

An important part of the neck exploration in HPT is to recognize or exclude the presence of *multiglandular disease or parathyroid hyperplasia*. Nodular chief cell hyperplasia is most common in this context, while multiple adenomas can be expected in 1-2% and water-clear cell hyperplasia is currently rare[43] (see chapter 3). Since the glandular enlargement in chief cell hyperplasia tends to be asymmetrical and most commonly affects two or three glands, it is important also in this respect not to terminate the exploration in HPT until four glands have been visualized if possible.[44-48]

Long term follow-up of patients with sporadic primary chief cell hyperplasia has demonstrated that generally it should be *sufficient to excise only the enlarged glands* in patients with asymmetrical, multiglandular involvement, and that clearly normal-sized glands may be left in the neck without increasing the risk of failure.[44-48] In patients with generalized sporadic parathyroid chief cell hyperplasia a classical *subtotal parathyroid resection*, implying excision of 3-3½ glands, is currently the most widely adopted treatment.[39,49-51] The subtotal resection has been reported to provide long-term cure in 85-90% of the patients with sporadic primary hyperplasia and failure resulting in persistent disease has been related mainly to the presence of overlooked supernumerary glands, and remnant recurrence has generally been rare.[39] Recurrence may thus essentially be due to intrinsic pathophysiological properties within the remaining parathyroid tissue as it has been difficult to prevent also by the more radical resections.[50] *Total parathyroidectomy and immediate autotransplantation* of parathyroid tissue to the forearm has been suggested as an alternative strategy in patients with sporadic primary parathyroid hyperplasia.[52,53] This procedure seems particularly suitable in rare cases with marked four gland enlargement, where it may be awkward to leave in the neck a remnant of a conspicuously enlarged and diseased gland. Recurrence of generally mild hypercalcemia have been encountered in up to one-third of the patients subjected to the total parathyroidectomy, and has apparently derived from graft hyperfunction possibly related to the transplantation of diseased tissue.[53] A state of prolonged hypocalcemia is, another general problem with this procedure. Irrespective of this, the subtotal resection and the total parathyroidectomy combined with autotransplantation are probably equally efficient in curing parathyroid hyperplasia, provided that the procedures are adequately performed. Whichever procedure is selected it should be imperative to choose the smallest parathyroid gland in an individual as the designated remnant when performing a subtotal resection or for grafting in association with total parathyroidectomy. A guide-line for the selection of strategy may be the fact that normal-sized, fat-rich glands lend themselves poorly to autotransplantation but should be excellent as remnants.

In patients with severe hypercalcemia the surgeon also has to emphasize the possibility that the patient may harbor parathyroid carcinoma, and typical features of a greyish-white hard and adherent tumor indicate extensive efforts to perform initially radical excision of the tumor and surrounding tissues (see chapter 10).

Unilateral exploration has been advocated even by experienced surgeons as an alternative surgical strategy in primary HPT.[54-57] However, this procedure should be less efficient in determining the pathology of the disease, considering that the glandular involvement in chief cell hyperplasia is almost invariably focal and asymmetrical.[44,46] Unilateral exploration may also fail to detect multiple parathyroid adenoma, which may occur in 1-3%, and it should be especially equivocal in the unrecognized MEN-1 patient, where enlarged glands, sometimes with criteria of adenoma may coexist with both diseased and histologically normal glands. Moreover, since excision of a normal-sized gland for histopathological examination often constitutes part of the unilateral procedure, it will be impossible to preserve the most appropriate "normal tissue" if two enlarged glands remain on the contralateral unexplored side. We and other surgeons, when occasionally performing unilateral exploration for primary HPT, as for instance after previously extensive thyroid surgery, have experienced persistent hypercalcemia due to the presence of a "second adenoma" on the contralateral side[58] (own unpublished observation).

Any patient with diagnosed parathyroid hyperplasia should be screened postoperatively for the presence of a MEN-1 syndrome. This syndrome will be present particularly in younger individuals, who exhibit multiglandular involvement often with unusually marked glandular enlargement. Such screening investigations have to be repeated during long term follow-up since parathyroid hyperplasia may precede other manifestations of this syndrome by many years (see chapter 7).

REFERENCES

1. Weller GL Jr. Development of the thyroid, parathyroid and thymus glands in man. Carneg. Inst. Washington Publ. No 443, Contrib Embryol 1933; 141: 93-139.
2. Boyd JD. Development of thyroid and parathyroid glands and the thymus. Ann R Coll Surg Engl 1950; 7: 455-71.
3. Gray SW, Skandalakis JE. Embryology for surgeons. Philadelphia, WB Saunders 1972.
4. Sedgwick CE, Cady B. Embryology and developmental abnormalities. Chapter 2. In Sedgwick, Cady, eds. Surgery of the thyroid and parathyroid glands. Philadelphia: WB Saunders 1980.
5. Kaplan EL, Yashiro T, Salti G. Primary hyperparathyroidism in the 1990s. Choice of surgical procedures for this disease. Ann Surg 1992; 215: 300-17.
6. Gilmour JR, Martin WJ. The weight of the parathyroid glands. J Pathol 1937; 44: 431-62.
7. Curley IR, Wheeler MH, Thompson NW et al. The challenge of the middle mediastinal parathyroid. World J Surg 1988; 12: 818-24.
8. Norris EH. The parathyroid glands and lateral thyroid in man: Their morphogenesis, histogenesis, topographic anatomy and perinatal growth. Carneg. Inst. Washington Publ. No 479. Contrib Embryol 1937; 159: 247-94.
9. Udekwu AO, Kaplan EL, Wu T-C et al. Ectopic parathyroid adenoma of the lateral triangle of the neck: report of two cases. Surgery 1987; 101: 114-8.
10. Edis AJ, Purnell DC, van Heerden JA. The undescended "parathymus": an occasional cause of failed neck exploration for hyperparathyroidism. Ann Surg 1979; 190: 64-8.
11. Thompson NW. Surgical anatomy of hyperparathyroidism. In Parathyroid surgery. Prog Surg Karger, Basel 1986; 18: 59-79.
12. Wheeler MH, Williams MA, Path FRC et al. The hyperfunctioning intrathyroidal parathyroid gland: a potential pitfall in parathyroid surgery. World J Surg 1987; 11: 110-4.
13. Gilmour JR. The gross anatomy of the parathyroid glands. J Pathol 1938; 46: 133-49.
14. Åkerström G, Malmaeus J, Bergström R. Surgical anatomy of human parathyroid glands. Surgery 1984; 95: 14-21.
15. Wang CA. The anatomic basis of parathyroid surgery. Surgery 1976; 183: 271-5.
16. Gilmour JR. The embryology of the parathyroid gland, the thymus and certain associated rudiments. J Pathol Bacteriol 1937; 45: 507-22.
17. Reddick RL, Costa JC, Marx SJ. Parathyroid hyperplasia and parathyromatosis. Lancet 1977; 1: 549.
18. Rattner DW, Marrone GC, Kadson E et al. Recurrent hyperparathyroidism due to implantation of parathyroid tissue. Am J Surg 1985; 149: 745-8
19. Åkerström G, Rudberg C, Grimelius L et al. Recurrent hyperparathyroidism due to peroperative seeding of neoplastic or hyperplastic parathyroid tissue. Acta Chir Scand 1988; 154: 549-52.
20. Fitko R, Roth SI, Hines JR et al. Parathyromatosis in hyperparathyroidism. Hum Pathol 1990; 21(2): 234-7.
21. Brennan MF, Brown EM, Marx SJ et al. Recurrent hyperparathyroidism from an autotransplanted parathyroid adenoma. N Engl J Med 1978; 299: 1057-9.
22. Frei U, Klempa I, Schneider M et al. Tumour-like growth of parathyroid autografts in uraemic patients. Proc Eur Dial Transpl 1981; 18: 548-55.
23. Welsh MA. Concerning the parathyroid glands. A critical anatomical and experimental study. Part II-anatomy. J Anat Physiol 1898; 2: 381-403.
24. Halsted WS, Evans HM. The parathyroid glandules. Their blood supply, and their preservation in operation upon the thyroid gland. Ann Surg 1907; 46: 489-506.
25. De Quervain F, Curtis GM. The operative treatment of goiter. Surg Gynecol Obstet 1926; 43: 498-503
26. Curtis GM. The blood supply of the human parathyroids. Surg Gynecol Obstet 1930; 51: 805-9.

27. Nobori MN, Saiki S, Tanaka N et al. Blood supply of the parathyroid gland from the superior thyroid artery. Surgery 1994; 115: 417-23.
28. Churchill ED, Cope O. Parathyroid tumors associated with hyperparathyroidism. Surg Gynecol Obstet 1934; 55: 25-71.
29. Åkerström G, Ljunghall S. Medical and radiologic evaluation and operative treatment of primary hyperparathyroidism. Curr Opinion Gen Surg; 1993: 130-8.
30. Thompson NW, Eckhauser FE, Harness JK. The anatomy of primary hyperparathyroidism. Surgery 1982; 92: 814-22.
31. Wang CA. The use of the inferior cornu of the thyroid cartilage in identifying the recurrent laryngeal nerve. Surg Gynecol Obstet 1975; 140; 91-4.
32. Hooghe L, Kinnaert P, van Geertuyden J. Surgical anatomy of hyperparathyroidism. Acta Chir Belg 1992; 92: 1-9.
33. Norton JA, Schneider PD, Brennan MF. Median sternotomy in reoperations for primary hyperparathyroidism. World J Surg 1985; 9: 807-13.
34. Black BK, Ackerman LV. Tumors of the parathyroid: A review of 23 cases. Cancer 1950; 3: 415-44.
35. Lack EE, Delay S, Linnoila I. Ectopic parathyroid tissue within the vagus nerve. Incidence and possible clinical significance. Arch Pathol Lab Med 1988; 112: 304-6.
36. Joseph MP, Nadol JB, Pilch BZ et al. Ectopic parathyroid tissue in the hypopharyngeal mucosa (pyriform sinus). Head Neck Surg 1982; 5: 70-4.
37. Liechty RD, Weil R. Parathyroid anatomy in hyperplasia. Arch Surg 1992; 127: 813-6.
38. Palmer JA. Importance of a fifth parathyroid gland in the treatment of hyperparathyroidism. Can J Surg 1978; 21: 350-1.
39. Edis JA, van Heerden JA. Results of subtotal parathyroidectomy for primary chief cell hyperplasia. Surgery 1979; 86: 462-4.
40. Wells SA, Stirman JA Jr, Bolman RM III. Parathyroid transplantation. World J Surg 1977; 1: 747-56.
41. Meakins JL, Milne CA, Hollomy DH et al. Total parathyroidectomy: parathyroid hormone levels and supernumerary glands in hemodialysis patients. Clin Invest Med 1984; 7: 21-5.
42. Edis AJ. Supernumerary parathyroid glands: implication for the surgical treatment of secondary hyperparathyroidism. World J Surg 1987; 11: 398-401.
43. Harness JK, Ramsburg SR, Nishiyama RH et al. Multiple adenomas of the parathyroids: do they exist? Arch Surg 1978; 114: 468-74.
44. Bruining HA, van Houten H, Juttman JR et al. Results of operative treatment of 615 patients with primary hyperparathyroidism. World J Surg 1981; 5: 85-90.
45. Scholz DA, Purnell DC, Edis AJ. Primary hyperparathyroidism with multiple parathyroid gland enlargement. Review of 53 cases. Mayo Clin Proc 1978; 53: 792-7.
46. Wallfelt C, Ljunghall S, Bergström R et al. Clinical characteristics and surgical treatment in primary hyperparathyroidism—with emphasis on chief cell hyperplasia. Surgery 1990; 107: 13-19.
47. Wells SA, Leight GS, Hensley M et al. Hyperparathyroidism associated with the enlargement of two or three parathyroid glands. Ann Surg 1985; 202: 533-8.
48. Roses DF, Karp NS, Sudarsky LA et al. Primary hyperparathyroidism associated with two enlarged parathyroid glands. Arch Surg 1989; 124: 1261-4.
49. Castleman B, Schantz A, Roth SI. Parathyroid hyperplasia in primary hyperparathyroidism: a review of 85 cases. Cancer 1976; 38: 1668-75.
50. Rudberg C, Åkerström G, Palmér M et al. Late results of operation for primary hyperparathyroidism in 441 patients. Surgery 1986; 99: 643-51.
51. Bondeson A-G, Bondeson L, Ljungberg O et al. Surgical strategy in nonfamilial primary parathyroid hyperplasia: long-term follow-up of thirty-nine cases. Surgery 1985; 97: 569-73.
52. Wells SA Jr, Ellis GJ, Gunnells JC et al. Parathyroid autotransplantation in primary parathyroid hyperplasia. N Engl J Med 1976; 295: 57-62.
53. Wells SA Jr, Farndon JR, Dale JK et al. Long-term evaluation of patients with primary parathyroid hyperplasia managed by total parathyroidectomy and heterotopic

autotransplantation. Ann Surg 1980; 192: 451-8.
54. Tibblin S, Bondeson A-G, Ljungberg O. Unilateral parathyroidectomy in hyperparathyroidism due to single adenoma. Ann Surg 1982; 195: 245-52.
55. Wang C. Surgical management of primary hyperparathyroidism. Curr Probl Surg 1985; 22: 1-50.
56. Lucas RJ, Welsh RJ, Glover JL. Unilateral neck exploration of primary hyperparathyroidism. Arch Surg 1990; 125: 982-5.
57. Worsey MJ, Carty SE, Watson CG. Success of unilateral neck exploration for sporadic primary hyperparathyroidism. Surgery 1993; 114: 1024-30.
58. van Heerden JA, Grant CS. Surgical treatment of primary hyperparathyroidism: An institutional perspective. World J Surg 1991; 15: 688-92.
59. Skaudalaleis JE, Gray SW. Embryology for surgeons (2nd ed.) Baltimore: Williams and Wilkins, 1994.

CHAPTER 5

Radiological Means of Parathyroid Localization and Ablation

Jonas Rastad

Most of the widely utilized techniques for preoperative localization of enlarged parathyroid glands are costly and time-consuming. Such examinations play a central role in the routine handling of patients scheduled for reoperation due to persistent or recurrent hyperparathyroidism despite the fact that most available techniques demonstrate meager specificity for parathyroid tissue and that randomized evaluation of their efficiency is lacking. It should also be born in mind that all these modalities require dedicated facilities staffed by physicians with thorough knowledge of parathyroid anatomy and pathology as well as close collaboration with the surgeon in order to ascertain an optimal outcome.

The problem of locating abnormal parathyroid glands prior to surgery has attracted considerable interest among surgeons and radiologists, and a host of methodologies has been evaluated for this purpose. This circumstance relates mainly to the difficulties associated with at least some parathyroid reoperations even in the hands of the most experienced surgeons, since hitherto there exists no unequivocal documentation substantiating favorable influence of successful preoperative localization on the outcome of parathyroid re-exploration with respect to neither short-term cure nor complications. Although the vast majority of referral centers including ours currently would attempt localization of pathological parathyroid tissue prior to re-exploration,[1-7] universal consensus is lacking on the indication for these investigations as well as for the choice of procedures. Most utilized means localization techniques are largely influenced by size and anatomical site of the enlarged glands, and the efficiency sometimes is more encouraging among the surgically less challenging glandular locations. The present chapter summarizing clinical aspects of widely applied techniques for pre- and intraoperative parathyroid localization, and

Current Controversy in Parathyroid Operation and Reoperation, edited by Göran Åkerström.

speculates on some future developments in this field. Attempts will be made to define indications for such radiologically assisted means of localization and therapy in patients with previously operated primary and secondary hyperparathyroidism (HPT).

HISTORICAL ASPECTS

Several techniques are of principally historical interest due mainly to their complicationsas well as to their limited sensitivity and specificity even for the more substantially enlarged parathyroid glands. In most instances these localization techniques have been replaced by more sensitive examinations (Table 5.1), which nevertheless are hampered by modest parathyroid tissue specificity and consequently are unsuitable for the clinical purpose of substantiating the diagnosis of HPT. The group of currently abandoned techniques postoperatively include cine esophagography, thermography, lymphography, and scintigraphy with ^{131}I, ^{57}Co-cyanocobolamine, as well as arterially and venously injected seleno-methionine.[8-13] Cervical palpation still is important in patients with HPT mainly for the purpose of establishing concomitant goiter, since this circumstance may contribute to the incidence of both false positive and negative findings with most of the currently techniques for parathyroid localization.[15-17] Increased risk of thyroid carcinoma also has been suggested in sporadic HPT,[17] and comprises a characteristic of the rare patients with HPT due to the multiple endocrine neoplasia type 2 syndromes. Parathyroid lesions nevertheless may be palpable in very rare patients with HPT, and these lesions preferentially should be suspected of representing parathyroid cysts or parathyroid carcinoma.[18-20]

Table 5.1. Current widely applied techniques of parathyroid localization

Non-invasive	
	Ultrasound
	Magnetic resonance imaging
Minimally invasive	
	Thallium-technetium subtraction scintigraphy
	Computed tomography
Invasive	
	Guided needle aspiration
	Selective arteriography
	Digital subtraction arteriography
	Venous sampling for parathyroid hormone determination
	Intraoperative ultrasound

PREOPERATIVE ULTRASOUND

TECHNICAL ASPECTS

Parathyroid ultrasonography was introduced in 1975 and comprises one of the most commonly utilized modes of noninvasive localization of parathyroid glands prior to re-exploration.[21] The patients are examined in the supine position with the neck hyperextended in order to elongate sonographic access mainly to superior retrosternal and parapharyngeal portions of the neck. Scanning is performed in both transverse, sagittal and oblique planes for the main purpose of attempting to visualize the often delicate fibrous tissue between the thyroid and adjacent parathyroid glands, and to reduce sonographically blind areas due to the trachea, clavicular head and manubrium sterni. Scanning should be repeated during swallowing and perhaps also a Valsalva maneuver, since this may assisit in visualizing caudally positioned lesions especially in patients with a short neck, assist in the identification of esophagus and vessels, and contribute to parathyroid recognition from asymmetric structural movements.[15,22-24] In order to fully appreciate different aspects of the central neck compartment and to identify location of suspected parathyroid glands, the sonographic examination should encompass bilateral identification of the thyroid, esophagus, trachea, carotid and internal jugular vessels, as well as the longus colli muscles posteriorly. The minor neurovascular bundle of the recurrent laryngeal nerve and inferior thyroid artery is also important in this respect. It has been suggested that ultrasound of even moderately high frequency may delineate the recurrent nerve as a thin hypoechoic tube in the neck.[25,26]

Parathyroid ultrasound should be conducted preferentially with linear array scanners of 10 MHz,[3,15,23] since this has been suggested to enhance sensitivity of glandular detection.[27] Relatively few institutions currently utilize this equipment, which is characterized by a visualized tissue depth of about 4 cm, as well as theoretical axial and lateral resolutions of about 0.5 and 1.5 mm, respectively. Lesions located mainly posteriorly in the neck may thus be more efficiently located with scanners of lower frequency, but at the cost of reduced resolution, and negative examinations consequently may become true positive upon analysis with equipments of 5-7.5 MHz. Ultrasound exhibits the distinct feature of being highly investigator dependent and unusually difficult to reconstruct in retrospect.[28,29] In order to acquire technical expertise, it may be necessary to practice on patients with surgically untreated HPT.

Parathyroid Appearance

Ultrasonically visualized parathyroid glands usually appear as oval to teardrop shaped and sharply marginated solid masses of low echogenicity (Fig. 5.1), which frequently exhibit the longest diameter in approximately the rostro-caudal direction. Naturally the size and shape of glands as well as their internal structure may vary considerably both within and between individual patients.[23,24,30-32] Occasional enlarged glands may exhibit tube-like, bi- and multilobular, globular, irregular or kidney-like shapes. The echolucency of characteristic parathyroids is substantially higher than both normal and most nodular thyroid glands. Very few parathyroids are isoechoic to the thyroid, although the Pse have been suggested to exceed 10% of the correctly visualized parathyroid glands, and the rare lipoadenomas may be hyperechoic.[33] Cystic or partly cystic parathyroids as well as calcifications may be encountered occasionally. About 10-15% of the ultrasonically

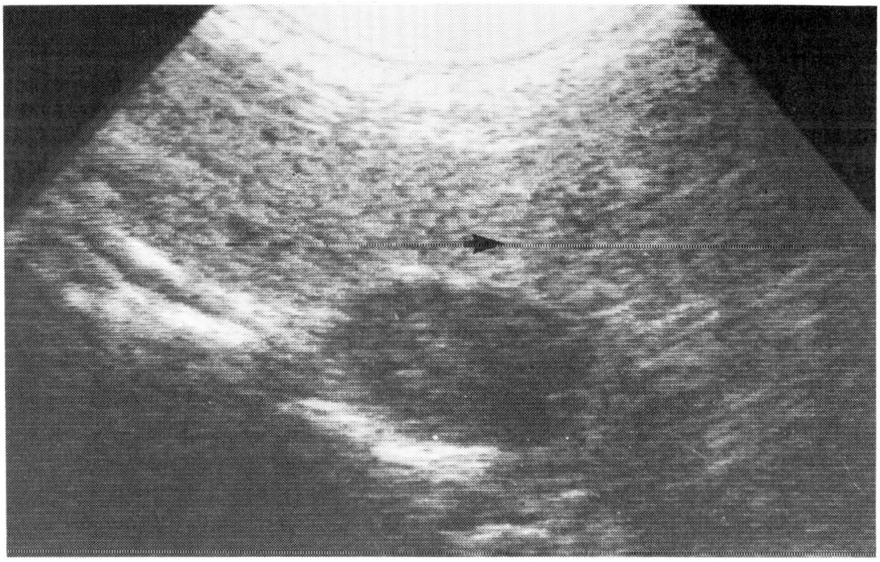

Fig. 5.1. Longitudinal ultrasonogram of a right-sided parathyroid adenoma located dorsal to the inferior portion of the thyroid lobe. The adenoma weighed 0.9 g and displays slightly ovoid shape, a well defined and rather echodense periphery, as well as a rather homogeneously sonolucent interior texture. This patient also demonstrated a follicular thyroid adenoma indicated by the arrow. The prominent scar tissue and adhesions from two previous neck explorations as well as a partial thyroid resection cannot be envisioned on the sonogram.

visualized parathyroid glands exhibit heterogeneous interior echogenicity, which renders the discrimination with thyroid nodules especially difficult (Fig. 5.2). This sonographic characteristic has been related to nodular or excessive acinar parenchymal arrangements, hemorrhage, fibrosis, and unevenly distributed structural fat within the glands. There seems to exist no consistent differences in sonographic appearance between adenomas and primary hyperplasias, and this possibly also explains ultrasonographical parathyroid carcinomas do not appear to invade adjacent structures.[24,32,34,35] In uremic HPT, however, tendencies for greater echodensity of the parathyroid glands frequently occur.[36-38]

Efficiency of Sonography

Normal parathyroid glands should not be expected to be visualized by ultrasound despite other observations in this regard.[23] Detection of pathological glands within surgically explored patients essentially seems to require mean glandular diameters of at least 5 mm and a weight exceeding about 100 mg for both adenomas and hyperplasias.[4,14,39,40] The accuracy of sonography alone has varied considerably between series of patients undergoing parathyroid reoperation. After the initial enthusiasm for this and indeed also other modes of preoperative localization, only about 50-60% of parathyroid adenomas have been found to undergo detection by ultrasound.[3,4,41-43] This rate of success is marginally less encouraging than in overtly careful analyses on previously unexplored individuals.[15,24,29,44-46] The fibrotic adherences, neovascularization, and distortion of anatomical relationships from parathyroid operations thus seem to exert minor influences on the outcome of sonography. This lack of obvious discrepancy in detection rate possibly relates to the circumstance that the majority of pathological glands are retrieved from anatomically normal positions during not only primary but also reoperative parathyroid surgery.[2,47] Glandular size also may be somewhat larger in the reoperative situation, since these explorations universally require the presence of unequivocal preoperative hypercalcemia.

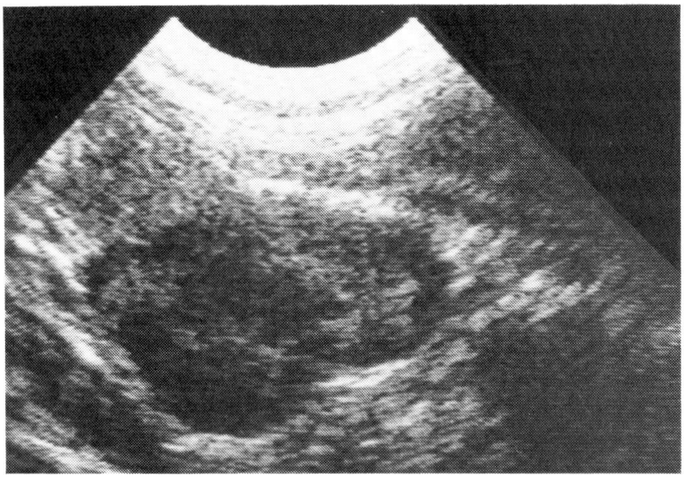

Fig. 5.2. Longitudinal sonogram of a left-sided parathyroid adenoma with less characteristic sonographic appearance in a patient with persistent primary HPT after parathyroid exploration revealing only two normal parathyroid glands. This adenoma of 1.4 g was located just dorsolateral to the middle portion of the thyroid lobe. It demonstrates a highly irregular contour, and a variably sonolucent interior structure. Histological examination of this gland displayed rather prominent regressive changes with fibrosis, necrosis and hemosiderin deposits, as well as an unusually prominent nodulation of the parenchyma.

Parathyroid hyperplasias especially of primary but also secondary HPT commonly are less efficiently located than adenomas, and this discrepancy has been related to the generally smaller size of hyperplastic glands.[3,36,38,42,48-50] The rate of detection of parathyroid glands in uremic HPT has been found to increase with duration and severity of the functional renal impairment as well as size of parathyroid glands and biochemical extent of HPT.[34,36-38,51] Ultrasound should not be expected to depict more than singularly enlarged glands of patients with hyperplasia whether this is primary or secondary. This clinically frequent finding is not surprising considering the markedly asymmetric extent of glandular enlargement that prevails in patients with sporadic and familiar primary hyperplasia as well as in those with HPT of uremia.[52-55]

The success of parathyroid ultrasound is highly sensitive to gland location (Table 5.2). Parathyroids situated in acoustic shadows of the trachea and bone cannot be visualized, so retropharyngeal, retroesophageal, paratracheal, tracheo-oesophageal groove, and retrosternal positions are more or less unfavorable. Lesions of substantial size within the mediastinum, however, may be sonographically located by intercostal examination. Surgically unrecognized parathyroids in paravascular positions, those located intrathyroidally and undescended glands in parathymus and perhaps also elsewhere in the neck may be visualized with essentially similar success as are glands in the more common immediate vicinity of the thyroid.[3,4,24,56,57] Sonographic visualization also seems to increase with glandular size,[15,24,36,58-60] although this relationship is complex and generally absent, weak or confined to parathyroid hyperplasia in some studies.[3,29,39,49] Particular circumstances relate to the visualization of recurrent HPT from intramuscular parathyroid autografts. Although such growth seems to be a truly rare cause of recurrence after total parathyroidectomy and brachioradial transplantation, sufficiently enlarged noduli of parathyroid tissue may be excellently visualized by ultrasound also in absence of externally palpable lesions.[61-64]

A variety of structures may be misinterpreted as enlarged parathyroid glands during ultrasonic examination of patients with HPT. These false positives principally have been found to encompass 10-25% of the patients undergoing reoperation.[3,4,41,43,65,66] The misinterpreted lesions mostly comprise structures of low to moderate echodensity such as thyroid nodules, hyperplastic lymph nodes, sympathetic ganglia, the longus colli muscle and tortuous vessels.[23,24,39,58] The thyroid is the main problem in this respect, and ultrasonic thyroid pathology indeed has been found in 40% of patients with HPT.[67] In many instances, however, no apparent

Table 5.2. Comparison of cutaneous ultrasound (US), thallium-technetium scintigraphy (TT), computed tomography (CT), and magnetic resonance imaging (MR) for preoperative parathyroid localization

Characteristic	US	TT	CT	MR
Availability	++[a]	+++	+++	++
Radiation exposure	–	++	+	–
Risks	–	–	+[c]	–
Operator dependency	+++	++	++	++
Resolution	+++[a]	++	+++	+++
Parathyroid tissue specificity	+	+	+	+
Detailed glandular positioning	++	+[b]	+++	+++
Cost	+	+	++	+++
Sensitivity to				
glandular size	++	+	++	+
cervical glands				
juxtathyroid	+++	++	++	++
intrathyroid	+++	+	++	+
ectopic	++	++	++	++
mediastinal glands	(–)	++	+++	+++

[a] 10 MHz scanners
[b] planar examination
[c] contrast mandatory

explanation for the occurrence of false positive parathyroid sonography can be provided upon re-exploration.

Improvements in Parathyroid Sonography

Attempts have been made to increase specificity of preoperative parathyroid ultrasound. The most commonly utilized improvement relates to the application of **guided biopsies** (Fig. 5.3), whereby the parathyroid nature of a sonographically visualized lesion may be established.[58,68,69] This procedure most frequently is conducted by means of a needle steering unit fitted onto the transducer head, which allows real-time analysis on progression of the needle tip along a predetermined sight line

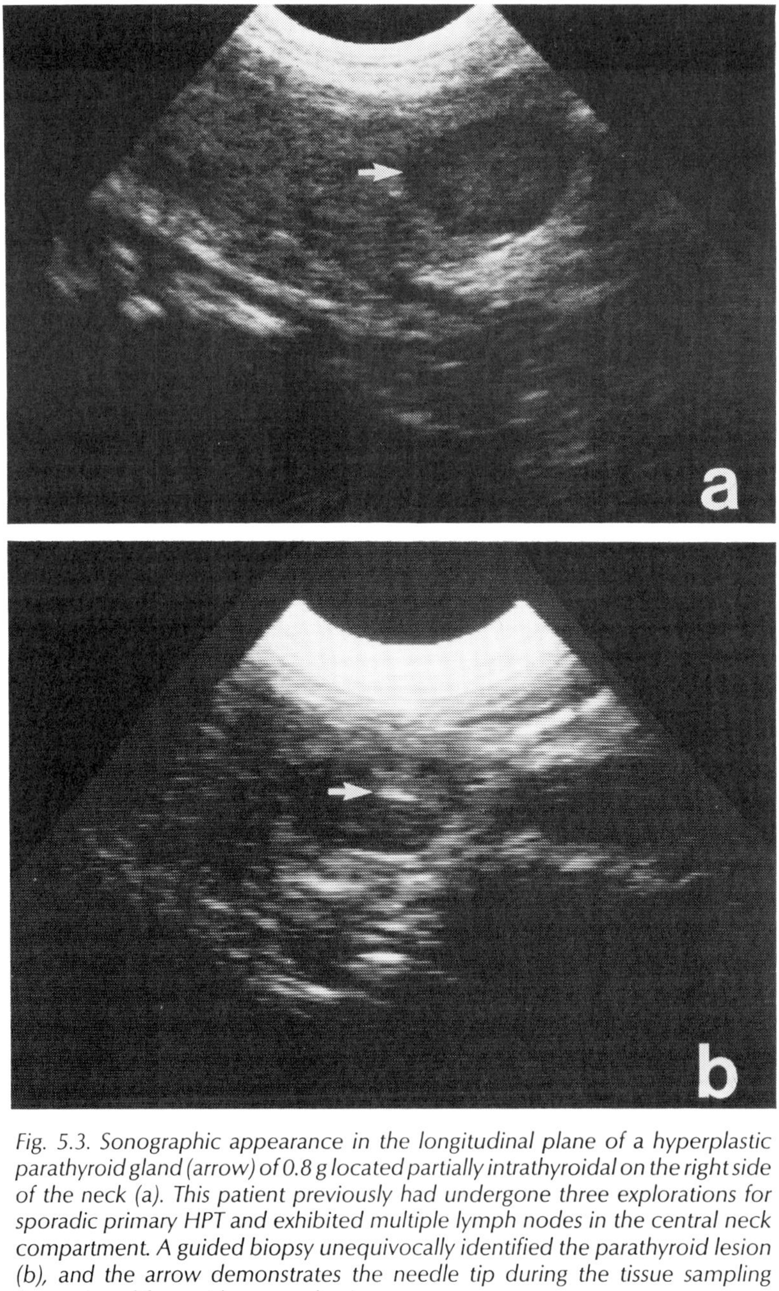

Fig. 5.3. Sonographic appearance in the longitudinal plane of a hyperplastic parathyroid gland (arrow) of 0.8 g located partially intrathyroidal on the right side of the neck (a). This patient previously had undergone three explorations for sporadic primary HPT and exhibited multiple lymph nodes in the central neck compartment. A guided biopsy unequivocally identified the parathyroid lesion (b), and the arrow demonstrates the needle tip during the tissue sampling (reproduced from video recording).

on the monitor display.[70] Aspirates from solid and cystic structures may be assayed for parathyroid hormone.[71,72] Conventional routine stainings of cytologic smears, however, seem insufficient for the recognition and discrimination of parathyroid cells;[69,73,74] argyrophilia and parathyroid hormone antibody stainings have been applied with enhanced specificity.[58,75-77] The efficiency of guided puncture in the identification of enlarged parathyroid glands varies considerably due mainly to the acquisition of non-diagnostic material. This difficulty has prompted application of small core biopsies.[78] We currently utilize cutting needles (Biopty-Cut™) of 1.0 mm external diameter[79] and staining of cryosectioned tissue cylinders with monoclonal antibodies specifically recognizing the human parathyroid tissue.[80] This procedure may be utilized to verify parathyroid glands exceeding about 8 mm in diameter, which should be located a minimum of roughly 5 mm from the carotid and internal jugular vessels as well as the great vessels of the mediastinum. Distinction between thyroid lesions and enlarged parathyroid glands by color **doppler imaging** has been evaluated without clinically useful success.[81] **Endoscopic sonography** have indicated possibilities for transpharyngeal and transoesophageal visualization of mainly posteriorly located parathyroid glands.[82]

THALLIUM-TECHNETIUM SUBTRACTION SCINTIGRAPHY

TECHNICAL ASPECTS

This examination relies on observations that human parathyroid and thyroid glands accumulate thallium chloride, that technetium pertechnetate is trapped by the thyroid rather than the parathyroid parenchyma, and that subtraction of scintigraphic images with these compounds may identify the location of parathyroid glands.[83-87] Thallium has a physical half-life of 73 hours, decays by electron capture, and exhibits about 90% photon energy in the range of 69-83 keV. Briefly the subtraction method generally involves anterior or oblique planar examination of the patient lying still with the neck extended and the head supported preferentially by a molded rest. Intravenous injection of 1-2mCi (~35-75 MBq) technetium-99m sodium pertechnetate is followed 10-20 minutes later by acquisition of a 5 minute image in the technetium window (~140 keV) utilizing a 4-6 mm pinhole or high resolution parallel-hole collimators. A technetium scatter image immediately is collected in the thallium window (~70 keV), 1-2 mCi thallium-201 chloride is injected intravenously, and dynamic scans are gathered in the thallium window for 25-30 minutes.

Subsequent computer processing of digital images includes background correction and subtraction of the technetium scan from the corrected and normalized composite thallium image, as well as motion adjustment usually by means of the thyroid as the region of interest.[85,86,88-90] Reversing the order of tracer injections, color image processing, modification of subtraction algorithms, and early thallium image acquisition due to rapid parathyroid clearance may improve outcome of the examination.[89,91-97] More recent attempts at technical refinement involve emission tomography and single photon emission tomography (SPECT) for thallium alone or combined with technetium.[98-101] These possibilities demonstrate that thallium/technetium scanning, as indeed all other studies of parathyroid localization, require dedicated physicians for optimization.

The ability of parathyroid glands to accumulate thallium has been related to regional blood flow and cellular uptake from potassium substitution in the Na/K-ATPase related exchange.[102-104] Such mechanisms possibly represent tissue nonspecific modes of trapping, and mainly reflect degrees of cellularity and vascularization. Similar parenchymal cell density, however, recently has been demonstrated in scintigraphically detected and undetected parathyroid glands.[90] Both the amplitude and temporal dynamics of thallium activity have been found to vary considerably between individual parathyroid glands, and short-term secretory stimulation from lowering of serum calcium has suggested enhanced uptake.[105-107] In partial analogy to cardiac myocytes, it has been hypothesized that thallium trapping may be coupled to functionally important Na^+/Cl^--transport as well as the Ca^{2+}-dependent Ca^{2+} uptake mediated principally through a cation receptor on the parathyroid cell surface.[90,108-111] The energy requirement of these mechanisms might be considered to coincide with demonstrations of efficient thallium accumulation in thyrocytes with abundant mitochondria.[112] This finding corroborates the demonstration of more efficient visualization by thallium/technetium scanning of parathyroid glands exhibiting high contents of oxyphil cells.[90] The mitochondria-rich oxyphil parathyroid cells increase with age and extent of functional renal impairment.[113-115] These cells, however, demonstrate meager Ca^{2+} regulated Ca^{2+} uptake and equivocal parathyroid hormone secretory capacity.[116,117]

Parathyroid Appearance

Scans usually are interpreted as positive when single or multiple foci of well-defined thallium concentrations appear on the subtracted images (Fig. 5.4). Although this methodology allows recognition of subtle lesions, intensity limits for unequivocal parathyroid identification have not been systematically investigated.[88,89] Moreover processing is hampered by the presence of abnormal thyroid glands upon palpation and pertechnetate imaging. Thyroid abnormalities coexisting with subtracted thallium excess as well as insufficient adjustment for patient movement consequently often leads to indeterminate findings, which are characterized by poorly circumscribed areas of thallium accumulation within and outside the thyroid gland.

Efficiency of Scintigraphy

Normal parathyroid glands are not demonstrable by thallium/technetium scintigraphy. Pathological parathyroids down to 60 mg have been reported to provide diagnostic scans,[91,118] but this represents a true exception from routine clinical use. In patients subjected to previous parathyroid exploration, subtraction scanning have been found to accurately locate about 40-60% of the pathological parathyroid glands.[3,4,42,43,49,90,119-122] With few exceptions these analyses each encompass 26 reoperative individuals or less,[4,90] so some caution on sensitivity seems applicable. On an average this result nevertheless is similar to the efficiency of subtraction scanning in previously unoperated individuals[29,43,44,49,123-127] provided that series describing the most exceptional results are omitted.[59,85,88,128-130] This notion is corroborated by studies concomitantly analyzing patients scheduled for primary and secondary operations.[49,88,90,91,121,123,131,132]

The success rate of dual isotope scanning has been related to glandular size (Table 5.2). Phantom studies and analyses in vivo have indicated that the lower limit of detection equals glandular weights of 0.3-0.8 g, which approaches resolution of the scanning procedure.[85,130,133,134] Although parathyroids above and below such an approximate limit demonstrate discrepancies in rates of in vivo detection, true positives may be obtained for occasional glands of smaller size and false negatives certainly are encountered among those being more conspicuously enlarged.[3,40,43,130,132-134] This inconsistency coincides with observations on variation in thallium accumulation per unit tissue weight for parathyroid glands of different size.[133] Detailed examination, including multivariate analysis on glands clearly exceeding the estimated limit of detection, has failed to demonstrate a correlation between the rate of true positive scans and parathyroid size.[90]

Subtraction scanning provides no detailed anatomic information on the location of lesions. It is even impossible to determine if visualized glands are inferior or superior parathyroids. The technique generally has been found to be most efficient for parathyroid glands located in the neck, and generally fails to demonstrate consistent discrepancies in the detection rate of

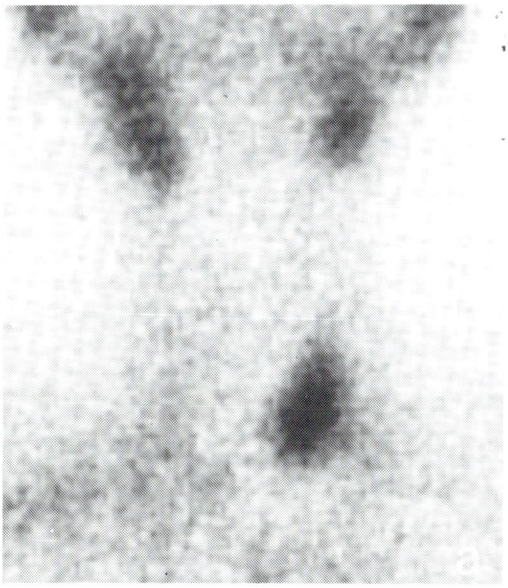

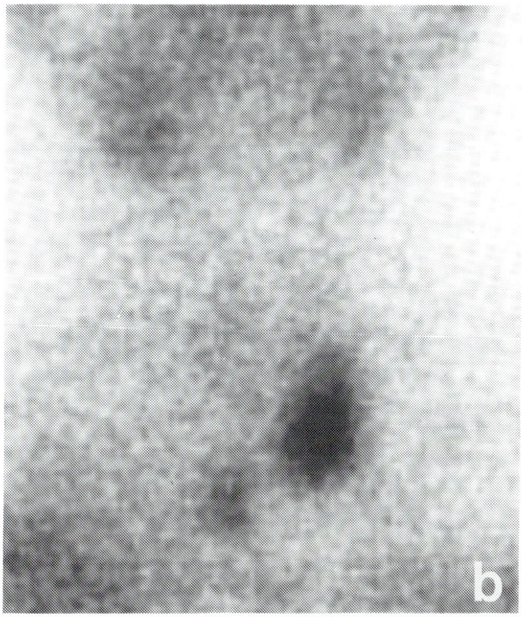

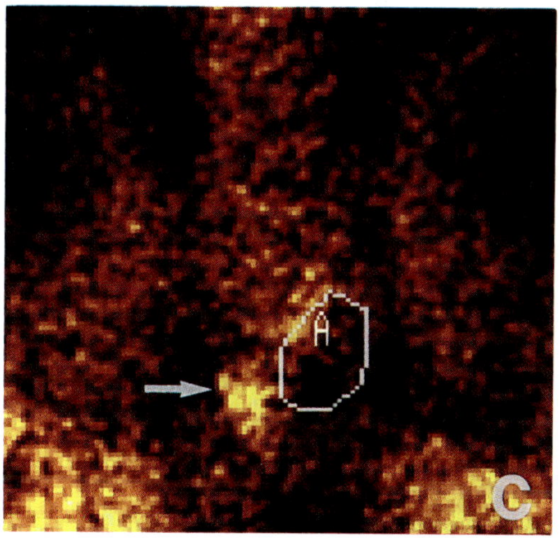

Fig. 5.4. Static scintigraphic images of the neck in the frontal plane 10 minutes after administration of technetium-99m (a) and thallium-201 (b), and image subtraction with the thyroid area outlined (c). This patient previously had been subjected to extirpation of two normal parathyroid glands together with the right thyroid lobe, and he was subsequently cured from his persistent primary HPT by extirpation of a 1.2 g adenoma located caudally on the right side of the neck (arrow in c). Images are collected with a total of 5x10^5 counts.

those in normal and ectopic positions.[4,36,44,91,120,123,132,135] Reduced sensitivities, however, have been reported for upper cervical glands located posteriorly and for those located intrathyroidally.[3,136] Mediastinal parathyroids located in the 'aorto-pulmonary' window have been visualized by subtraction scanning,[42,44,100,121,132,137] but the limited number of observations even in combined patient series prevents conclusions on sensitivity for the glands in different portions of the mediastinum. Moreover the limited resolution and energy of emitted photons can prevent diagnostic images of mediastinal parathyroids.[137] The scanning procedure rarely has been used to demonstrate recurrent HPT due to growth of forearm autografts.[138]

Adenomas generally have been found to yield localizing dual isotope scans more often than the hyperplastic glands of sporadic and familiar primary HPT.[44,49,50,60,86,87,91,96,97,131,139] The true positive rates of detection for these glandular types commonly have been reported to differ by a ratio approaching 2.0 in individual patient series,[123,133,140] but this evaluation is hampered by variable criteria of histological diagnosis. Closer inspection of this discrepancy, however, has supported that the reduced efficiency in chief cell hyperplasia can be related to the less conspicuous extent of glandular enlargement. Thallium uptake standardized for tissue weight thus seems to be the same in adenomas and primary hyperplasias, and the detection rate of hyperplastic glands equals that of adenomas upon examination within defined ranges of glandular weight.[123,133] Moreover multivariate analysis has failed to disclose significant differences in the detection of these glandular types when other factors like size are included in the examination.[90]

The efficiency of thallium/technetium scintigraphy has been less explored in secondary HPT. True positive localization has been obtained for about 40-80% of operatively verified parathyroid glands in patients with different extent of uremic HPT, and the success rate has been reported to increase with the size of the glands.[36,91,129,134,141,142] Analysis of the parathyroid tissue in secondary HPT has denstrated levels of thallium accumulation similar to those in the glands of primary HPT upon standardization for weight.[133] On the basis of expectations from true positive rates and the common variation in glandular size in parathyroid hyperplasia,[53-55,143] subtraction scanning cannot be utilized to demonstrate all enlarged parathyroids within individuals harboring multiple gland enlargement of primary or secondary HPT.

Goiters contribute significantly to the incidence of negative subtractions scans in patients with HPT. This circumstance mainly relates to masking of the parathyroids from diffusely enhanced thallium uptake within an enlarged thyroid gland. Investigations in the presence of goiter may thus be of meager diagnostic value unless ectopic parathyroids exist. Moreover neck muscles and myocardium exhibit thallium trapping, making more difficult the detection of small glands.[122,134] Caution also is mandatory in hyperthyroidism, endogenous or exogenous thyroid suppression, and recent exposure to iodinated contrast agents from computed tomography or invasive studies of parathyroid location.

Thallium-technetium scanning generally has provided false positive parathyroid localization in 10-20% of patients undergoing reoperation for HPT, and this frequency roughly equals that of individuals without previous explorations.[4,42,43,49,66,127] Thyroid lesions account for most of the known causes of these failures. Thallium seems to accumulate more rapidly and sometimes more efficiently in the abnormal thyroid than parathyroid tissues, and this finding in itself has been used to predict limitations on diagnostic yield of the scanning procedure.[133,134,144] A main cause of false positive scans relates thyroid lesions trapping thallium relatively more efficiently than technetium. These lesions mainly comprise nodular goiters, thyroid adenomas, and papillary carcinoma, although follicular carcinoma and perhaps also lymphocytic thyroiditis may exhibit similar uptake characteristics.[88,131,145-148] Consistent with findings on considerable thallium accumulation in oxyphil cell-rich parathyroid glands, eosinophilic thyroid lesions have been found to provide intense thallium scans.[112] Enlarged lymph nodes and aberrant thyroid tissue in the mediastinum comprise other causes of falsely positive parathyroid subtraction scans.[14,149]

Developments in Parathyroid Scintigraphy

Technetium-sestamibi (^{99m}Technetium hexakis 2-methoxyisobutyl isonitrile) recently has been introduced as a substitute for thallium chloride during subtraction scanning of enlarged parathyroid glands. This cationic compound was introduced for cardiac imaging and exhibits superior physical characteristics in relation to thallium, which allows reduced dosages of radiation and improved image processing.[150,151] It accumulates more efficiently and with less temporal decay in the adenomatous and hyperplastic parathyroid tissues compared to the thyroid gland. Upon subtraction with iodine-123, this agent has been found to localize enlarged and even a few normal-sized parathyroid glands of a limited number of patients with primary and secondary HPT.[151-153] As with thallium/technetium scanning, false positives occur preferentially with thyroid adenomas. The role of this scanning technique and its efficiency for preoperative parathyroid localization awaits clarification; lessons from other techniques suggest that enthusiasm for this technique will wane.

Toluidine blue is a thiazide dye binding to nucleic acids and mucopolysaccharides, which has been omitted for vital staining of parathyroid glands due mainly to toxic side effects.[154,155] But radioiodination of this freshly prepared compound and subtraction scanning preferentially with technetium pertechnetate allows reduction of the administered dose and absence of complications.[156-161] Systematic analysis of the accuracy of this localizing agent has not been presented in reoperative parathyroid surgery, and widespread use has not been attained. In primary explorations, however, substantial localizing ability has been demonstrated without appreciable relationship to glandular size above 100 mg, as well as efficient visualization of a limited number of ectopic parathyroid glands and reduced sensitivity for hyperplasia of primary HPT.

Monoclonal antibodies may become useful for preoperative localization in patients with persistent or recurrent HPT, although tentative usefulness of such compounds awaits clinical exploration. The BB5-G1 switch antibody selectively recognizes a hitherto unidentified structure of human parathyroid cells.[162] In particular the Fab'2 fragment of this antibody has demonstrated an interesting ability to immunolocalize human parathyroid tissues transplanted into nude mice after labeling with Indium-111 rather than radioiodine.[163,164] A panel of other monoclonal antibodies has been generated by immunization of mice with intact human parathyroid cells.[165] These antibodies recognize an exceptionally large glycoprotein on the parathyroid cell surface, which mediates calcium regulation of parathyroid hormone release and may account for the relative hormone excess as well as the hypercalcemia of HPT.[111,166] This target structure demonstrates highly restricted tissue distribution,[80,165] which suggests possibilities for specific targeting in vivo. Examination of mice harboring pieces of human parathyroid adenoma and carcinoma has indicated substantial antibody accumulation especially in the tissue of parathyroid cancer.[167] Several problems, however, have to be attended to prior to human use and these particularly include characterization of antibody preparations as well as optimal radiolabeling of the immunoglobulins.

COMPUTED TOMOGRAPHY

Technical Aspects

Computed tomography is a widely utilized technique, and modern equipment with high resolution and favorable signal to noise ratios is required for parathyroid analysis. The patient should be examined with the neck hyperextended. A positioning device depressing the shoulders and immobilizing the neck, chin and shoulders has been found to increase the yield of parathyroid investigation and to reduce streak artifacts related to shoulder position and mobility.[168,169] The patient should be encouraged to take shallow breaths and to refrain from swallowing. Scanning mostly encompasses 5 mm thick slices from the epiglottis to the sternal notch, and mostly 10 mm slices down to the carina. Scans are obtained prior to intravenous contrast administration and as a dynamic examination during such infusion. Prospective image targeting conventionally is used to improve resolution and picture element size, and to decrease artifacts. Selected sections may be gathered during oral contrast ingestion to facilitate identification of the esophagus, which especially on the left side of the neck may produce false positive parathyroid localizations.[169-172] Conventional metallic clips severely distort interpretation of local tomograms.

Parathyroid Appearance

Enlarged parathyroids exhibit no unequivocally characteristic appearance on the tomograms, and recognition of these glands thus requires familiarity with the common and uncommon sites of their location (Fig. 5.5). Enlarged parathyroids typically consist of round to ovoid or elongated soft tissue masses, which rather frequently exhibit irregular contours.[168,171,173-178] Prior to contrast exposure, parathyroid attenuation commonly is similar to muscle (~35-45 HU) and higher than the thyroid gland. Contrast enhancement is common but not obligatory, and has occasionally been reported to comprise only 25% of the glands.[169] The extent of this enhancement may differ greatly and be more intense in larger glands and heterogeneous especially in those containing extensive regressive changes. Many enlarged parathyroids are at least partially surrounded by hypodense fat and connective tissue, which may distiguish them from the commonly adjacent thyroid gland. Rare parathyroids contain cysts and calcifications offering additional difficulties in differentiating it from the thyroid.[19,172,176]

Efficiency of Computed Tomography

Normal parathyroid glands are not visualized by computed tomography. Enlarged parathyroids of patients subjected to previous parathyroid exploration have been correctly localized in mainly 40-50%.[2-4,43,66,169,179,180] Corresponding proportions of only 10-15% have been registered in some series containing substantial number of reoperative individuals.[1,181] In contrast to some suggestions,[45] visualization of enlarged parathyroid glands in reoperative cases mostly has been somewhat less encouraging than in unoperated individuals.[29,43,44,50,60,127,168,171,172,177,178,182] Actual glandular diameters may be underestimated by computed tomography, and parathyroid size has been suggested to influence the detection rate in some[3,44,50,60,169,172] but not all studies.[4,29,43,168,170,183] Parathyroid adenoma and hyperplasia cannot be distinguished by computed tomography. Primary hyperplasia might be detected less frequently than adenomas, which has been related to discrepancies in glandular size.[44,60] Multifactorial analysis including size and parathyroid tissue type, however, has not been reported for computed tomography in primary HPT. Parathyroids of uremic HPT have been correctly localized with essentially similar efficiency as adenomas prior to primary operation, and seem to exhibit size-related proportions of true positive examinations.[36,50,141,169,178]

Computed tomography has been found to image superior parathyroids in their common position adjacent to the thyroid gland more effectively than the inferior ones situated especially some distance below the inferior thyroid pole.[3,29,50,141] In addition ectopic parathyroids have been suggested to be accurately detected to a greater extent than those in juxtathyroid position.[14,45,173,184] In the neck this might encompass lesions in the tracheo-esophageal groove, paravascular position and perhaps also undescended glands (Table 5.2), but probably not those located intrathyroidally nor in the parathymus.[1,3,4,44,50,56,57,169,179,182] Analysis of the rather limited number of currently presented individuals indicates that computed tomography can be expected to visualize about 50% of mediastinal parathyroid glands.[4,44,100,173,182,185]

False positive parathyroid localizations have occurred in 15-25% of patients subjected to computed tomography prior to parathyroid reoperation.[3,43,44,50,66,127,169,178] These principally relate to thyroid lesions, lymph nodes, tortuous vessels, and unidentified structures. Scanning under contrast exposure and comparison with unenhanced images may contribute to reducing the number of false positives and negatives. Computed tomography rarely has been used to obtain **fine needle aspirates** for verification of the parathyroid nature of localized glands.[71]

MAGNETIC RESONANCE IMAGING

Technical Aspects

Magnetic resonance imaging has been introduced relatively recently in the preoperative localization of enlarged parathyroid glands, and optimal study designs with respect to a variety of physical parameters remain to be evaluated. The neck seems suitable for high resolution magnetic

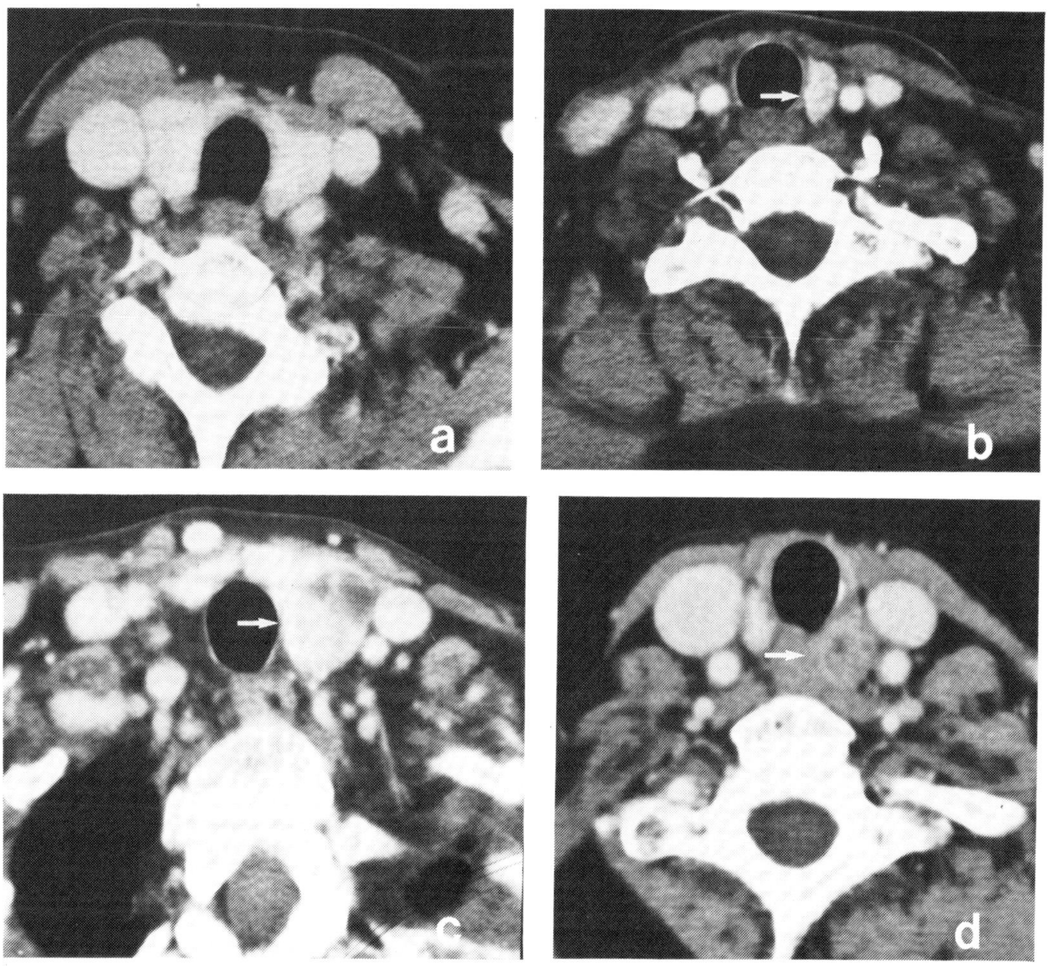

Fig. 5.5. Transverse tomograms of the neck demonstrating contrast enhancement of the normal thyroid gland (A), and enlarged parathyroids located around the lower thyroid pole on the left side of the neck in patients subjected to second or third parathyroid procedures (B-D, arrows). A parathyroid adenoma of 0.65 g displays fairly homogeneous and intense contrast accumulation (B) while a partially intrathyroidal parathyroid adenoma of 2.7 g is characterized by heterogeneous enhancement due to its prominent cystic portions (C). A previously uremic patient with recurrent hypercalcemia despite a functioning kidney graft and subtotal parathyroid resection shows a nodular hyperplastic parathyroid gland with meager contrast accumulation (D).

resonance imaging.[186] The magnetic resonance signal of routine examinations depends on the interaction of radiowaves with atomic nuclei exhibiting an odd number of protons. The single proton-containing hydrogen nucleus is the most abundant of such atoms and provides a strong signal, which is utilized to obtain computerized tomographic images. Imagers of high field strength (1.5 Tesla) are associated with superior resolution, which essentially depends on spatial abilities of the equipment, contrast characteristics of tissues and signal to noise ratios. A variety of surface coils of different sizes and shapes have been utilized mainly in direct contact with or wrapped around anterior portions of the neck; in this way intense images of low signal to noise ratio have been obtained at sites common for the parathyroid glands.[182,187-190] Problems with such equipment may arise, however, due mainly to distance-related inhomogeneities in image intensity and contrast as well as visualized tissue depth. The lower limit of detection for parathyroid glands in vivo consequently by far exceeds the impressive theoretical resolution (<1 mm) of modern equipment for magnetic resonance imaging. Patients may experience claustrophobic symptoms preventing analysis in body coils, while metallic implants, apart from cardiac pacemakers are not contraindication to the investigation.

Parathyroid imaging with surface coils usually encompasses examination from the hyoid bone down to the upper thoracic aperture, while mediastinal analysis generally requires conventional body coils. Parathyroid glands preferentially have been investigated in 3-5 mm thick transverse multisections utilizing interslice intervals of single or few millimeters. Artifacts from blood flow, respiration and swallowing may be reduced with presaturation pulses, chest images can be gated by electrocardiography, and streak artifacts from movement generally pose negligible problems.[188,191-194] Variable images of magnetic resonance may be obtained by altering the times for repetition of spin echo pulse sequences (TR) and inversion delays (TE), whereby T1-weighted images usually encompass short TR/TE and T2-weighted images long TR/TE times. Tissues with different water content may be distinguished by magnetic resonance imaging and vessels containing moving fluid can easily be distinguished from solid parenchyma. Normal structures of the neck sometimes can be differentiated from neoplastic lesions on the basis of magnetic resonance signals alone, but malignant processes should generally not be expected to be distinguished with certainty from adenomas.[195] Contrast enhancement of T1-weighted parathyroid images has been recorded with Gadopentate dimeglumine, but without appreciable improvement in localization.[196,197] Such images, however, are less prone to degradation by swallowing and patient motion and thereby comprise a useful complement to T2-weighted analysis. Fat suppression sequences in combination with T1-weighted images have been attempted in limited patient series in order to improve diagnostic yield.[198,199]

Parathyroid Appearance

Enlarged parathyroid glands characteristically provide signals of low to moderate intensity on T1-weighted images and of high intensity upon T2-weighting.[66,121,182,187,188,190,200,201] T2-weighted images thus seem to provide greater parathyroid sensitivity, but T1-weighted images are important by providing superior resolution and glandular delineation as well as contrast towards structural fat, which commonly surrounds at least portions of all extrathyroidal parathyroid glands.[189-191] About half the parathyroids identified preoperatively by magnetic resonance imaging have exhibited signals being isointense either to neck muscles or the thyroid gland on T1-weighted images, and the majority demonstrates T2-weighted signal intensities exceeding fat.[188] Consistent discrepancies in imaging appearance have not been recorded between adenomas, hyperplasias and parathyroid carcinomas.[188,191,200]

The characteristics of enlarged parathyroid glands may vary considerably, however, no single combination of signal intensities provide unequivocal recognition of all glands (Fig. 5.6). Knowledge on common and uncommon sites for parathyroid location thus comprises a requisite for their identification. About one–third of visualized parathyroid glands display heterogeneous interior signal intensities, and majority show asymmetrical contours on transaxial imaging.[178] Classical parathyroid appearances characterized by low signals on short TR/TE sequences and intense signals on long TR/TE images have been associated with high parenchymal cellularity of adenomas, while acute hemorrhage and chronic regressive changes (fibrosis, hemosiderin deposits, infiltrating leukocytes) may cause high and low intensities on both T1- and T2-weighted images.[201] Naturally the parathyroid glands with less common signal characteristics are particularly difficult to identify prior to operation.

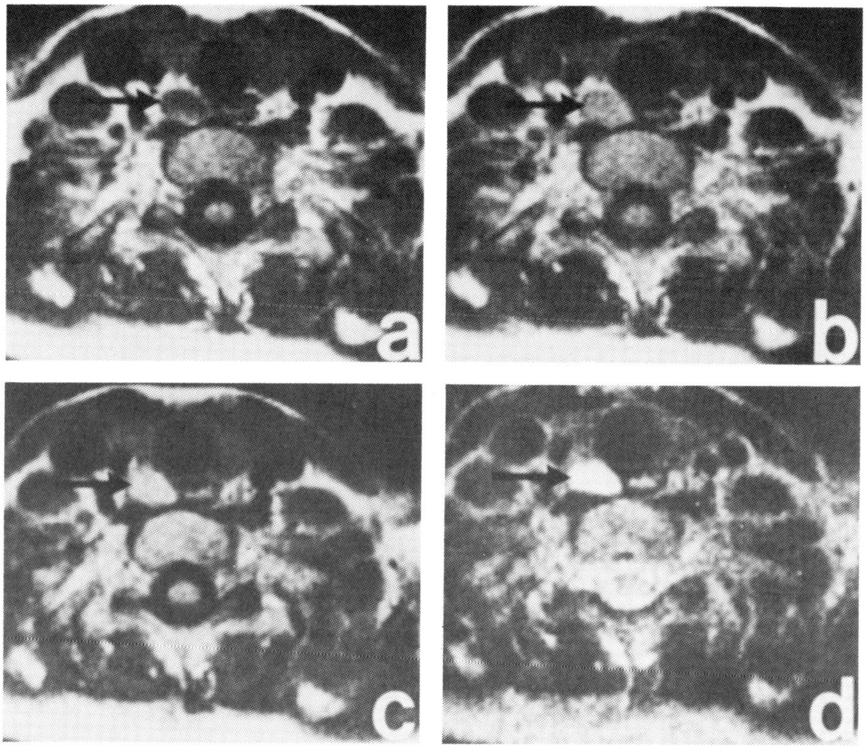

Fig. 5.6. Transverse slices of the neck with magnetic resonance imaging demonstrating a hyperplastic parathyroid gland (arrow) weighing 1.4 g and located dorsal to the right thyroid lobe. This patient had undergone excision of the contralateral upper parathyroid gland during previous surgery for HPT of the multiple endocrine neoplasia type 1 syndrome. The reoperation displayed two enlarged parathyroids, one of which could not be located preoperatively with magnetic resonance imaging. The relaxation time for the visualized parathyroid gland was 2 470 ms and 310 ms for T1- and T2-weighted images, respectively. Repetition and echo times were 500 and 35 ms (A), 500 and 70 ms (B), 1 500 and 35 ms (C), and 1 500 and 120 ms (D), respectively.

Efficiency of Magnetic Resonance Imaging

Normal parathyroid glands may be visualized by magnetic resonance imaging.[189,190,194] This imaging modality generally has been associated with 60-70% true positive localization of enlarged parathyroid glands in patients with persistent or recurrent HPT.[4,42,43,66,121,190,196] This seems to be slightly lower than modest estimates of the efficiency of magnetic resonance imaging within previously unexplored patients.[43,44,124,187,188,202] Hyperplasias of primary HPT might be detected with similar efficiency as single adenomas, and the limited information on secondary HPT suggests no substantial variation in sensitivity.[42,50,178,182,188,190,191] Multiple enlarged glands rarely are visualized in patients harboring parathyroid hyperplasia. The location of parathyroids may be accurately related to surrounding structures including the minor neurovascular bundle, which might be delineated by its adjacent structural fat.

Conflicting results have been recorded with respect to the sensitivity of magnetic resonance imaging to glandular size (Table 5.2). Some reports, but not others, display absence of both threshold size and weight-related increase in the proportion of true positive localizations.[44,50,188,190,202] Parathyroids confined to the neck seem to be visualized with similar accuracy whether they represent upper or lower glands in normal and ectopic positions.[4,42,50,182,188,190]

Although the investigated number of parathyroids in unusual cervical locations is limited, a substantial percentage of enlarged glands has been correctly located in cervical thymus, tracheo-esophageal groove, carotid sheath, and to a lesser degree also intrathyroidally. Moreover magnetic resonance imaging generally has located 40-80% of mediastinal parathyroids in series exceeding three patients.[42,44,66,121,190,203]

False positive parathyroid localizations have been reported with magnetic resonance imaging in up to 30% of patients with primary or secondary parathyroid explorations.[42,43,121,124,178,187,188,190,202] Coexistant thyroid diseases, like nodules, adenomas and cysts, as well as enlarged lymph nodes and large cervical sympathetic ganglia seem to explain most of the demonstrable causes for such failure, but many of these inaccuracies cannot be accounted for. Other recognized difficulties in this respect include partial volume effects from apparently normal tissues.

VENOUS SAMPLING FOR PARATHYROID HORMONE DETERMINATION

Venous catheterization for parathyroid effluents and localization of enlarged glands from acquired gradients in serum concentrations of parathyroid hormone was introduced decades ago.[204-207] Although this method initially included sampling from large veins of the neck and upper mediastinum, selective catheterization of mainly thyroid, internal mammary, thymic, and vertebral veins, and in some instances even their upstream branches, has been advocated for the purpose of enhancing sensitivity.[208-211] Such cannulations, however, are technically difficult, time consuming, and require determination of thyroid vein anatomy preferentially through arterial rather than venous digital subtraction angiography or selective arteriography.[181,208,212-215]

VENOUS ANATOMY

Preoperative and postoperative venous blood flow in the region of the thyroid and parathyroid glands varies considerably.[204,208,211,216-220] Briefly ipsilateral drainage of the parathyroid glands occurs in the vast majority of patients with and without previous neck explorations, although midline anastomoses certainly exist and may be visualized by retrograde, but rarely antegrade venous contrast administration. The majority of upper and lower parathyroids of the unexplored neck drain via the ipsilateral inferior thyroid vein, although some upper and very few lower glands also send tributaries to middle and superior thyroid veins. Rare inferior glands in the neck seem to empty into the internal mammary vein or its branches. Mediastinal parathyroids characteristically drain directly or via the internal mammary and inferior thyroid veins into the left brachiocephalic vein. Blood from parathyroid glands in the mediastinum also can enter the azygos preferentially via thymic tributaries. Moreover the middle thyroid vein constitutes the most inconsistent, variably large, and unpredictable vein of the thyroid-parathyroid complex, which may empty high to low in the internal jugular vessel. The inferior thyroid vein may comprise one, two or multiple vessels preferentially draining into the left innominate in addition to or exclusively to its contralateral counterpart.

Neck surgery mostly encompasses division of the middle thyroid vein, although its outflow may remain open due to contributaries lateral to the field of operation. Ligation of inferior thyroid veins rarely is performed intentionally during parathyroid exploration unless thyroid procedures or excision of pre- and paratracheal fat and cervical thymus have been performed, or the vein empties laterally into the internal jugular vein. In these instances drainage from even mediastinal glands can occur preferentially through the superior thyroid vein, as well as thymic, azygos, and internal mammary veins. Rare cervical glands also may contribute to substantial hormone gradients in subclavian, vertebral, intercostal and anterior jugular veins. Serum from subclavian veins may be particularly interesting in patients experiencing recurrent HPT after brachioradial parathyroid autotransplantation.

Technical Aspects

Transfemoral catheterization under local anesthesia, premedication and intravenous fluids conventionally are utilized. Contrast exposure from venous sampling alone poses no serious problem unless severe renal impairment exists, while concomitant selective arteriography or digital subtraction angiography considerably increases this exposure.[213] True retrograde venograms may be performed for analysis of thyroid drainage as well as to verify sites of actual sampling, but this procedure in itself exhibits low parathyroid sensitivity.[28,48,221,222] In most instances selective aspiration from all three thyroid veins is attempted bilaterally together with sampling from three levels in the internal jugular and left brachiocephalic veins, the right brachiocephalic, superior cava, both subclavian veins, azygos and internal mammary veins. In order to calculate the background level of circulating parathyroid hormone, blood is drawn from at least two sites within the inferior cava. Samples of 2 ml blood are more than sufficient for modern assays of parathyroid hormone.

In our hands selective cannulation of the inferior thyroid and mammary veins is successful in less than half the patients subjected to previous parathyroid surgery. This observation may be considered to be consistent with the meager information on the actual rate of selective aspirations from small target veins of high priority in reports on parathyroid venous sampling.[208,216,219,220,221] Moreover some studies have utilized junior radiologists for this purpose and others state unsuccessful cannulations only due to failures in entering the internal jugular vein.[28,48] In addition it has recently been reported that sampling from large veins of the neck and upper mediastinum together with analyses of intact (1-84) parathyroid hormone values may be sufficient for parathyroid localization,[223] although knowledge on venous flow suggests that, at best, this can be sensitive at diagnostic hormone gradients in the internal jugular veins.

Adverse effects are rare during selective venous catheterization, and generally include local discomfort, hematoma and thrombosis. The procedure of selective aspiration frequently takes around 3 hours, while large vein cannulations alone generally can be completed within 1 hour.

Interpretation of Parathyroid Hormone Gradients

Peripheral concentrations of parathyroid hormone is estimated as the mean of at least two measurements gathered well away from the expected site of excess and preferentially spaced in time to partly adjust for fluctuations during the sampling procedure. Systematic evaluation on the minimal ratio of true positive localizations as well as the corresponding maximum of false positives have not been presented. A step-up amounting to twice the periphery usually has been considered as significant, while others require four standard deviations above the mean of 4-6 background values.[4,179,181,208,211] Similar ranges of values seem applicable upon analysis of bioactive and intact parathyroid hormone levels.[223,224] Venous sampling cannot provide information on exact sites for hyperfunctioning parathyroids, but rather should be expected to lateralize and indicate cervical or mediastinal location of such glands. Selective versus large vein sampling has been suggested to exhibit considerably higher specificity, although the difference toward values in middle and superior thyroid veins compared to the internal jugular seems clinically less striking. Significant ratios in the brachiocephalic veins alone, however, cannot be expected to predict cervical or mediastinal glandular location nor comprise a basis for accurate lateralization. Similar difficulties, but to a lesser extent, also exist with selective sampling. Moreover venous sampling cannot determine the number of enlarged glands in unilateral neck or mediastinal positions, and hyperplasia generally may be suggested from more than a single step-up in jugular or brachiocephalic contributaries.[1,28,48,208,215,220,225,226]

Efficiency of Venous Sampling

Selective venous sampling generally has been reported to lateralize cervical and demonstrate mediastinal location of enlarged parathyroid glands in 70-80% of patients subjected to previous parathyroid exploration.[4,14,208,213,223,226,227] In the clinical evaluation venous sampling commonly is performed as a last resort, whereby over representation of patients with 'technically complicated' glandular localizations should prevail. Evaluation of results from this mode of preoperative visualization also may become biased by the circumstance that many modern series utilize venous sampling in immediate succession to arteriograms. Considerably lower rates of success thus have been found in other series of reoperative patients, so that the utility and specificity of venous sampling have been questioned.[1,181,225,228] In our own hands one out of about every third reoperative patient with HPT currently is subjected to venous sampling. Utilizing analyses of intact serum parathyroid hormone values, lateralization in the neck comprises a true positive finding in 35% of these individuals and somewhat less than 30% of those with enlarged mediastinal parathyroid glands (unpublished data).

The efficiency of venous sampling seems unrelated to the size of residual parathyroid glands.[4,14,215] Singularly enlarged glands are demonstrated with similar sensitivity irrespective of histological diagnosis of adenoma or hyperplasia, and the result in patients harboring multiple enlarged glands has been found to be less encouraging.[28,48,208,210] Systematic analyses in this respect is lacking for patients demonstrating persistent or recurrent secondary HPT. The occurrence of more than a single step-up in ratios of parathyroid hormone values mostly is confusing and rarely a true aid in surgical planning. Knowing the limitations of sampling, the extent of this problem increases with the number of such ratios. Moreover the level of parathyroid hormone values generally decreases gradually downstream to the site of maximal excess, whereby complicated distributions of enhanced hormone ratios can be obtained in patients with multiple gland enlargement. Venous sampling probably is less sensitive for glands in the mediastinum,[4,210,215] which generally coincides with suggestions that the absence of significant hormone ratios indicates the presence of mediastinal disease.[14] In contrast to some studies,[4,215] false positives seem to occur in about 10% of patients subjected to venous sampling.[28,179,181,220,225,226] Traceable causes of these failures comprise midline anastomoses of thyroid blood flow.

ARTERIOGRAPHY

Arteriography for parathyroid localization will only be briefly discussed, since most centers including ourselves have ceased to employ at least the technique of selective arteriography. This decision relates to the risk of serious complications mainly involving permanent visual disturbances including blindness, as well as hemiplegia, tetraplegia, seizures and, in older series, even death.[225,229-233] In experienced hands such serious side effects rarely occur by avoiding cannulation of the costocervical trunk and vertebral vessels, unnecessary manipulation in the carotids during search for the superior thyroid arteries, and by limiting the contrast load.[215,222]

Inferior parathyroid glands virtually always are supplied by the inferior thyroid artery. This vessel most commonly arises from the thyreocervical trunk, sometimes from the subclavian artery, and rarely from ectopic positions in vertebral, carotid or brachiocephalic vessels.[234-238] The inferior thyroid arteries commonly supply most inferior parathyroids in the mediastinal position, which also may receive blood from thymic branches of the internal mammary system. The inferior thyroid artery frequently anastomoses with its superior counterpart and thereby comprises the principal blood supply also to the upper glandular pair. Parathymic lesions frequently connect to the superior thyroid artery and vein, while truly paravascular parathyroids embedded within the carotid sheath seem to be supplied mainly from the inferior thyroid artery.[56,57]

Enlarged parathyroid glands visualized by **selective arteriography** characteristically are supplied by a single, short vessel connecting to an oval blush mostly retaining its opacification longer than thyroid and muscle.[222,228,239,240] The investigation primarily attempts selective cannulation of the inferior thyroid artery, followed by mammary and rarely the superior thyroid or ima arteries. Venous phases are assessed to facilitate subsequent sampling for parathyroid hormone determination. Failure of such cannulations are accompanied by reduced sensitivity, and the selective procedure has yielded true positive parathyroid localization in 40-60% of patients subjected to previous parathyroid exploration.[1,14,208,213,219,225,227] False positives generally occur in less than 10% of patients and mainly relate to misinterpretations of thyroid lesions, lymph nodes and focal muscular contrast accumulation.

Digital subtraction angiography comprises a more recently introduced alternative for parathyroid localization. This method relies on computerized subtraction of images, and may depend on non-selective venous and non-selective or selective arterial contrast administrations. Venous digital subtraction angiography[212] has been investigated in relatively small series of patients requiring parathyroid reoperation.[213,214,241] It involves caval contrast administrations; 29-75% true positive localizations have been obtained. The success rate, however, seems to be below this range, and direct comparison in individual patient series with selective angiography has demonstrated no diagnostic improvement. Non-selective digital subtraction arteriography involves contrast injection into mainly the ascending aorta, innominate or subclavian arteries, or the common carotids.[213,215,242] Although this technique might comprise a safer and less technically demanding procedure in comparison with conventional selective arteriography and the success rate has been superior to venous subtraction angiography, the accuracy cannot match that of conventional selective arteriography.[213,215] Selective digital subtraction arteriography involves bilateral cannulation of internal mammary, inferior thyroid and common carotid arteries.[227] Utilizing this technique on patients with previously unsuccessful parathyroid surgery has improved localization of parathyroid adenomas especially in anterior mediastinum. Selective arteriography also has been utilized for **guided biopsy** under fluoroscopic control.[243]

SELECTION OF PROCEDURES AND PATIENTS

From the above mentioned multitude of available means for preoperative localization and their roughly similar rates of sensitivity and specificity, it might be difficult to envision an optimal flow chart for the application of these investigations. Since all techniques are more or less investigator dependent, it seems important primarily to emphasize that only familiar techniques should be employed and that the investigating physician must be competent in parathyroid gland anatomy. If these requisites cannot be fulfilled within the hospital, outside expertise must be recruited for the purpose of obtaining optimal handling of the patient. The same line of reasoning applies to the preoperative analysis as indeed to the performance of parathyroid reoperation. Moreover the extent and number of previous operations, the skill of surgeon(s), and to some extent also duration from the latest exploration influence the need and extent of preoperative investigation for parathyroid localization. In our hands, well explored patients subjected to more than a single recent operative procedure would be most carefully examined, while less emphasis would be utilized in instances where surgical ability seems less impressive. The application of these localizing techniques must be individualized, since concurrent demonstration by two different modalities of an enlarged parathyroid gland at the same site generally should lead to cessation of further investigations. It also is necessary to stress that all attempts at routine preoperative localization should be reserved for individuals subjected to previous thyroid and/or parathyroid procedures, and that surgeons feeling uncomfortable with primary exploration in the absence of such visualizations probably should refrain from performing parathyroid surgery.

Several studies have demonstrated that the currently available means of preoperative localization complement each other with respect both to the occurrence of false positives and negatives.[3,4,36,42-44,50,66,127,178,182,215] We would begin with ultrasonography and include guided biopsy for equivocal findings with possible biopsy. Further attempts at localization cease upon the demonstration of unequivocal parathyroid tissue. Otherwise the sequence of thallium-technetium subtraction scintigraphy, computed tomography, and magnetic resonance imaging would follow. The absence of confirmatory findings of parathyroid localization subsequently would lead to large and small vein sampling for parathyroid hormone determination.

Patients previously treated with brachioradial autotransplantation of parathyroid tissue primarily would be examined by analysis of intact serum parathyroid hormone values in antecubital veins of the grafted arm in comparison with another location in the peripheral circulation. Although the results of this investigation have been incompletely evaluated, adequately functioning grafts may produce hormone levels 20 that of normal values in the systemic circulation. Moreover recurrent hypercalcemia from residual parathyroid tissue in the neck characteristically is accompanied by elevated systemic hormone values. Graft recurrences are truly rare and seem to be indistinguishable with respect to the hormone ratio alone, but are asociated with high systemic hormone values in combination with an elevated ratio (see chapter 9 for details). Moreover patients with signs of graft related excess would be examined for influences on the systemic parathyroid hormone values from ischemia of the grafted arm[61,244] as well as ultrasound and scintigraphy of the site of grafting.

We recently have had the opportunity of analyzing **positron emission tomography** in the investigation of patients with persistent or recurrent HPT. This procedure is potentially valuable, since positron emitting nuclides of exceptionally short half-life might be chemically included in a variety of substances like peptides, metabolites and pharmaceuticals. Unique applications for dynamic studies in vivo on several aspects of cell function and tumor response might be developed. The dose of radiation approximately equals 10 mSv. In a primary analysis employing carbon-11-labeled L-methionine, (Fig. 5.7) patients scheduled for reoperative parathyroid surgery have demonstrated more efficient localization of enlarged parathyroid glands and accidental implants than with the above mentioned modalities taken together. The success, however, seems related to gland size, and the occurrence of false negatives is due mainly to tracer uptake in adjacent thyroid gland.[245] Studies in progress will reveal the clinical applicability of positron emission tomography, and hopefully the contribute to the development of parathyroid tissue specific tracers.

INTRAOPERATIVE ADJUNCTS OF LOCALIZATION

Intraoperative ultrasound rather recently has been utilized as an adjunct to visualization of enlarged parathyroid glands in patients undergoing parathyroid reoperation.[3,41,215,246,247] The utility of this localizing modality suggests that reoperative parathyroid surgery should not be conducted without access to intraoperative ultrasound. This examination conventionally includes analysis of the neck medially, dorsally and laterally after extensive dissection of the cutaneous-platysma flaps and incision of the strap muscles medial to the sternocleidomastoid muscles. High-frequency real-time scanners and dedicated transducers are mandatory. Lesions should be viewed in at least two planes; saline may simplify acoustic contact along the incision. Intraoperative ultrasound can also aid in localizing mediastinal glands, although tissue depth and cardiac movement may offer some difficulty. The procedure takes roughly 15 minutes and might considerably reduces the duration of parathyroid reoperation.

Analyses of the efficiency of intraoperative ultrasound have demonstrated 80% true positive localizations without detectable relationship to glandular size.[3,41,215] Normal parathyroids cannot reliably be recognized on the echograms, whereas enlarged glands demonstrate characteristics similar to lesions viewed by preoperative ultrasonography, and false positives occur very rarely. Intraoperative ultrasound is less efficient for superior glands, even in the juxtathyroid position, than their inferior counterparts, although this knowledge partly may be compensated for by exceptional care during the investigation of common and uncommon sites of the upper glandular pair. Intrathyroid parathyroids have posed no serious problem despite the circumstance that ultrasound does not distinguish between thyroid and parathyroid lesions.

Vital staining of parathyroid tissue with methylene blue has been recommended in parathyroid surgery for primary and secondary HPT.[248-254] This phenothiazide dye is given as an intravenous infusion over 1 hour at the dosage of 5-7.5 mg per kg body weight, which is terminated at the time of parathyroid dissection. It has been associated with few side effects mainly including nausea and local discomfort at the site of injection. It stains the vast majority of enlarged parathyroid glands deeply blue and normal parathyroids less deeply. In addition some thyroid nodules and enlarged lymph nodes may stain. The technical difficulties of reoperative parathyroid surgery, however, may necessitate several administrations due to rapid clearance, in which case staining of non-parathyroid tissues may increase.[1] When scar tissue from previous explorations conceal pathological glands making macroscopic identification nevertheless in unequivocal, vital staining may have limited applicability during reoperative surgery.

NON-SURGICAL PARATHYROID ABLATION

Parathyroid cysts comprise uncommon causes of primary HPT, and additional cysts may be considered nonfunctioning due to absence of concomitant hypercalcemia.[255-258] These cysts classically contain water-clear fluid, although sanguinous contents similar to thyroid cysts and degenerations also may occur. The fluid has been found to exhibit high concentrations of parathyroid hormone with modern assays for the intact peptide.[259-262] **Fine needle aspiration** of this fluid may lead to reversal of local discomfort and hypercalcemia.[258,262-265] Sclerosing agents may be utilized preferentially upon recurrence after aspiration.[260,262,266] Due to the frequency of such recurrences, we would prefer conventional excision in these patients unless strong contraindications to surgery prevail.

Preoperatively localized parathyroid glands at accessible sites in the neck may be percutaneously punctured, preferentially under ultrasonic guidance, and subjected to intraglandular **ethanol instillation**.[267-274] The rather limited cure rate with this method during currently available short-term follow-up, the necessity for repeat injections, and the significant risk of transient and permanent vocal cord paralyses restrict the application of such therapy. There may exist a very narrow subgroup of patients with extensive HPT and ultrasonically visualized sites of hormone excess, definite contraindications to conventional surgery even under local anesthesia, and failure to respond with lowered serum calcium upon pharmacological therapy—preferentially with bisphosphonates, in whom ethanol instillation could be the treatment of choice.

Angiographic ablation constitutes another means of radiological treatment for HPT, the clinical application of which recently has been excellently reviewed.[7] This modality naturally requires comfort with parathyroid angiography, although rather severe limitations on its utility currently exist. Such ablation requires wedging a catheter into the feeding vessel of an enlarged parathyroid gland in patients subjected to previous parathyroid operation in order to infuse ionic contrast material, rarely ethanol alone, and most recently a mixture of ethanol and Lipiodol.[275-281] Provided that contrast material is chosen, the resulting parathyroid blush is impressive, and superior results have been achieved when contrast trapping persists for at least 24 hours. Transient lowering of serum calcium values persisting for several days and permanent reversal of hypercalcemia have been associated with partial to complete parathyroid necrosis.[278,282,283] The success rate with angiographic ablation in series followed for more than 2.5 years has been around 70%.[277-279] Adverse effects mainly include transient thyroiditis, bradycardia, a single case of respiratory arrest, hoarseness and hiccups. These complications mainly have occurred upon cannulation of the inferior thyroid artery and theoretically have been related to vagal and phrenic nerve stimulation.[7,278,279] As a consequence of these findings, ablation has been recommended only for mediastinal glands supplied by the internal mammary vessel.[7]

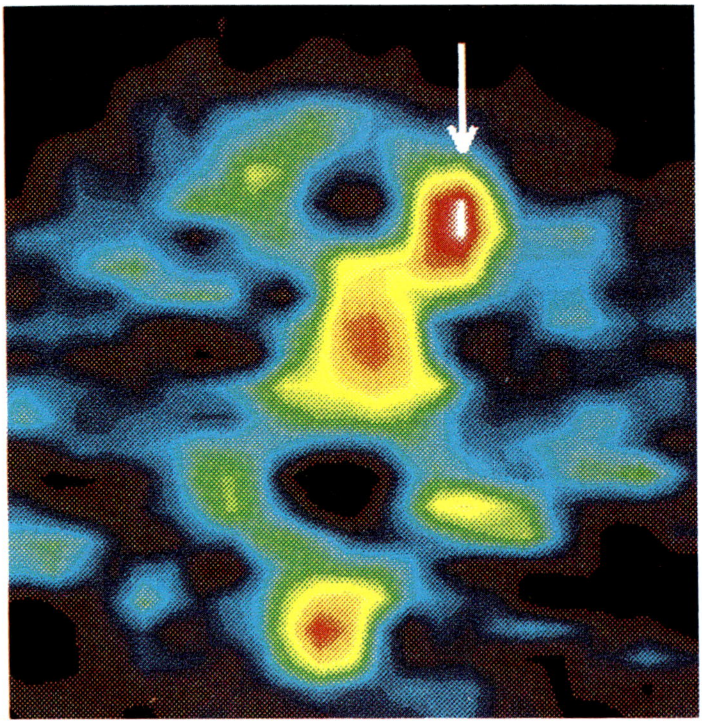

Fig. 5.7. Transverse section of the neck (anterior is upwards) with positron emission tomography utilizing ^{11}C-labeled L-methionine. This tracer preferentially accumulates in relation to protein synthesis and amino acid turnover; the vertebral bone marrow, esophagus and right thyroid lobe are depicted in green through yellow to light red. The highest uptake (deep red to white) is seen centrally in a local recurrence from parathyroid carcinoma (arrow). This lesion weighed 1.4 g and it was situated at the site where the primary tumor previously had been excised together with the left thyroid lobe.

REFERENCES

1. Brennan MF, Norton JA. Reoperation for persistent and recurrent hyperparathyroidism. Ann Surg 1985; 201: 40-4.
2. Grant CS, van Heerden JA, Charboneau JW et al. Clinical management of persistent and/or recurrent primary hyperparathyroidism. World J Surg 1986; 10: 555-65.
3. Kern KA, Shawker TH, Doppman JL et al. The use of high-resolution ultrasound to locate parathyroid tumors during reoperations for primary hyperparathyroidism. World J Surg 1987; 11: 579-85.
4. Levin KE, Gooding GAW, Okerlund M et al. Localizing studies in patients with persistent or recurrent hyperparathyroidism. Surgery 1987; 102: 917-25.
5. Rothmund M, Wagner PK. Reoperations for persistent and recurrent secondary hyperparathyroidism. Ann Surg 1988; 207: 310-4.
6. Thompson NW. Localization studies in patients with primary hyperparathyroidism. Br J Surg 1988; 75: 97-8.
7. Miller DL. Pre-operative localization and interventional treatment of parathyroid tumors: When and how? World J Surg 1991; 15: 706-15.
8. DiGiulio W, Beierwaltes WH. Parathyroid scanning with selenium labelled methionine. J Nucl Med 1964; 5: 417-27.
9. Stevens AC, Jackson CE. Localization of parathyroid adenomas by esophageal cineroentgenography. Am J Roentgenol 1967; 99: 233-7.
10. Mailliard JA. Localization of a parathyroid by ^{131}I scintiscan. JAMA 1968; 204: 177-8.
11. Kato T, Hattori T, Miura K et al. Application of thyroid lymphography to preoperative localization of hyperfunctioning parathyroid adenomas. Ann Surg 1974; 179: 378-81.
12. Samuels BI. The present status of parathyroid thermography. JAMA 1975; 233: 907-8.
13. Waldorf JC, van Heerden JA, Gorman CA et al. [^{75}Se]Selenomethionine scanning for parathyroid localization should be abandoned. Mayo Clin Proc 1984; 59: 534-7
14. Clark OH, Okerlund MD, Moss AA et al. Localization studies in patients with persistent or recurrent hyperparathyroidism. Surgery 1985; 98: 1083-93.
15. van Heerden JA, James EM, Karsell PR et al. Small-part ultrasonography in primary hyperparathyroidism. Ann Surg 1982; 195: 774-80.
16. Rastad J, Lindgren PG, Ljunghall S et al. Ultrasound scanning for preoperative location of parathyroid tumours. Acta Chir Scand 1984; 150: 199-204.
17. Lever EG, Refetoff S, Straus FH et al. Coexisting thyroid and parathyroid disease—are they related? Surgery 1983; 94: 893-900.
18. Holmes EC, Morton DL, Ketcham AS. Parathyroid carcinoma: A collective review. Ann Surg 1969; 169: 631-40.
19. Krudy AG, Doppman JL, Shawker TH et al. Hyperfunctioning cystic parathyroid glands: CT and sonographic findings. Am J Roentgenol 1984; 142: 175-8.
20. Fujimoto Y, Obara T, Ito Y et al. Localization and surgical resection of metastatic parathyroid carcinoma. World J Surg 1986; 10: 539-47.
21. Arima M, Yokoi H, Sonoda T. Preoperative identification of tumor of the parathyroid by ultrasonotomography. Surg Gynecol Obstet 1975; 141: 242-4.
22. Barraclough BH, Reeve TS, Duffy PJ et al. The localization of parathyroid tissue by ultrasound scanning prior to surgery in patients with hyperparathyroidism. World J Surg 1981; 5: 91-5.
23. Simeone JF, Mueller PR, Ferrucci Jr JT et al. High-resolution real-time sonography of the parathyroid. Radiology 1981; 141: 745-51.
24. Reading CC, Charboneau JW, James EM et al. High-resolution parathyroid sonography. Am J Roentgenol 1982; 139: 539-46.
25. Sample WF, Mitchell SP, Bledsoe RC. Parathyroid ultrasonography. Radiology 1978; 127: 485-90.
26. Solbiati L, De Pra L, Ierace T et al. High-resolution sonography of the recurrent laryngeal nerve: Anatomic and pathologic considerations. Am J Roentgenol 1985; 145: 989-93.
27. Duh Q-Y, Sancho JJ, Clark OH. Parathyroid localization. Acta Chir Scand 1987; 153: 241-54.

28. Lloyd MNH, Lees WR, Milroy EJG. Preoperative localisation in primary hyperparathyroidism. Clin Radiol 1990; 41: 239-43.
29. Udén P, Aspelin P, Berglund J et al. Preoperative localization in unilateral parathyroid surgery. A cost-benefit study on ultrasound, computed tomography and scintigraphy. Acta Chir Scand 1990; 156: 29-35.
30. Rastad J, Fransson A, Lindgren PG et al. Ultrasonic appearance of adenomatous and hyperplastic parathyroid glands. Acta Radiol Diagn 1984; 25: 471-5.
31. Kinoshita Y, Fukase M, Uchihashi M et al. Significance of preoperative use of ultrasonography in parathyroid neoplasms: Comparison of sonographic textures with histologic findings. J Clin Ultrasound 1985; 13: 457-60.
32. Randel SB, Gooding GAW, Clark OH et al. Parathyroid variants: US evaluation. Radiology 1987; 165: 191-4.
33. Graif M, Itzchak Y, Strauss S et al. Parathyroid sonography: Diagnostic accuracy related to shape, location and texture of the gland. Br J Radiol 1987; 60: 439-43.
34. Clark OH, Stark DA, Duh Q-Y et al. Value of high resolution real-time ultrasonography in secondary hyperparathyroidism. Am J Surg 1985; 150: 9-17.
35. Edmonson GR, Charboneau JW, James EM et al. Parathyroid carcinoma: High-frequency sonographic features. Radiology 1986; 161: 65-7.
36. Takagi H, Tominaga Y, Uchida K et al. Evaluation of image-diagnosing methods of enlarged parathyroid glands in chronic renal failure. World J Surg 1986; 10: 605-11.
37. Takebayashi S, Matsui K, Onohara Y et al. Sonography for early diagnosis of enlarged parathyroid glands in patients with secondary hyperparathyroidism. Am J Roentgenol 1987; 148: 911-4.
38. Diederich S, Wernecke K, Möller U et al. Sonographie der nebenschilddrüsen bei langzeitdialysetherapie. Radiologe 1991; 31: 339-43.
39. Krudy AG, Shawker TH, Doppman JL et al. Ultrasonic parathyroid localisation in previously operated patients. Clin Radiol 1984; 35: 113-8.
40. Yao M, Jamieson C, Blend R. Magnetic resonance imaging in preoperative localization of diseased parathyroid glands: A comparison with isotope scanning and ultrasonography. Can J Surg 1993; 36: 241-4.
41. Norton JA, Shawker TH, Jones BL et al. Intraoperative ultrasound and reoperative parathyroid surgery: An initial evaluation. World J Surg 1986; 10: 631-9.
42. Auffermann W, Gooding GAW, Okerlund MD et al. Diagnosis of recurrent hyperparathyroidism: Comparison of MR imaging and other imaging techniques. Am J Roentgenol 1988; 150: 1027-33.
43. Erdman WA, Breslau NA, Weinreb JC et al. Noninvasive localization of parathyroid adenomas: A comparison of x-ray computerized tomography, ultrasound, scintigraphy and MRI. Magn Res Imaging 1989; 7: 187-94.
44. Krubsack AJ, Wilson SD, Lawson TL et al. Prospective comparison of radionuclide, computed tomographic, sonographic, and magnetic resonance localization of parathyroid tumors. Surgery 1989; 106: 639-46.
45. Doppman JL, Miller DL. Localization of parathyroid tumors in patients with asymptomatic hyperparathyroidism and no previous surgery. J Bone Min Res 1991; 6 (suppl 2): S153-8.
46. Serpell JW, Campbell PR, Young AE. Preoperative localization of parathyroid tumors does not reduce operating time. Br J Surg 1991; 78: 589-90.
47. Åkerström G, Rudberg C, Grimelius L et al. Causes of failed primary exploration and technical aspects of re-operation in primary hyperparathyroidism. World J Surg 1992; 16: 562-9.
48. Manhire AR, Anderson PN, Milroy E. Parathyroid venous sampling and ultrasonography in primary hyperparathyroidism due to multigland disease. Br J Radiol 1984; 57: 375-80.
49. Gooding GAW, Okerlund MD, Stark DD et al. Parathyroid imaging: Comparison of double-tracer (TI-201, Tc-99m) scintigraphy and high-resolution US. Radiology 1986; 161: 57-64.
50. Kohri K, Ishikawa Y, Kodama M et al.

Comparison of imaging methods for localization of parathyroid tumors. Am J Surg 1992; 164: 140-5.

51. Brzac HT, Pavlovic D, Halbauer M et al. Parathyroid sonography in secondary hyperparathyroidism: Correlation with clinical findings. Nephrol Dial Transplant 1989; 4: 45-50.
52. Bruining HA, van Houten M, Juttman JR et al. Results of operative treatment of 615 patients with primary hyperparathyroidism. World J Surg 1981; 5: 85-90.
53. Hellman P, Åkerström G, Ljunghall S et al. Surgical findings and results of subtotal and total parathyroidectomy in hypercalcemic patients with uremic hyperparathyroidism. Acta Chir Scand 1989; 155: 573-82.
54. Hellman P, Skogseid B, Juhlin C et al. Findings and long-term results of parathyroid surgery in multiple endocrine neoplasia type 1. World J Surg 1992; 16: 718-23.
55. Wallfelt C, Ljunghall S, Bergström R et al. Clinical characteristics and surgical treatment of sporadic primary hyperparathyroidism with emphasis on chief cell hyperplasia. Surgery 1990; 107: 13-9.
56. Doppman JL, Shawker TH, Krudy AG et al. Parathymic parathyroid: CT, US, and angio-graphic findings. Radiology 1985; 157: 419-23.
57. Fraker DL, Doppman JL, Shawker TH et al. Undescended parathyroid adenoma: An important etiology for failed operations for primary hyperparathyroidism. World J Surg 1990; 14: 342-48.
58. Rastad J, Johansson H, Lindgren PG et al. Ultrasonic localization and cytologic identification of parathyroid tumors. World J Surg 1984; 8: 501-8.
59. Winzelberg GG, Hydovitz JD, O'Hara KR et al. Parathyroid adenomas evaluated by Tl-201/Tc-99m pertechnetate subtraction scintigraphy and high-resolution ultrasonography. Radiology 1985; 155: 231-5.
60. Kobayashi S, Miyakawa M, Kasuga Y et al. Parathyroid imaging: Comparison of ^{201}Tl-^{99m}Tc subtraction scintigraphy, computed tomography and ultrasonography. Jpn J Surg 1987; 17: 9-13.
61. Casanova D, Sarfati E, De Francisco A et al. Secondary hyperparathyroidism: Diagnosis of site of recurrence. World J Surg 1991; 15: 546-50.
62. Karsenty G, Petraglia A, Bordeau A et al. Evaluation of parathyroid autograft growth and function in hemodialysis patients. Am J Kidney Dis 1986; 8: 43-50.
63. Takebayashi S, Matsui K, Nozawa T et al. Hyperplasia of autotransplanted parathyroid in the forearm. Clin Nucl Med 1990; 15: 354-5.
64. Winkelbauer F, Ammann ME, Längle F et al. Diagnosis of hyperparathyroidism with US after autotransplantation: Results of a prospective study. Radiology 1993; 186: 255-7.
65. Reading CC, Charboneau JW, James EM et al. Postoperative parathyroid high-frequency sonography: Evaluation of persistent or recurrent hyperparathyroidism. Am J Roentgenol 1985; 144: 399-402.
66. Miller DL, Doppman JL, Shawker TH et al. Localization of parathyroid adenomas in patients who have undergone surgery: Part I. Noninvasive imaging methods. Radiology 1987; 162: 133-7.
67. Stark DD, Clark OH, Gooding GAW et al. High-resolution ultrasonography and computed tomography of thyroid lesions in patients with hyperparathyroidism. Surgery 1983; 94: 863-8.
68. Clark OH, Gooding GAW, Ljung BM. Locating a parathyroid adenoma by ultrasonography and aspiration biopsy cytology. Western J Med 1981; 135: 154-8.
69. Solbiati L, Montali G, Croce F et al. Parathyroid tumors detected by fine-needle aspiration biopsy under ultrasonic guidance. Radiology 1983; 148: 793-7.
70. Lindgren PG. Ultrasonically guided punctures: A modified technique. Radiology 1980; 137: 235-7.
71. Doppman JL, Krudy AG, Marx SJ et al. Aspiration of enlarged parathyroid glands for parathyroid hormone assay . Radiology 1983; 148: 31-5.
72. Karstrup S, Glenthøj A, Torp-Pedersen S et al. Ultrasonically guided fine nedle aspiration of suggested enlarged parthyroid glands. Acta Radiol 1988; 29: 213-6.
73. Gooding GAW, Clark OH, Stark DD et al.

Parathyroid aspiration biopsy under ultrasound guidance in the postoperative hyperparathyroid patient. Radiology 1985; 155: 193-6.
74. Glenthøj A, Karstrup S. Parathyroid identification by ultrasonically guided aspiration cytology. APMIS 1989; 97: 497-502.
75. Winkler B, Gooding GAW, Montgomery CK et al. Immunoperoxidase confirmation of parathyroid origin of ultrasound-guided fine needle aspirates of the parathyroid glands. Acta Cytol 1987; 31: 40-4.
76. Halbauer M, Crepinko I, Brzac HT et al. Fine needle aspiration cytology in the preoperative diagnosis of ultrasonically enlarged parathyroid glands. Acta Cytol 1991; 35: 728-35.
77. Sardi A, Bolton JS, Mitchell Jr WT et al. Immunoperoxidase confirmation of ultrasonically guided fine needle aspirates in patients with recurrent hyperparathyroidism. Surg Gynecol Obstet 1992; 175: 563-8.
78. Karstrup S, Glenthøj A, Hainau B et al. Ultrasound-guided, histological, fine-needle biopsy from suspect parathyroid tumours: Success-rate and reliability of histological diagnosis. Br J Radiol 1989; 62: 981-5.
79. Lindgren PG. Percutaneous needle biopsy. A new technique. Acta Radiol Diagn 1982; 23: 653-6.
80. Juhlin C, Rastad J, Klareskog L et al. Parathyroid histology and cytology with monoclonal antibodies recognizing a calcium sensor of parathyroid cells. Am J Pathol 1989; 135: 321-8.
81. Gooding GAW, Clark OH. Use of color doppler imaging in the distinction between thyroid and parathyroid lesions. Am J Surg 1992; 164: 51-6.
82. Henry J-F, Audiffret J, Denizot A et al. Endosonography in the localization of parathyroid tumors: A preliminary study. Surgery 1990; 108: 1021-5.
83. Fukuchi M, Hyodo K, Tachibana K et al. Marked thyroid uptake of thallium 201 in patients with goiter: A case report. J Nucl Med 1977; 18: 1199-201.
84. Fukunaga M, Morita R, Yonekura Y et al. Accumulation of 201 Tl-chloride in a parathyroid adenoma. Clin Nucl Med 1979; 4: 229-30.
85. Ferlin G, Borsato N, Camerani M et al. New perspectives in localizing enlarged parathyroids by technetium-thallium subtraction scan. J Nucl Med 1983; 24: 438-41.
86. Young AE, Gaunt JI, Croft DN et al. Location of parathyroid adenomas by thallium-201 and technetium-99^m subtraction scanning. Br Med J 1983; 286: 1384-6.
87. MacFarlane SD, Hanelin LG, Taft DA et al. Localization of abnormal parathyroid glands using thallium-201. Am J Surg 1984; 148: 7-13.
88. Basarab RM, Manni A, Harrison TS. Dual isotope subtraction parathyroid scintigraphy in the preoperative evaluation of suspected hyperparathyroidism. Clin Nucl Med 1985; 10: 300-14.
89. Blue PW, Crawford G, Dydek GJ. Parathyroid subtraction imaging- Pitfalls in diagnosis. Clin Nucl Med 1989; 14: 47-57.
90. Sandrock D, Merino MJ, Norton JA et al. Ultrastructural histology correlates with results of thallium-201/technetium-99m parathyroid subtraction scintigraphy. J Nucl Med 1993; 34: 24-9.
91. Okerlund MD, Sheldon K, Corpuz S et al. A new method with high sensitivity and specificity for localization of abnormal parathyroid glands. Ann Surg 1984; 200: 381-8.
92. Greenberg SB, Park CH, Intenzo C. Dynamic or early imaging in dual-tracer parathyroid scintigraphy. Clin Nucl Med 1986; 11: 627-8.
93. Krubsack AJ, Wilson SD, Lawson TL et al. Prospective comparison of radionuclide, computed tomographic, and sonographic localization of parathyroid tumors. World J Surg 1986; 10: 579-85.
94. Fine EJ. Parathyroid imaging: Its current status and future role. Sem Nucl Med 1987; 17: 350-9.
95. Liehn J-C, Amico S, Delisle M-J et al. Improvement of parathyroid Tl-Tc scintigraphy by using a new image subtraction method. Eur J Nucl Med 1988; 14: 184-9.
96. Sandrock D, Dunham RG, Neumann RD. Simultaneous dual energy acquisition for $^{201}Tl/^{99}Tc^m$ parathyroid subtraction scintigraphy: Physical and physiological considerations. Nucl Med Commun 1990; 11:

503-10.

97. Erwin WD, Groch MW, Ali A et al. Image normalization and background subtraction in TI-201/Tc-99m parathyroid subtraction scintigraphy. Effect on lesion detection. Clin Nucl Med 1992; 17: 81-9.
98. Jenkins BJ, Newell MS, Goode AW et al. Impact of conventional and three-dimensional thallium-technetium scans on surgery for primary hyperparathyroidism. J Royal Soc Med 1990; 83: 427-9.
99. Ziffer JA, Fajman WA. Ectopic parathyroid gland localization with thallium-201 SPECT. Clin Nucl Med 1987; 12: 617-9.
100. Obara T, Fujimoto Y, Tanaka R et al. Mid-mediastinal parathyroid lesions: Preoperative localization and surgical approach in two cases. Jpn J Surg 1990; 20: 481-6.
101. Neumann DR. Simultaneous dual-isotope SPECT imaging for the detection and characterization of parathyroid pathology. J Nucl Med 1992; 33: 131-4.
102. Strauss HW, Harrison K, Pitt B. Thallium-201: Noninvasive determination of the regional distribution of cardiac output. J Nucl Med 1977; 18: 1167-70.
103. Ito Y, Muranaka A, Harada T et al. Experimental study on tumor affinity of ^{201}Tl-chloride. Eur J Nucl Med 1978; 3: 81-6.
104. Oster ZH, Strauss HW, Harrison K et al. Thallium-201 distribution in the thyroid: Relationship to thyroidal trapping function. Radiology 1978; 126: 733-4.
105. Gupta SM, Belsky JL. Use of oral phosphate to enhance visualization of enlarged parathyroids on scanning. J Nucl Med 1985; 26: 100-1.
106. Gallacher SJ, Fraser WD, Logue FC et al. Augmentation of parathyroid ^{201}Tl/^{99}Tc^{m} scanning by infusion of trisodium edetate. Nucl Med Commun 1991; 12: 793-7.
107. Bergenfelz A, Tennvall J, Ahrén B. Thallium-technetium subtraction scintigraphy of enlarged parathyroid glands after calcitonin stimulation of parathyroid hormone secretion. Acta Radiol 1992; 33: 319-22.
108. Sessler MJ, Geck P, Maul F-D et al. New aspects of cellular thallium uptake: Tl^{+}-Na^{+}-$2Cl^{-}$ -cotransport is the central mechanism of ion uptake. Nuclearmedizin 1986; 25: 24-7.
109. Wallfelt C, Larsson R, Johansson H et al. Stimulus-secretion coupling of parathyroid hormone release: Studies of ^{45}Ca and ^{86}Rb fluxes. Acta Physiol Scand 1985; 124: 239-45.
110. Gylfe E, Johansson H, Larsson R et al. Activation of Ca^{2+} influx into parthyroid cells by external cation binding. In: Cohn DV, Martin TJ, Meunier PJ, eds. Calcium Regulation and Bone Metabolism: Basic and Clinical Aspects. New York: Elsevier Science Publishers. 1987; 9: 33-8.
111. Juhlin C, Klareskog L, Nygren P et al. Hyperparathyroidism is associated with reduced expression of a parathyroid calcium receptor mechanism defined by monoclonal antiparathyroid antibodies. Endocrinology 1988; 122: 2999-3001.
112. Müller SP, Guth-Tougelidis B, Piotrowski B et al. Tl-201 scintigraphy in the follow-up of eosinophilic thyroid carcinoma. J Nucl Med 1990; 31: 767.
113. Malmaeus J, Grimelius L, Johansson H et al. Parathyroid pathology in hyperparathyroidism secondary to chronic renal failure. Scand J Urol Nephrol 1984; 18: 157-66.
114. Åkerström G, Malmaeus J, Grimelius L et al. Histological changes in parathyroid glands in subclinical and clinical renal disease. Scand J Urol Nephrol 1984; 18: 75-84.
115. Åkerström G, Rudberg C, Grimelius L et al. Histologic parathyroid abnormalities in an autopsy series. Hum Pathol 1986; 17: 520-7.
116. Johansson H, Rastad J, Bjerneroth G et al. Microfluorometric measurements of cytoplasmic calcium in chief and oxyphil parathyroid cells of adenomatous and hyperplastic glands and of normal-sized glands associated with adenomas Surgery 1989; 106: 517-24.
117. Rudberg C, Grimelius L, Johansson H et al. Alteration in density, morphology and parathyroid hormone release of dispersed parathyroid cells from patients with hyperparathyroidism. Acta Pathol Microbiol Immunol Scand (A) 1986; 94: 253-61.
118. Basarab RM. The evolving role of parathyroid scintigraphy. Clin Nucl Med 1989; 14: 58-60.

119. Skibber JM, Reynolds JC, Spiegel AM et al. Computerized technetium/thallium scans and parathyroid reoperation. Surgery 1985; 98: 1077-82.
120. Hauty M, Swartz K, McClung M et al. Technetium-thallium scintiscanning for localization of parathyroid adenomas and hyperplasia. Am J Surg 1987; 153: 479-86.
121. Peck WW, Higgins CB, Fisher MR et al. Hyperparathyroidism: Comparison of MR imaging with radionuclide scanning. Radiology 1987; 163: 415-20.
122. Wilson NM, Gaunt J, Nunan TO et al. Role of thallium-201/technetium-99m subtraction scanning in persistent or recurrent hypercalcaemia following parathyroidectomy. Br J Surg 1990; 77: 794-5.
123. McCall A, Henkin R, Calendra D et al. Routine use of the thallium-technetium scan prior to parathyroidectomy. Am Surg 1987; 53: 380-4.
124. Attie JN, Khan A, Rumancik WM et al. Preoperative localization of parathyroid adenomas. Am J Surg 1988; 156: 323-6.
125. Sandrock D, Merino MJ, Norton JA et al. Failure of parathyroid scintigraphy: 180 patient studies. J Nucl Med 1988; 29: 860.
126. Maltby C, Russel CFJ, Laird JD et al. Thallium-technetium isotope subtraction scanning in primary hyperparathyroidism. J R Coll Surg Edinb 1989; 34: 40-3.
127. Roses DF, Sudarsky LA, Sanger J et al. The use of preoperative localization of adenomas of the parathyroid glands by thallium-technetium subtraction scintigraphy, high-resolution ultrasonography and computed tomography. Surg Gynecol Obstet 1989; 168: 99-106.
128. Fogelman I, McKillop JH, Bessent RG et al. Successful localisation of parathyroid adenomata by thalllium-201 and technetium-99m subtraction scintigraphy: Description of an improved techique. Eur J Nucl Med 1984; 9: 545-7.
129. Pauwels EKJ, Bolk JH, Heslinga JM. Scintigraphic detection of adenoma in primary hyperparathyroidism. Eur J Nucl Med 1985; 10: 403-5.
130. Park CH, Intenzo C, Cohn HE. Dual tracer imaging for localization of parathyroid lesions. Clin Nucl Med 1986; 11: 237-41.
131. Manni A, Basarab RM, Plourde PV et al. Thallium-technetium parathyroid scan. A useful noninvasive technique for localization of abnormal parathyroid tissue. Arch Intern Med 1986; 146: 1077-80.
132. Basso LV, Keeling C, Goris ML. Parathyroid imaging. Use of dual isotope scintigraphy for the localization of adenomas before surgery. Clin Nucl Med 1992; 17: 380-3.
133. Blake GM, Percival RC, Kanis JA. Thallium-pertechnetate subtraction scintigraphy: A quantitative comparison between adenomatous and hyperplastic parathyroid glands. Eur J Nucl Med 1986; 12: 31-6.
134. Gimlette TMD, Brownless SM, Taylor WH et al. Limits to parathyroid imaging with thallium-201 confirmed by tissue uptake and phantom studies. J Nucl Med 1986; 27: 1262-5.
135. Ott R, Lawrence AM, Jorgensen R et al. Localization of ectopic parathyroid adenomas by the technetium-thalllium subtraction scan. Am Surg 1985; 51: 344-8.
136. Harding LK, de Bolla A, Everett K et al. Problems with detection of upper pole parathyroid adenomas using TC/TL imaging. Nuclearmedizin 1987; 24(suppl): 670-3.
137. Picard D, D'Amour P, Carrier L et al. Localization of abnormal parathyroid gland(s) using thallium-201/iodine-123 subtraction scintigraphy in patients with primary hyperparathyroidism. Clin Nucl Med 1987; 12: 60-4.
138. Fronistas O, Stavraka-Kakavaki A, Giougi A et al. Evaluation of parathyroid tissue transplants by TI-201 scintigraphy. Clin Nucl Med 1992; 17: 954-7.
139. Katz AD, Formichella D. Fifty-three reoperations for hyperparathyroidism. Am J Surg 1989; 158: 385-7.
140. Gimlette TMD, Taylor WH. Localization of enlarged parathyroid glands by thallium-201 and technetium-99m subtraction imaging. Gland mass and parathormone levels in primary hyperparathyroidism. Clin Nucl Med 1985; 10: 235-9.
141. Takagi H, Tominaga Y, Uchida K et al. Comparison of imaging methods for diagnosing enlarged parathyroid glands in chronic renal failure. J Comput Assist

Tomogr 1985; 9: 733-7.
142. Moolenaar W, Heslinga JM, Arndt JW et al. ^{201}Tl-^{99m}Tc subtraction scintigraphy in secondary hyperparathyroidism of chronic renal failure. Nephrol Dial Transplant 1988; 2: 166-8.
143. Bonjer HJ, Bruining HA, Birkenhager JC et al. Single and multigland disease in primary hyperparathyroidism: Clinical follow-up, histopathology, and flow cytometric DNA analysis. World J Surg 1992; 16: 737-44.
144. Blake GM. A simple objective method of recognizing goitre during parathyroid scintigraphy. Nucl Med Commun 1986; 7: 489-96.
145. Harada T, Ito Y, Shimaoka K et al. Clinical evaluation of ^{201}thallium chloride scan for thyroid nodule. Eur J Nucl Med 1980; 5: 125-30.
146. Tonami N, Bunko H, Michigishi T et al. Clinical application of 201Tl scintigraphy in patients with cold thyroid nodules. Clin Nucl Med 1978; 3: 217-21.
147. Ochi H, Sawa H, Fukuda T et al. Thallium-201-chloride thyroid scintigraphy to evaluate benign and/or malignant nodules: Usefulness of the delayed scan. Cancer 1982; 50: 236-40.
148. Percival RC, Blake GM, Urwin GH et al. Thallium-technetium subtraction scintigraphy as an aid to parathyroid surgery. Br J Urol 1985; 57: 133-6.
149 Asp A, Hasbargen J, Blue P et al. Ectopic thyroid tissue on thallium/technetium parathyroid scan. Arch Intern Med 1987; 147: 595-6.
150. Coakley AJ, Kettle AG, Wells CP et al. ^{99m}Tc^{m}-sestamibi- A new agent for parathyroid imaging. Nucl Med Commun 1989; 10: 791-4.
151. O'Doherty MJ, Kettle AG, Wells P et al. Parathyroid imaging with technetium-99m-sestamibi: Preoperative localization and tissue uptake studies. J Nucl Med 1992; 33: 313-8.
152. Wei JP, Burke GJ, Mansberger AR. Prospective evaluation of the efficacy of technetium 99m sestamibi and iodine 123 radionuclide imaging of abnormal parathyroid glands. Surgery 1992; 12: 1111-7.
153. Taillefer R, Boucher Y, Potvin C et al. Detection and localization of parathyroid adenomas in patients with hyperparathyroidism using a single radionuclide imaging procedure with technetium-99m-sestamibi (double-phase study). J Nucl Med 1992; 33: 1801-7.
154. Hurvitz RJ, Perzik SL, Morgenstern L. In vivo staining of the parathyroid glands. A clinical study. Arch Surg 1968; 97: 722-6.
155. Yeager RM, Krementz ET. Toluidine blue in identification of parathyroid glands at operation. Ann Surg 1969; 169: 829-38.
156. Larose JH, Whitaker RH, Reba RC. Radioiodinated toluidine blue: An unsatisfactory scanning agent. J Nucl Med 1970; 11: 731-2
157. Skretting A, Aas M, Normann E et al. Clinical results with ^{131}I-toluidine blue and triple radionuclide subtraction for preoperative localization of enlarged parathyroid glands. Eur J Nucl Med 1978; 3: 5-9.
158. Normann E, Bøhmer T, Otnes B et al. Clinical radionuclide-imaging of enlarged parathyroids with ^{131}I-toluidine blue. Acta Chir Scand 1974; 140: 517-22.
159. Blower PJ, Carter NJ. Rapid preparation of ^{123}I-labelled methylene blue and toluidine blue: Potential new agents for parathyroid scintigraphy. Nucl Med Commun 1990; 11: 413-20.
160. Czerniak A, Zwas ST, Shustik O et al. The use of radioiodinated toluidine blue for preoperative localization of parathyroid pathology. Surgery 1991; 110: 832-8.
161. Zwas ST, Czerniak A, Boruchowsky S et al. Preoperative parathyroid localization by superimposed iodine-131 toluidine blue and technetium-99m pertechnetate imaging. J Nucl Med 1987; 28: 298-307.
162. Cance WG, Wells SA, Dilley WG et al. Human parathyroid antigen: Characterization and localization with monoclonal antibodies. Proc Natl Acad Sci USA 1986; 83: 6112-6.
163. Cance WG, Otsuka FL, Dilley WG et al. A potential new radiopharmaceutical for parathyroid imaging: Radiolabeled parathyroid-specific monoclonal antibody-I. Evaluation of ^{125}I-labeled antibody in a nude mouse model system. Nucl Med Biol 1988; 15:

299-303.
164. Otsuka FL, Cance WG, Dilley WG et al. A potential new radiopharmaceutical for parathyroid imaging: Radiolabeled parathyroid-specific monoclonal antibody- II. Comparison of ^{125}I- and ^{111}In-labeled antibodies. Nucl Med Biol 1988; 15: 305-11.
165. Juhlin C, Holmdahl R, Johansson H et al. Monoclonal antibodies with exclusive reactivity against parathyroid cells and tubule cells of the kidney. Proc Natl Acad Sci USA 1987; 84: 2990-4.
166. Juhlin C, Lundgren S, Johansson H et al. 500-kilodalton calcium sensor regulating cytoplasmic Ca^{2+} in cytotrophoblast cells of human placenta. J Biol Chem 1990; 265: 8275-9.
167. Bjerneroth G, Juhlin C, Arnberg H et al. Distribution of monoclonal antiparathyroid antibody E11 in mice grafted with human parathyroid adenoma and carcinoma. Surgery 1991; 110: 839-46.
168. Stark DD, Moss AA, Gooding GAW et al. Parathyroid scanning by computed tomography. Radiology 1983; 148: 297-9.
169. Stark DD, Gooding GAW, Moss AA et al. Parathyroid imaging: Comparison of high-resolution CT and high-resolution sonography. Am J Roentgenol 1983; 141: 633-8.
170. Adams JE, Adams PH, Mamtora H et al. Computed tomography and the localisation of parathyroid tumours. Clin Radiol 1981; 32: 251-4.
171. Krebs FJ, Archer CR, Awwad EE et al. Preoperative computerized tomographic imaging in hyperparathyroidism. Otolaryngol Head Neck Surg 1987; 97: 351-5.
172. Cates JD, Thorsen MK, Lawson TL et al. CT evaluation of parathyroid adenomas: Diagnostic criteria and pitfalls. J Comput Assist Tomogr 1988; 12: 626-9.
173. Doppman JL, Brennan MF, Koehler JO et al. Computed tomography for parathyroid localization. J Comput Assist Tomogr 1977; 1: 30-6.
174. Kovarik J, Willvonseder R, Küster W et al. Localization of parathyroid tumors by computed tomography. N Engl J Med 1980; 303: 885.
175. Whitley NO, Bohlman M, Connor TB et al. Computed tomography for localization of parathyroid adenomas. J Comput Assist Tomogr 1981; 5: 812-7.
176. Lineaweaver W, Clore F, Mancuso A et al. Calcified parathyroid glands detected by computed tomography. J Comput Assist Tomogr 1984; 8: 975-7.
177. Awwad EE, Archer CR, Krebs FJ. Parathyroid adenomas; computed tomographic imaging and the importance of preoperative localization. Comput Med Imaging Graph 1988; 12: 305-14.
178. von Schulthess GK, Weder W, Goebel N et al. 1.5 T MRI, CT, ultrasonography and scintigraphy in hyperparathyroidism. Eur J Radiol 1988; 8: 157-64.
179. Clark OH, Stark DD, Gooding GAW et al. Localization procedures in patients requiring reoperation for hyperparathyroidism. World J Surg 1984; 8: 509-21.
180. Vogl T, Hefele B, Hahn D et al. A comparative study of MR, CT and sonography in patients with primary hyperparathyroidism. Fortschr Röntgenstr 1986; 145: 167-72.
181. Brennan MF, Doppman JL, Kurdy AG et al. Assessment of techniques for preoperative parathyroid gland localization in patients undergoing reoperation for hyperparathyroidism. Surgery 1982; 91: 6-11.
182. Kneeland JB, Krubsack AJ, Lawson TL et al. Enlarged parathyroid glands: High-resolution local coil MR imaging. Radiology 1987; 162: 143-6.
183. Roza AM, Wexler MJ, Stein L et al. Value of high-resolution computerized tomography in localizing diseased parathyroid glands. Can J Surg 1984; 27: 334-6.
184. May GR, James EM, Johnson CM. The radiologist's role in acute endocrine problems. World J Surg 1982; 6: 725-34.
185. Krudy AG, Doppman JL, Brennan MF et al. The detection of mediastinal parathyroid glands by computed tomography, selective arteriography, and venous sampling. Radiology 1981 140: 739-44.
186. Stark DD, Moss AA, Gamsu G et al. Magnetic resonance imaging of the neck. Part I: Normal anatomy. Radiology 1984; 150: 447-54.
187. Kier R, Blinder RA, Herfkens RJ et al.

MR imaging with surface coils in primary hyperparathyroidism. J Comput Assist Tomogr 1987; 11: 863-8.
188. Spritzer CE, Gefter WB, Hamilton R et al. Abnormal parathyroid glands: High-resolution MR imaging. Radiology 1987; 162: 487-91.
189. Higgins CB, Auffermann W. MR imaging of thyroid and parathyroid glands: A review of current status. Am J Roentgenol 1988; 151: 1095-106.
190. Stevens SK, Chang J-M, Clark OH et al. Detection of abnormal parathyroid glands in postoperative patients with recurrent hyperparathyroidism: Sensitivity of MR imaging. Am J Roentgenol 1993; 160: 607-12.
191. Stark DD, Moss AA, Gamsu G et al. Magnetic resonance imaging of the neck. Part II: Pathologic findings. Radiology 1984; 150: 455-61.
192. Felmlee JP, Ehman RL. Spatial presaturation: A method for suppressing flow artifacts and improving depiction of vascular anatomy in MR imaging. Radiology 1987; 164: 559-64.
193. Gefter WB, Spritzer CE, Eisenberg B et al. Thyroid imaging with high-field-strength surface-coil MR. Radiology 1987; 164: 483-90.
194. Hamilton B, Greenberg BM, Gefter W et al. Successful localization of parathyroid adenomas by magnetic resonance imaging. Am J Surg 1988; 155: 370-3.
195. Russell P, Lean CL, Delbridge L et al. Proton magnetic resonance and human thyroid neoplasia. I: Discrimination between benign and malignant neoplasms. Am J Med 1994; 96:383-8.
196. Seelos KC, DeMarco R, Clark OH et al. Persistent and recurrent hyperparathyroidism: Assessment with gadopentetate dimeglumine-enhanced MR imaging. Radiology 1990; 177: 373-8.
197. von Peiß J, Füzesi L, Bohndorf K et al. Das Signalverhalten von Nebenschilddrüsenadenomen in der MRT-kontrastverhalten zu Schilddrüse und Fettgewebe. Fortschr Röntgenstr 1992; 156: 130-4.
198. Wright AR, Goddard PR, Nicholson S et al. Fat-suppression magnetic resonance imaging in the preoperative localization of parathyroid adenomas. Clin Radiol 1992; 46: 324-8.
199. Noguchi Y, Takashima S, Ikezoe J et al. Hyperparathyroidism- Comparison of flash imaging with spin echo MR imaging. Acta Radiol 1993; 34: 625-30.
200. Hemmingsson A, Ericsson A, Ljunghall S et al. Technical aspects of magnetic resonance imaging in parathyroid gland lesions. Acta Radiol Diagn 1986; 27: 595-7.
201. Auffermann W, Guis M, Tavares NJ et al. MR signal intensity of parathyroid adenomas: Correlation with histopathology. Am J Roentgenol 1989; 153: 873-6.
202. Whelan PJ, Rotstein LE, Rosen IB et al. Do we really need another localizing technique for parathyroid glands? Am J Surg 1989; 158: 382-4.
203. Kang YS, Rosen K, Clark OH et al. Localization of abnormal parathyroid glands of the mediastinum with MR imaging. Radiology 1993; 189: 137-41.
204. Doppman JL, Melson GL, Evens RG et al. Selective superior and inferior thyroid vein catheterization. Venographic anatomy and potential applications. Invest Radiol 1969; 4: 97-9.
205. Reitz RE, Pollard JJ, Wang C-A et al. Localization of parathyroid adenomas by selective venous catheterization and radioimmunoassay. N Engl J Med 1969; 281: 348-51.
206. O'Riordan JLH, Kendall BE, Woodhead JS. Preoperative localization of parathyroid tumours. Lancet 1971; 2: 1172-5.
207. Powell D, Shimkin PM, Doppman JL et al. Primary hyperparathyroidism. Preoperative tumor localization and differentiation between adenoma and hyperplasia. N Engl J Med 1972; 286: 1169-75
208. Bilezikian JP, Doppman JL, Shimkin PM et al. Preoperative localization of abnormal parathyroid tissue. Cumulative experience with venous sampling and arteriography. Am J Med 1973; 55: 505-14.
209. Tomlinson S, Clements VR, Smith MJG et al. Selective catheterization of the thyroid veins for preoperative localization of parathyroid tumours. Br J Surg 1974; 61: 633-7.

210. Monchik JM, Doppman JL, Earl JM et al. Localization of hyperfunctioning parathyroid tissue. Radioimmunoassay of parathyroid hormone on samples from the large veins of the neck and thorax and selectively catheterized thyroid veins. Am J Surg 1975; 129: 413-20.
211. Mallette LE, Gomez L, Fisher RG. Parathyroid angiography: A review of current knowledge and guidelines for clinical application. Endocr Rev 1981; 2: 124-35.
212. Levy JM, Hessel SJ, Dippe SE et al. Digital subtraction angiography for localization of parathyroid lesions. Ann Intern Med 1982; 97: 710-2.
213. Krudy AG, Doppman JL, Miller DL et al. Work in progress: Abnormal parathyroid glands. Comparison of nonselective arterial digital arteriography, selective parathyroid arteriography, and venous arteriography as methods of detection. Radiology 1983; 148: 23-9.
214. Obley DL, Winzelberg GG, Jarmolowski CR et al. Parathyroid adenomas studied by digital subtraction angiography. Radiology 1984; 153: 449-51.
215. Miller DL, Doppman JL, Krudy AG et al. Localization of parathyroid adenomas in patients who have undergone surgery. Part II. Invasive procedures. Radiology 1987; 162: 138-41.
216. Doppman JL, Hammond WG. The anatomic basis of parathyroid venous sampling. Radiology 1970; 95: 603-10.
217. Doppman JL, Wells SA, Shimkin PM et al. Parathyroid localization by angiographic techniques in patients with previous neck surgery. Br J Radiol 1973; 46: 403-18.
218. Shimkin PM, Doppman JL, Pearson KD et al. Anatomic considerations in parathyroid venous sampling. Am J Roentgenol 1973; 118: 654-62.
219. Eisenberg H, Pallotta J, Sherwood LM. Selective arteriography, venography and venous hormone assay in diagnosis and localization of parathyroid lesions. Am J Med 1974; 56: 810-20.
220. Dunlop DAB, Papapoulos SE, Lodge RW et al. Parathyroid venous sampling: Anatomic considerations and results in 95 patients with primary hyperparathyroidism. Br J Radiol 1980; 53: 183-91.
221. Shimkin PM, Doppman JL, Powell D et al. Demonstration of parathyroid adenomas by retrograde thyroid venography. Radiology 1972; 103: 63-7.
222. Doppman JL. Parathyroid localization. Arteriography and venous sampling. Radiol Clin North Am 1976; 14: 163-88.
223. Nilsson BE, Tisell L-E, Jansson S et al. Parathyroid localization by catheterization of large cervical and mediastinal veins for determination of serum concentrations of intact parathyroid hormone. World J Surg, in press.
224. Hsu FSF, Clark OH, Serata TY et al. Rapid localization of parathyroid tumors by selective venous catheterization and parathyroid hormone bioassay. Surgery 1983; 94: 873-6.
225. Edis AJ, Sheedy PF, Beahrs OH et al. Results of reoperation for hyperparathyroidism, with evaluation of preoperative localization studies. Surgery 1978; 84: 384-93.
226. Granberg P-O, Hamberger B, Johansson G et al. Selective venous sampling for localization of hyperfunctioning parathyroid glands. Br J Surg 1986; 73: 118-20.
227. Miller DL, Chang R, Doppman JL et al. Localization of parathyroid adenomas: Superselective arterial DSA versus superselective conventional angiography. Radiology 1989; 170: 1003-6.
228. Doppman JL, Mallette LE, Marx SJ et al. The localization of abnormal mediastinal parathyroid glands. Radiology 1975; 115: 31-6.
229. Seldinger SI. Localization of parathyroid adenomata by arteriography. Acta Radiol 1954; 42: 353-66.
230. Krementz ET, Yeager R, Hawley W et al. The first 100 cases of parathyroid tumor from Charity Hospital of Louisiana. Ann Surg 1971; 173: 872-83.
231. Bradley EL, McGarity WC. Surgical evaluation of parathyroid arteriography. Am J Surg 1973; 126: 67-73.
232. Mishkin MM, Baum S, Di Chiro G. Emergency treatment of angiography-induced paraplegia and tetraplegia. N Engl J Med 1973; 288: 1184-5.

233. Rothmund M, Diethelm L, Brünner H et al. Diagnosis and surgical treatment of mediastinal parathyroid tumors. Ann Surg 1976; 183: 139-45.
234. Daseler EH, Anson BJ. Surgical anatomy of the subclavian artery and its branches. Surg Gynecol Obstet 1959; 108: 149-74.
235. Doppman JL, Hammond WG, Melson GL et al. Staining of parathyroid adenomas by selective arteriography. Radiology 1969; 92: 527-30.
236. Doppman JL, Marx SJ, Brennan MF et al. The blood supply of mediastinal parathyroid adenomas. Ann Surg 1977; 185: 488-90.
237. Jelenko C, Teeslink CR, Herndon JR et al. Localization of parathyroid adenomata by selective arteriography. Am Surg 1971; 37: 25-33.
238. Kuntz CH, Goldsmith RE. Selective arteriography of parathyroid adenomas. Radiology 1972; 102: 21-8
239. Newton TH, Eisenberg E. Angiography of parathyroid adenomas. Radiology 1966; 86: 843-50.
240. Jander HP, Diethelm AG, Russinovich NAE. The parathyroid artery. Am J Roentgenol 1980; 135: 821-8.
241. Esselstyn CB, Buonocore E. The use of digital subtraction angiography and computed tomography scanning in localization of parathyroid adenomas in secondary parathyroid operations: Preliminary observations. Surgery 1983; 94: 869-72.
242. Lacombe P, Foster D, Dubost C et al. Selective intraarterial DSA of the parathyroid glands in patients with hyperparathyroidism after parathyroidectomy. Am J Roentgenol 1987; 149: 479-83.
243. Krudy AG, Doppman JL, Marx SJ et al. Parathyroid aspiration directed by angiography: An alternative to venous sampling. Radiology 1984; 152: 207-8.
244. de Francisco ALM, Amado JA, Casanova D et al. Recurrence of hyperparathyroidism after total parathyroidectomy with autotransplantation: A new technique to localize the source of hormone excess. Nephron 1991; 58: 306-9.
245. Hellman P, Ahlström H, Bergström M et al. Positron emission tomography with ^{11}C-methionine in hyperparathyroidism. Surgery, in press.
246. Sigel B, Kraft AR, Nyhus LM et al. Identification of a parathyroid adenoma by operative ultrasonography. Arch Surg 1981; 116: 234-5.
247. Charboneau JW, Grant CS, James EM et al. High-resolution ultrasound-guided percutaneous needle biopsy and intraoperative ultrasonography of a cervical parathyroid adenoma in a patient with persistent hyperparathyroidism. Mayo Clin Proc 1983; 58: 497-500.
248. Dudley NE. Methylene blue for rapid identification of the parathyroids. Br Med J 1971; 3: 680-1.
249. Gordon DL, Airan MC, Thomas W et al. Parathyroid identification by methylene blue infusion. Br J Surg 1975; 62: 747-9.
250. Wheeler MH, Wade JSH. Intraoperative identification of parathyroid glands: Appraisal of methylene blue staining. Am J Surg 1982; 143: 713-6.
251. Devine RM, van Heerden JA, Grant CS et al. The role of methylene blue infusion in the management of persistent or recurrent hyperparathyroidism. Surgery 1983; 94: 916-8.
252. Bland KI, Tidwell S, von Fraunhofer JA et al. Intraoperative localization of parathyroid glands using methylthionine chloride tetramethylthionine chloride in secondary hyperparathyroidism. Surg Gynecol Obstet 1985; 160: 42-8.
253. Kobayashi S, Miyakawa M, Sugenoya A et al. An evaluation of the intraoperative staining technique using methylene blue for the detection of hyperplastic parathyroid glands. Jpn J Surg 1988; 18: 729-31.
254. Derom AF, Wallaert PC, Janzing HM et al. Intraoperative identification of parathyroid glands with methylene blue infusion. Am J Surg 1993; 165: 380-2.
255. Stoffer SS, Szpunar WE, Hawker CD. Differentiation of thyroid from parathyroid cysts. JAMA 1980; 233: 1427.
256. Rosenberg J, Orlando R, Ludwig M et al. Parathyroid cysts. Am J Surg 1982; 143: 473-80.

257. Calandra DB, Shah KH, Prinz RA et al. Parathyroid cysts: A report of eleven cases including two associated with hyperparathyroid crisis. Surgery 1983; 94: 887-92.
258. Kodama T, Obara T, Fujimoto Y et al. Eleven cases of nonfunctioning parathyroid cyst- Significance of needle aspiration in diagnosis and management. Endocrinol Japon 1987; 34: 769-77.
259. Clark OH. Parathyroid cysts. Am J Surg 1978; 135: 395-402.
260. Silverman JF, Khazanie PG, Norris HT et al. Parathyroid hormone (PTH) assay of parathyroid cysts examined by fine needle aspiration biopsy. Am J Clin Pathol 1986; 86: 776-80.
261. Ramos-Gabatin A, Mallette LE, Bringhurst FR et al. Functional mediastinal parathyroid cysts. Dynamics of parathyroid hormone secretion during cyst aspirations and surgery. Am J Med 1985; 79: 633-9.
262. Prinz RA, Peters JR, Kane JM et al. Needle aspiration of nonfunctioning parathyroid cysts. Am Surg 1990; 56: 420-2.
263. Ginsberg J, Young JEM, Walfish PG. Parathyroid cysts. Medical diagnosis and treatment. JAMA 1978; 240: 1506-7.
264. Katz AD, Dunkleman D. Needle aspiration of nonfunctioning parathyroid cysts. Arch Surg 1984; 119: 307-8.
265. Oertel YC, Wargotz ES. Diagnosis of parathyroid cysts. Am J Clin Pathol 1987; 88: 252-3.
266. Takeichi N, Dohi K, Matsumoto H et al. A parathyroid cyst effectively treated with a sclerosing agent. Jpn J Surg 1985; 15: 405-7.
267. Solbiati L, Giangrande A, De Pra L et al. Percutaneous ethanol injection of parathyroid tumors under US guidance: Treatment for secondary hyperparathyroidism. Radiology 1985; 155: 607-10.
268. Karstrup S, Holm HH, Torp-Pedersen S et al. Ultrasonically guided percutaneous inactivation of parathyroid tumours. Br J Radiol 1987; 60: 667-70.
269. Karstrup S, Transbøl I, Holm HH et al. Ultrasound-guided chemical parathyroidectomy in patients with primary hyperparathyroidism: A prospective study. Br J Radiol 1989; 62: 1037-42.
270. Karstrup S, Holm HH, Glenthøj A et al. Nonsurgical treatment of primary hyperparathyroidism with sonographically guided percutaneous injection of ethanol: Results in a selected series of patients. Am J Roentgenol 1990; 154: 1087-90.
271. Charboneau JW, Hay ID, van Heerden JA. Persistent primary hyperparathyroidism: Successful ultrasound-guided percutaneous ethanol ablation of an occult adenoma. Mayo Clin Proc 1988; 63: 913-7.
272. Futh U, Hofereiter F, Fröhling PT. Methodik und erste Ergebnisse der perkutanen ultraschallgezielten Verödung von Nebenschilddrüsenadenomen bei sekundärem order tertiärem Hyperparathyreoidimus. Z Urol Nephrol 1989; 82: 437-41.
273. Verges B, Cercueil JP, Pfitzenmeyer P et al. Percutaneous ethanol injection of parathyroid adenomas in primary hyperparathyroidism. Lancet 1991; 337: 1421-2.
274. Giangrande A, Castiglioni A, Solbiati L et al. Ultrasound-guided percutaneous fine-needle ethanol injection into parathyroid glands in secondary hyperparathyroidism. Nephrol Dial Transplant 1992; 7: 412-21.
275. Doppman JL, Marx SJ, Spiegel AM et al. Treatment of hyperparathyroidism by percutaneous embolization of a mediastinal adenoma. Radiology 1975; 115: 37-42.
276. Doppman JL, Brown EM, Brennan MF et al. Angiographic ablation of parathyroid adenomas. Radiology 1979; 130: 577-82.
277. Geelhoed GW, Krudy AG, Doppman JL. Long-term follow-up of patients with hyperparathyroidism treated by transcatheter staining with contrast agent. Surgery 1983; 94: 849-62.
278. Miller DL, Doppman JL, Chang R et al. Angiographic ablation of parthyroid adenomas: Lessons from a 10-year experience. Radiology 1987; 165: 601-7.
279. Pallotta JA, Sacks BA, Moller DE et al. Arteriographic ablation of cervical parathyroid adenomas. J Clin Endocrinol Metab 1989; 69: 1249-55.
280. Doherty GM, Doppman JL, Miller DL et al. Results of a multidisciplinary strategy for management of mediastinal parathyroid adenoma as a cause of persistent primary

hyperparathyroidism. Ann Surg 1992; 215: 101-6.

281. Reidy JF, Ryan PJ, Fogelman I et al. Ablation of mediastinal parthyroid adenomas by superselective embolization of the internal mammary artery with alcohol. Clin Radiol 1993; 47: 170-3.

282. Doppman JL, Popovsky M, Girton M. The use of iodinated contrast agents to ablate organs: Experimental studies and histopathology. Radiology 1981; 138: 333-40.

283. Krudy AG, Doppman JL, Marx SJ et al. Failure of ablation of a mediastinal parathyroid adenoma by repeated contrast staining. Radiology 1981; 140: 63-5.

CHAPTER 6

Clinics of Sporadic Primary Hyperparathyroidism

Göran Åkerström, Sverker Ljunghall,
Jonas Rastad, Claes Juhlin

Awareness that primary HPT may cause subtle but incapacitating symptoms of fatigue and psychiatric disability has led to a general liberal attitude towards surgery, but still the patients who undergo operation seem to comprise only 10% of the affected population.

Only a few decades ago primary hyperparathyroidism (HPT) was considered a rare disorder associated with severe bone symptoms, and many of the early patients finally deteriorated with pronounced neuromuscular weakness and fatigue in progressive renal failure. Subsequently it was demonstrated that a considerable number of patients also suffered from a more or less severe renal stone disorder, and it was in fact suggested that the patients were prone to develop either the bone or the renal stone complications of the disease.[1] In more recent years primary HPT has been diagnosed with increased frequency, due to the general introduction of liberal measurements of serum calcium into the clinical evaluation, and fewer patients are now found to be afflicted with the severe "classical" symptoms.[2,3] Instead many patients present with only moderate hypercalcemia, and the majority of them have vague complaints of fatigue or psychiatric disability or are apparently asymptomatic. Concomittantly, and particularly due to the introduction of new methods for measurement of intact serum parathyroid hormone (PTH), the diagnosis of HPT catheter become simplified and may now be settled with considerable certainty even in cases with borderline elevation of serum calcium. A main concern in currently diagnosed primary HPT has then been to establish the appropriate indications for surgery, and this should be especially important in patients scheduled for reoperation.

Current Controversy in Parathyroid Operation and Reoperation,
edited by Göran Åkerström.

PREVALENCE

Primary HPT is now one of the most common endocrine disorders, following only diabetes and thyroid disease in prevalence. The disease occurs about three times as often in females as in males. It occurs in all age groups, but shows a marked age-related increase in incidence, and is particularly common in females after menopause. A health survey in Sweden comprising more than 16,000 individuals of all age groups, subjected to repeat serum calcium determination, revealed an overall prevalence of primary HPT of 1% and presented figures as high as 3% among females above 60 years of age[4] (Fig. 6.1). This is higher than was previously anticipated in studies with limited inclusion of older age groups where HPT is most prevalent.[5] These findings emphasize that prevalence figures depend largely on the age and sex of the population, as well as on the chosen normal limits of serum calcium.[4] Lower prevalence figures may thus represent less efficient screening for mild disease, but could also be due to geographical variation in disease distribution.[5,6] This possibility, however, still awaits proper study, since prevalence data are not available for most countries. An autopsy investigation has indeed confirmed the high prevalence of HPT in the elderly Swedish population, since it demonstrated parathyroid adenoma in 2.4%, and mainly subclinical, micronodular hyperplasia in another 7%.[7] A majority of the hypercalcemic individuals detected at health screening will exhibit only mild or moderate elevations of serum calcium, but cases with severe hypercalcemia may occasionally also be encountered.[4] The disease has to be actively searched for, since symptoms occur silently, and even fortuitously detected patients may exhibit irreversible complications. The number of operations for HPT has increased markedly during recent years due mainly to widely adopted liberal indications for treatment, but the patients undergoing surgery still seem to comprise only 10% of the expected patient population.[4,8] Considering the high prevalence of clinically undetected mild HPT, it appears appropriate to continue to recommend surgery for individuals with more significant hypercalcemia, who obviously are at risk to experience symptoms or complications of the disease, while the indications for surgery in the really mild cases still awaits clarification.

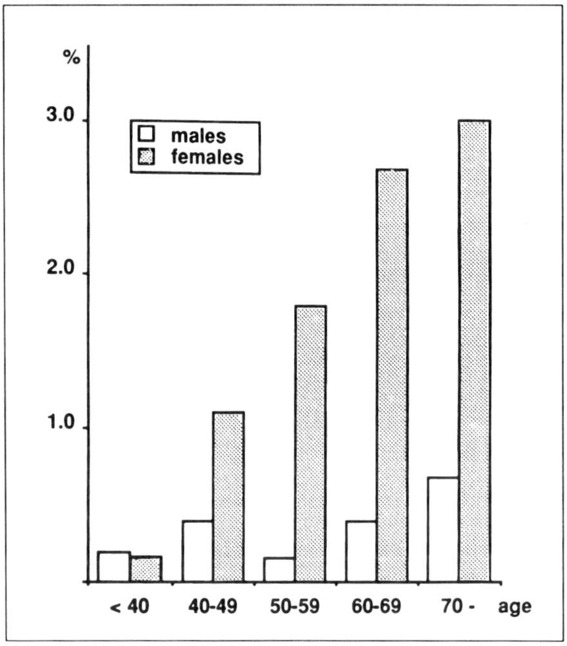

Fig 6.1. Prevalence of hypercalcemia (defined as a value > 2.60 mmol/l on two separate accounts with an interval of 2 years) in a Swedish health survey. Reprinted with permission from Palmér M et al.[4]

ETIOLOGY

The etiology of non-familial primary HPT is thus far largely unknown. Exceptiontionally, the disease has in some patients developed as a result of previous neck irradiation, often given as treatment for childhood neck adenitis.[9-11] These patients have generally been afflicted with parathyroid adenoma. A history of irradiation has in some series comprised 15-25% of the diagnosed population, but in our experience the association is more unusual. Only rarely has HPT been reported to occur as a result of ^{131}I treatment for thyroid disease.[12]

Circumstantial evidence has indicated that insufficient levels of active vitamin D may be related to increased incidence of subclinical and clinical parathyroid disease in elderly individuals.[7] The prevalence of HPT thus seems to be unusually high in Scandinavia, where elderly persons are more prone to develop slightly decreased levels of $1,25(OH)_2D_3$ due to insufficient sunshine exposure in combination with age-related diminished renal tubular mass.[4,7,13] It has also been suggested that the vitamin D status may influence the clinical expression of primary HPT.[14] It is claimed that patients with low vitamin D levels more easily develop marked parathyroid gland enlargement, severe hypercalcemia as well as advanced bone symptoms of the disease.[13-16] Consistent with this hypothesis recurrent renal stones and hypercalciuria are more prevalent in young persons with HPT.[13] Nowadays when the parathyroid bone disease is rare, the psychiatric and neuromuscular disturbances more commonly affect the elderly, with supposedly lower vitamin D levels.[13-17] Although these distinct differences in symptom distribution have been disputed,[17] the recognition that vitamin D exerts a principal regulation of the PTH secretion as well as the parathyroid cell proliferation, and that it could also influence the symptoms associated with the disease, may possibly provide important clues to treatment and prophylaxis in the future.

DIAGNOSIS

Serum calcium. Consistent with the principal role of the parathyroid to maintain tight regulation of the serum calcium concentration, HPT is generally diagnosed by the demonstration of hypercalcemia. The majority of clinically detected patients has moderately elevated serum calcium values. Short-term fluctuations in these values are common, but during longer periods of observation the measures tend to remain stable or increase slowly.[4,18]

Measurements of the *ionized calcium concentration* should be particularly sensitive for detection of border-line hypercalcemia, but the general clinical utilization of such measurements has been restrained by comparatively large inter-laboratory variation.[19] Determination of the *total serum calcium concentration* has shown better precision, allowing standardization between laboratories and consensus about reference limits (the upper limit generally being 2.60 mmol/l), and is therefore often preferred in the clinical setting.[19,20] Major errors associated with the total serum calcium measurements are non-analytical, caused by inappropriate sampling or variation in posture, which tend to cause falsely elevated values. In order to minimize such imprecision, samples should be drawn without stasis in a fasting, resting patient.[19,20] The accuracy of the total serum calcium measurements is increased if adjustments are made for alteration in plasma albumin, by approximately 0.02 mmol/l for each gram the prevailing serum albumin concentration deviates from the normal mean of the laboratory.[19,20] Although these formulas are of clinical value, it has to be appreciated that they more accurately correct larger plasma protein variations than the borderline deviations.[20]

Parathyroid hormone (PTH) is rapidly degraded in the circulation and exhibits a half-life of 5-10 minutes. Carboxyterminal peptide fragments depend on maintained renal function for their clearance, while aminoterminal fragments are responsible for the principal biological activity of the hormone.[21] The assay of serum PTH has been notoriously difficult, and as biologically active PTH circulates in low concentrations, a variable renal clearance of carboxyterminal fragments has made measurements difficult to interpret in the presence of renal impairment. The PTH determinations have also been influenced by heterogeneity of fragments as well as an increased release of hormone fragments in HPT.[21] Recently developed sensitive immunometric assays for detection of intact PTH utilizing two populations of region specific antibodies have proven considerably more sensitive and specific than previously used PTH assays, and have also lacked the nonspecific serum effects of the older radioimmunoassays.[21] The routine use of intact PTH measurements has therefore greatly simplified the diagnostic discrimination in hypercalcemia, and the vast majority of patients with primary HPT will exhibit increased concentrations of intact PTH.[20-27] The remaining patients with mild HPT, tend to have values in the upper normal range. Considering the inverse relationship between serum calcium and intact PTH in the normal population the HPT patients then exhibit inappropriately elevated serum PTH values for the prevailing serum calcium concentration.[20,21] A remaining overlap between patients with very mild HPT and normal individuals however, may occasionally necessitate some time of follow-up in order to obtain repeat measurements and confidently establish the abnormal levels of both serum calcium and PTH. The urinary calcium excretion tends to be moderately elevated and more occasionally within upper normal limits in patients with primary HPT.

The patients with HPT also tend to exhibit low normal serum phosphate, as well as slightly increased serum chloride concentrations.[28] Discriminant analyses have utilized serum estimates of calcium, phosphate and chloride as well as hematocrit, alkaline phosphatases and albumin, so that diagnostic accuracy can be improved. Such calculations seem to be rarely needed in the current diagnosis of HPT.[20,28]

DIFFERENTIAL DIAGNOSIS

Before the introduction of the intact PTH measurements the diagnosis of HPT was generally settled by exclusion of other causes of hypercalcemia. To ensure this discrimination the patients frequently had to undergo more or less complicated metabolic and radiological studies. The diagnosis is nowadays rarely associated with problems, since patients with hypercalcemia due to other causes than HPT should exhibit suppressed values of intact serum PTH.[20,21] Besides HPT the principal differential diagnosis to consider in patients with hypercalcemia is *malignancy,* and together these two diagnoses account for 80-90% of all hypercalcemias[20,28,29] (Table 6.1). In this respect, primary HPT is known to comprise a majority of hypercalcemic individuals detected in outpatient populations, while malignancy generally predominates among hospitalized patients.[4,5,30] The hypercalcemia of malignancy occurs most often in patients with already diagnosed, advanced malignancy. Moreover, it tends to develop and progress rapidly, in contrast to the generally benign and chronic course of serum calcium in primary HPT.[28,29] Carcinoma of the bronchus, breast, head and neck, urogenital tract, and multiple myeloma are the most prevalent malignancies associated with hypercalcemia.[31] Skeletal metastases, which cause hypercalcemia mainly by local osteolysis, will be present in approximately 20% of these malignancies, and preferentially includes patients with multiple myeloma and breast carcinoma.[31] In the remaining 80% the malignancy-associated hypercalcemia is related to the release of humoral factors from the tumors, and may occur also in the absence of skeletal metastases. The most important of these humoral factors is the recently discovered PTH-like peptide (PTHrp). This peptide exhibits aminoterminal homology with PTH, and thus has the ability to bind and activate PTH receptors in bone and kidney, whereby its effects mimic the metabolic consequences of HPT.[32-34] PTHrp values may now be directly measured by immunoassay to make a diagnosis of malignancy-associated hypercalcemia.[34] Values of intact PTH should be low in such circumstances, as ectopic PTH release by a non-parathyroid tumor are most unusual, and has only occasionally been described.[35] Raised levels of intact PTH in patients with malignancy is, however, not uncommon, and more or less invariably relate to concomitant HPT.[20,21]

Thyrotoxicosis is sometimes associated with moderate hypercalcemia, but adequate treatment will invariably normalize the serum calcium values, unless the patient also has HPT (Table 6.1). Other differential diagnoses, that have to be considered, are *granulomatous diseases* (sarcoidosis, tubercu-

Table 6.1. Differential diagnosis of hypercalcemia

Common causes (80-90% of patients with hypercalcemia):
Primary hyperparathyroidism (albumin corrected s-Ca, intact PTH-repeat measurements)
Malignancy
Humoral hypercalcemia of malignancy (PTHrP)
Metastatic bone disease (local osteolytic factors, radiology, bone scintigraphy)
Lymphoproliferative diseases (malignant lymphoma-1,25$(OH)_2D_3$, blood count, bone marrow biopsy)
Uncommon causes
Thyreotoxicosis (TSH)
Granulomas (sarcoidosis, tuberculosis - 1,25$(OH)_2D_3$, ACE)
Familial hypocalciuric hypercalcemia (urinary calcium/creatinine, family studies)
Immobilization
Milk/alkali syndrome
Vitamin D intoxication
Rare causes
Lithium therapy
Adrenal insufficiency
Pheocromocytoma
Vipoma
Hypothyroidism
Vitamin A intoxication
Sepsis

losis) and *lymphoproliferative disorders* (lymphoma), but also these disorders characteristically exhibit low intact PTH values. The hypercalcemia of the latter conditions is related to high values of 1,25$(OH)_2D_3$, due to presence of 1-α hydroxylase within the granuloma/lymphoid cells, and typically responds to steroid suppression.[28-29] A diagnosis of sarcoidosis may also be supported by the demonstration of increased levels of angiotensin converting enzyme (ACE), which may be elevated in approximately 50% of the patients.

FAMILIAL HYPOCALCIURIC HYPERCALCEMIA

An important diagnosis to consider in patients planned for reoperative parathyroid surgery is familial hypocalciuric hypercalcemia (FHH), which also has been named familial benign hypercalcemia (FBH).[36-40] This is an autosomal, dominant condition, which is inherited with high penetrance. Close relatives within these kindreds will usually exhibit raised serum calcium values and many of them may in fact have been subjected to unsuccessful parathyroid surgery.[38] The hypercalcemia is thought to be present from birth, and severe neonatal hypercalcemia is a rare complication in some families.[39,41] The serum calcium, and especially the ionized calcium values tend to be moderately elevated. This derangement classically is associated with no symptoms, for this reason FHH needs to be carefully excluded in all younger (< 50 years) patients with overtly asymptomatic hypercalcemia.[36,39,42] The condition should be particularly suspected when hypercalcemia is detected in children, since HPT is unusual in these age groups and other familial forms such as the multiple endocrine neoplasia type 1 (MEN-1) associated disease rarely develops before the age of 20.[39] Patients with FHH characteristically exhibit low urinary calcium, normal to slightly elevated values of serum magnesium, and normal levels of intact PTH, although occasionally these values may be slightly raised.[36,39,43,44] The parathyroid glands seem to be grossly and histologically normal.[45,46] Diagnosis should rely on the presentation of a typical family history, demonstration of hypercalcemia in other probands, and determination of the 24-hour urinary calcium and creatinine quotient, whereby a ratio < 0.01 indicates FHH. There may, however, be an overlap between occasional patients with primary HPT, who exhibit unusually low urinary calcium.[39,44] The discrimination is crucially important even before the primary parathyroid operation, since the patients with FHH should not be surgically explored.

SYMPTOMS

The symptoms of primary HPT are principally related to effects of the excess PTH secretion, which increases the serum calcium concentration. One of the effects is to enhance calcium mobilization from the skeleton; more or less pronounced demineralization of bone appears as an inevitable complication. PTH also stimulates calcium reabsorption in the kidney tubule, but since the filtered calcium load is increased, the net effect tends to be moderate hypercalciuria, with a resulting propensity for renal stones. It is likely, however, that the raised serum calcium concentration per se also is the cause of adverse effects, which preferentially seem to encompass the less distinct symptoms of HPT such as neuromuscular weakness and psychiatric disability. The stimulatory effect of PTH on conversion in the proximal kidney tubule of vitamin D to the active hormone $1,25(OH)_2D_3$, will raise serum calcium indirectly by enhancing gastrointestinal calcium absorption and further substantiates the close interaction between the vitamin D metabolism and the parathyroids. In patients with vitamin D deficiency HPT may be masked, and these patients may exhibit weakness, bone pain, elevation of alkaline phosphatases and a normal serum calcium concentration, typically together with low serum phosphate.[47,48] Whether relative vitamin D deficiency and concomitant HPT in elderly individuals may be the cause of a similarly confusing clinical picture, with respect both to diagnosis and symptomatic impairment, remains to be addressed by appropriate study. However, elderly patients are certainly less prone to develop a renal stone disorder. The severity of symptoms in HPT is related to the level and rate of rise in serum calcium, but apparently different patient groups are more likely to develop either bone, renal stone, or vague symptomatology. Even patients with moderate hypercalcemia, however, will generally exhibit symptoms which are clearly associated with the disease provided these are actively sought.

Bone Disease

Parathyroid bone disease, osteitis fibrosa cystica, characterized by advanced demineralization and cystic lesions, bone pain and pathological fracture, is today an extreme rarity in patients with primary HPT.[1] The bone disease used to occur in patients with unusually large parathyroid tumors, markedly raised PTH values, low $1,25(OH)_2D_3$ levels, and also consequently a tendency to decreased intestinal calcium absorption.[14,16,49,50] More subtle skeletal changes may be radiologically evident in somewhat less than 20% of currently diagnosed patients, and mainly in those with more pronounced hypercalcemia and increased levels of alkaline phosphatases.[51,52] In such cases typical subperiostal erosions may be revealed, especially on the radial side of the middle phalanges and the distal clavicles. A condition where the skull exhibits a "salt and pepper" pattern and bone cysts are present will very rarely be encountered and then only in the most severely compromised cases.[51] The more common contemporary patient with HPT will lack the typical radiological bone changes, and instead tends to exhibit generalized, nonspecific skeletal demineralization. Enhanced bone-turnover with increased activation of remodeling cycles may be demonstrated by histological examination of bone biopsy, whereby the cortical bone tends to be reduced in thickness while cancellous bone may be more or less preserved.[53,54] Bone density measurements by dual energy x-ray absorptiometry (DEXA) may also reveal loss of bone mineral in the more general patient with HPT.[55-58] The reduced bone mineral content has often developed insidiously over long periods of time before the disease is detected. It tends to be most pronounced in patients with marked hypercalcemia, but may be revealed also in those with moderate elevation of serum calcium.[55,56,59] The bone loss is most extensive at sites rich in cortical bone such as the distal radius, while cancellous bone, like in the lumber spine, tends to be well preserved.[55] Pathological fracture used to be a common feature in primary HPT but is currently rare.[59] Slightly increased risk of forearm fragility fracture has been observed, but it is still controversial whether such risk enhancement is valid also for the femoral neck or the vertebral fracture incidence.[56,60-63] Some, yet incomplete, recovery of bone mineral can be expected after successful parathyroid surgery.[55] In the typically elderly, postmenopausal female with mild HPT, loss of bone mineral may have other causes than the parathyroid disorder, such as estrogen deficiency and impaired intestinal calcium absorption due to reduced levels of active vitamin D.[64,65] The bone loss associated with estrogen deficiency should preferentially affect the cancellous bone of the spine, and it is yet uncertain if parathyroidectomy may influence this bone loss or if the cancellous bone in fact is protected by the parathyroid disease if appropriate vitamin D levels are maintained.[66-68]

Renal Complications

In the early reports *renal stones* used to affect up to 80% of patients with primary HPT,[1] and later on many series commonly reported stone incidence of 50% or more.[69,70] However, an increased diagnosis of the disease among the elderly has been coupled to a considerably lower frequency, and nowadays renal stones may be encountered in 10-20% of the patients or less.[3,20,52,71] Several authors have reported that the bone and stone complications of HPT do not occur in the same patients and that the individuals with renal stones display higher levels of active vitamin D and thereby increased intestinal calcium absorption.[15-17,72] However, hypercalciuria due to increased bone resorption could apparently contribute to stone formation in some patients. Renal stones in HPT are generally made up of calcium oxalate, and only to some extent mixed with calcium phosphate.[73] Younger individuals and particularly males are more prone to develop the stone disorder, and may experience recurrent renal stones even in mild hypercalcemia.[74] Among the elderly, postmenopausal female patients with HPT, renal stones tend to be less prevalent, although some of them have sporadic and generally asymptomatic stones. However, since renal stones are an unusual finding in this group, their presence should make the clinician particularly aware of the parathyroid disease. *Hypercalciuria* is considered as the most important risk factor for stone formation in patients with primary HPT, and is present when the 24-hour urinary calcium excretion exceeds 250 mg for women and 300 mg for men.[15,74-76] After successful parathyroidectomy in patients with HPT and renal stones the increased urinary calcium excretion decreases markedly and the formation of renal stones generally ceases completely.[20,70,74,75] Primary HPT may be detected in 5-7% of all patients with renal stones or less.[77] In any case, this disease should be actively sought in every patient experiencing a verified stone attack, since efficient treatment may be provided to these patients.

Nephrocalcinosis with diffusely scattered calcium salt precipitations in the renal parenchyma is nowadays a relatively uncommon feature in HPT, and is in fact more likely to result from sarcoidosis or a tubular dysfunction with acidification defect.[78] When nephrocalcinosis is present in HPT it is generally associated with significant renal function impairment and parathyroidectomy is considered important in order to prevent progression of the renal dysfunction.[20]

Renal function impairment leading to renal insufficiency used to be a frequent complication of primary HPT, but is only occasionally encountered among current patients with marked hypercalcemia. Slight reduction in the creatinine clearance is more common and may represent an irreversible complication of long-standing hypercalcemia.[79] Patients with border-line hypercalcemia, however, rarely exhibit clinically significant renal function impairment.[80]

Neuromuscular Weakness

Marked *neuromuscular weakness* together with atrophy of proximal muscle groups used to be a prominent symptom of patients with primary HPT a few decades ago, but is currently rarely or ever encountered.[81,82] Less pronounced weakness or a general fatigue, however, is a typical complaint of the contemporary patients with HPT.[82-87] Reduced muscle strength and muscle contraction defects may be objectively demonstrated to affect various muscle groups also in apparently asymptomatic patients.[83-87] The weakness tends to improve significantly after successful parathyroid surgery, and this sometimes occurs unexpectedly when insidious development of the powerlessness has been unnoticed by the patient.[84-87]

Psychiatric Symptoms

Physicians involved in the treatment of patients with primary HPT have commonly recognized that psychiatric disability may be an important part of the symptomatology.[88-90] More detailed psychiatric evaluation by different protocols has revealed a relatively frequent occurrence of general fatigue and mainly depressive-like disturbances. Symptoms like easy fatiguability, lassitude, failing memory and concentration difficulty are prevalent, and have often gone unnoticed by the patient.[90,91] The psychiatric disability and in particular the fatigue and tendency to confusion generally have been more impressive in patients with higher serum calcium values, but the ailment has been demonstrated also in patients with mild hypercalcemia.[90,91] Especially elderly patients may be sensitive in this respect and exhibit impaired mental capacity and confusion even at moderate elevation of the serum calcium concentration.[92] Due to its insidious development this disturbance may have been regarded as an effect of normal aging.[92] Differential but clear improvement of the HPT-related psychiatric symptoms can be expected after parathyroid surgery, with positive effects particularly evident in patients with fatigue, depression, concentration difficulty and confusion.[90] Sometimes HPT patients present with dementia-like states, or the elevated serum calcium concentration causes further confusion in a patient with organic brain syndrome.[92] Impressive improvement has been reported in some of these patients and especially those who have had less extensive mental derangement of limited duration.[92,93] This issue needs further evaluation, however, since the improvement after parathyroid surgery has not been invariable and certainly the dementia of elderly individuals may have many causes.[94] It is interesting in this context that the psychiatric symptoms of HPT have been related to elevated calcium concentrations and reduced levels of monoamine metabolites in the cerebrospinal fluid, mimicking the biochemical disturbances of patients with endogenous depression.[95] The monoamine levels tend to normalize after successful parathyroid surgery.[95] Although the neurobehavioral disturbances often appear subtle and nonspecific compared to the classical symptoms of HPT, the mental impairment may for the patient indeed be one of the more serious consequences of the disease.

Cardiovascular Disease

Patients with primary HPT have enhanced risk to develop *cardiovascular disease*, and they also exhibit a tendency to impaired glucose tolerance as well as disturbed lipid and urate metabolism.[80,96-100] The lipid and urate disturbances tend to normalize after successful parathyroid surgery, while some of the other cardiovascular risk factors remain uneffected and may be indirectly related to the disease. Hypertension is thus overrepresented in primary HPT, especially in patients with renal impairment, but is inconsistently improved by parathyroid surgery.[101-106] Significantly increased mortality in cardiovascular diseases has been revealed by long-term follow-up studies of individuals with unattended, generally mild hypercalcemia, and also in patients who have undergone surgery for primary HPT.[80,100,107,108,109] Successful surgery for HPT tends to normalize the increased death-rate, but higher mortality seems to remain if patients are operated upon at more advanced stages of the disease.[109]

Gastrointestinal Disturbance

Primary HPT has frequently been claimed as a cause of *gastrointestinal disturbances,* essentially peptic ulcer disease and pancreatitis.[110-112] A clear association between HPT and peptic ulcer disease is virtually only present in the Zollinger-Ellison syndrome of MEN-1, and the parathyroid disease is then known to adversely affect the ulcer disease. In patients with sporadic primary HPT the relationship between HPT and peptic ulcer is probably circumstantial and represents the fortuitous occurrence of two common disorders. Symptoms compatible with non-ulcer dyspepsia are, however, frequently encountered in primary HPT. They tend to be aggravated by more severe hypercalcemia, whereby disease progression may be subjectively experienced. Pancreatitis is only rarely caused by HPT, but it may be a serious complication of extensive hypercalcemia.[112-114] However, if other obvious causes of pancreatitis are absent the presence of this complication in a patient with primary HPT generally constitutes an indisputable indication for parathyroid surgery.

MEDICAL TREATMENT

Estrogens and progestins have been suggested as a possible treatment of postmenopausal females with mild HPT, as these agents may reduce the skeletal effects of the PTH excess and lower the serum calcium concentration.[115,116] However, these effects are moderate and somewhat inconsistent, and the expected benefit as compared to the risks of this therapy are presently not well documented.[115,116] Oral diphosphonates may prevent bone resorption and lower serum calcium in HPT, but the effect is generally transient.[117,118] Intravenous pamidronate (APD) has been used to lower serum calcium mainly in patients with hypercalcemic crisis or in patients where surgery has been postponed because of intercurrent disease.[119,120] The drug has also been commonly applied in the therapy of patients with parathyroid carcinoma. Moreover, recently developed vitamin D analogs without hypercalcemic effects, seem to constitute a possible future therapy in HPT.[121] Awaiting further development of such different, but in some respects, rather promising modes of medical therapy and their proper evaluation, parathyroid surgery is currently the accepted treatment in HPT.

SURVEILLANCE

A recent NIH Consensus Conference suggested that a group of HPT patients with mildly elevated serum calcium values and no evident symptoms, could be expected to follow a benign disease course, and possibly could be managed nonoperatively as part of a research program.[122] Mild hypercalcemia in this context was defined as serum calcium values below 2.85-3.0 mmol/l.[122] In the opinion of many colleagues this level of serum calcium may be too high to justify mere surveillance without operation.[123] Slight renal function impairment and bone mineral loss are then relevant complications, and the patients will often be found to exhibit symptoms if examined more closely.[58,61,123-125] Moreover, the long-term surveillance of patients with surgically unattended primary HPT hitherto has been seriously hampered by lack of compliance.[126-128] Fatal hypercalcemic crisis has occasionally been reported to develop unexpectedly during follow-up of patients with HPT, and the patients who progress more rapidly seem to lack specific features at early stages of the disease.[129,130] Non-operative follow-up might entail a significant risk to result finally in physically and intellectually reduced capacity or even confusion in elderly patients, and seems to contribute to premature death in cardiovascular disease.[90,100,107-109] The costs associated with the repeated laborious investigations, being necessary for safe monitoring, seem to soon outweigh the inconveniences and costs associated with surgery.[126] Although long-term follow-up of individuals with unattended borderline hypercalcemia have disclosed significant psychiatric disturbances, these patients have rarely shown progressive disease or more compromised renal function, and the serum calcium concentration tends to remain stable for years.[18,80] Considering that patients with mild hypercalcemia constitute a major proportion of HPT patients detected at population survey, it seems appropriate to restrict the nonoperative surveillance to elderly patients clearly without symptoms or complications, who exhibit only borderline elevations of serum calcium.[123] In our opinion this would arbitrarily imply serum calcium values below or around 2.70 (-2.80) mmol/l. It is essential in these circumstances that the neurobehavioral symptoms commonly associated with HPT are evaluated, as also the vague symptoms like muscle weakness, fatigue or confusion, may markedly limit the activity of especially elderly individuals.[79] An argument in favor of non-operative surveillance and follow-up in patients with borderline hypercalcemia is that these individuals tend to exhibit increased incidence of micronodular parathyroid hyperplasia and tiny adenomas, which implies increased difficulties during parathyroid operation, concerning both the glandular visualization and the histopathological interpretation.[130] A prospective controlled study is indeed warranted to evaluate whether surveillance is equivalent to parathyroid surgery in truly asymptomatic mild HPT,[79] but it will certainly still be difficult to reveal long-term, silent effects on the mental condition or on the incidence of cardiovascular disease in the elderly. In the absence of an effective alternate therapy, it seems reasonable at present to refer patients with HPT liberally to operation, but require excellent results of surgery.

SURGERY

Comprehensive series of patients with primary HPT, where surgery has been performed by experienced colleagues, have demonstrated 95-98% postoperative normocalcemia.[79,131-141] Considerably less favorable results have been obtained when the operation has been performed by less experienced surgeons.[142] The results of surgery also relate to the prevailing histopathology, since the cure rate is higher in adenomatous disease, while multiglandular involvement and particularly the MEN-1-associated HPT are associated with considerably increased rates of both persistent and recurrent disease.[79,131,143-147] The classical complications, recurrent laryngeal nerve paralysis and hypoparathyroidism, used to occur in up to 5% of operations or more, but is now frequently reported in the range of 1% or less.[139,140] The neck exploration in HPT is very rarely associated with mortality. Elderly patients and those with complicating diseases, essentially cardiac or respiratory insufficiency, constitute higher risks, but can often be expediently managed if appropriate considerations concerning the preoperative management and the anesthesia are undertaken. In high risk patients the operation may be performed under local anesthesia, but this is rarely necessary, and makes adequate surgery more difficult.[148] Older individuals need to be protected by appropriate measures against thromboembolism. Moreover, those elderly patients who exhibit marked hypercalcemia prior to surgery should be liberally provided with postoperative calcium (and occasionally vitamin D) in order to prevent cardiac arrhythmia which may otherwise result from pronounced hypocalcemia.[123]

The high success rate of parathyroid surgery is a strong argument in favor of a liberal attitude towards active treatment in primary HPT, provided that the operation can be performed by an experienced parathyroid surgeon. In our opinion, *the indications for surgery* (Table 6.2) of primary HPT should comprise all patients with evident symptoms or complications to the disease, as well as those with serum calcium con-

Table 6.2. Indications for surgery in primary HPT

Parathyroid bone disease –
  typical radiographic features
  significant reduction of bone mineral content
  elevated alkaline phosphatases
    (bone isoenzymes)

Nephrolithiasis/nephrocalcinosis
  –hypercalciuria (relative indication)

Renal function impairment

Pancreatitis –without other obvious causes

Muscle weakness/psychiatric disturbance
  –confusion in elderly patients*

Serum calcium concentration >2.70 (–2.80) mmol/l**

* if the confusional state is likely to be related to the parathyroid disorder
** higher serum calcium values or evident symptoms are needed to justify operation in older patients or those with associated illness, who constitute surgical risks.

centrations above 2.70-2.80 mmol/l. This should include patients with significantly reduced bone mineral content, renal stones, nephrocalcinosis and/or marked hypercalciuria and renal function impairment, as well as those with a neuromuscular or psychiatric disturbance. An expectant attitude may be chosen in clearly asymptomatic individuals with border-line elevation of serum calcium (< 2.65-2.70 mmol/l). Advanced age (> 80 years) as well as associated illness, which may involve increased surgical risk, will generally require higher serum calcium values or evident symptoms, so that the expected improvement clearly justifies the increased risks of surgery. Patients with borderline hypercalcemia, who may be submitted to surgery because of a renal stone disorder, as well as patients with familial or MEN-1-associated HPT can be expected to constitute intraoperatively difficult cases and should be referred to centers with more considerable experience.

The high success rate of surgery also has another important implication. Radiological methods for preoperative visualization of parathyroid glands generally have a sensitivity of 50-70% or less, and are afflicted by a significant rate of false positive results. The radiological studies also frequently fail to localize less conspicuously enlarged parathyroid glands, multiglandular disease, and in some instances also glands in ectopic positions, which indeed represent the more difficult surgical cases.[149,150] Since the experienced surgeon will localize parathyroid glands considerably more effectively, these studies are not indicated prior to the initial parathyroid operation, nor should they be used to establish or confirm the diagnosis. An exception to this rule are the patients with hypercalcemic crisis, or those who represent unusually high operative risks, where routine means of localization may be used to facilitate the subsequent surgery.

REFERENCES

1. Albright F, Reifenstein EC. The parathyroid glands and metabolic bone disease. Baltimore: Williams & Wilkins. 1948.
2. Mundy GR, Cove DR, Fisken R. Primary hyperparathyroidism; changes in the pattern of clinical presentation. Lancet 1980; 1: 1317-20.
3. Heath III H, Hodgson SF, Kennedy MA. Primary hyperparathyroidism: incidence, morbidity and potential economic impact in a community. N Engl J Med 1980; 302: 189-93.
4. Palmér M, Jakobsson S, Åkerström G et al. Prevalence of hypercalcemia in a health survey: a 14-year follow-up of serum calcium values. Eur J Clin Invest 1988; 118: 39-46.
5. Christensson T, Hellström K, Wengle B et al. Prevalence of hypercalcemia in a health screening in Stockholm. Acta Med Scand 1976; 200: 131-7.
6. Boonstra CE, Jackson CE. Serum calcium survey for hyperparathyroidism: results in 50,000 clinic patients. Am J Clin Pathol 1971; 55: 523-6.
7. Åkerström G, Rudberg C, Grimelius L et al. Histologic parathyroid abnormalities in an autopsy series. Hum Pathol 1986; 17: 520-7.
8. Melton LJ. Epidemiology of primary hyperparathyroidism. J Bone Mineral Res 1991; 6 (suppl 2): 25-30.
9. Prinz RA, Paloyan E, Lawrence AM et al. Radiation-associated hyperparathyroidism: A new syndrome? Surgery 1977; 82: 296-302.
10. Tissel LE. Hyperparathyroidism in persons treated with X-rays for tuberculous cervical adenitis. Cancer 1977; 40: 846-54.
11. Cohen J, Gierlowski TC, Schneider AB. A prospective study of hyperparathyroidism in individuals exposed to radiation in childhood. JAMA 1990; 264: 581-4.
12. Bondeson AG, Bondeson L, Thompson NW. Hyperparathyroidism after treatment with radioactive iodine: not only a coincidence? Surgery 1989; 106: 1025-7.
13. Broadus AE. Primary hyperparathyroidism. J Urol 1989; 141: 723-30.
14. Kleeman CR, Norris K, Coburn JW. Is the clinical expression of primary hyperparathyroidism a function of the long-term vitamin D status of the patient. Min Electrol Metab 1987; 13: 305-10.
15. Broadus AE, Horst RL, Lang R et al.The importance of circulating $1,25(OH)_2D_3$ in the pathogenesis of hypercalciuria and renal stone formation in primary hyperparathyroidism. N Engl J Med 1980; 302: 421-6.
16. Patron P, Gardin J-P, Paillard M. Renal mass and reserve of vitamin D. Determinants in primary hyperparathyroidism. Kidney Int 1987; 31: 1174-80.
17. Pak CYK, Nicar MJ, Peterson et al. Lack of unique pathophysiologic background for nephrolithiasis in primary hyperparathyroidism. J Clin Endocrinol Metab 1981; 53: 536-42.
18. Christensson T. Primary hyperparathyroidism-pathogenesis, incidence and natural history. Progr Surg 1986; 18: 34-44.
19. Ladenson JH. Calcium determination in primary hyperparathyroidism. J Bone Mineral Res 1991; 6 (suppl 2): 33-41.
20. Ljunghall S, Hellman P, Rastad J et al. Primary hyperparathyroidism: Epidemiology, diagnosis and clinical picture. World J Surg 1991; 15: 681-7.
21. Nussbaum SR, Potts JT. Immunoassays for parathyroid hormone 1-84 in the diagnosis of hyperparathyroidism. J Bone Mine Res 1991; 6 (suppl 2): 43-50.
22. Brown RC, Aston JP, Weeks I et al. Circulating intact parathyroid hormone measured by a two-site immunochemiluminometric assay. J Clin Endocrinol Metab 1987; 65: 407-14.
23. Nussbaum SR, Zahradnik R, Lavigne J et al. Highly sensitive two-site immunoradiometric assay for parathyrin and its clinical utility in evaluating patients with hypercalcemia. Clin Chem 1987; 33: 1364-7.
24. Blind E, Schmidt-Gayk H, Scarla S et al. Two-site assay of intact parathyroid hormone in the investigation of primary hyperparathyroidism and other disorders of calcium metabolism compared with a midregion assay. J Clin Endocrinol Metab 1988; 67: 353-60.
25. Logue FC, Perry B, Chapman RS et al. A

two-site immunoradiometric assay for PTH (1-84) using N and C terminal specific monoclonal antibodies. Ann Clin Biochem 1991; 28: 160-6.
26. Endres DB, Villanueva R, Sharp CF et al. Immunochemiluminometric and immunoradiometric determinations of intact and total immunoreactive parathyrin: performance in the differential diagnosis of hypercalcemia and hypoparathyroidism. Clin Chem 1991; 37: 162-8.
27. Williams JG, Wheeler MH, Aston JP et al. The relationship between adenoma weight and intact (1-84) parathyroid hormone level in primary hyperparathyroidism. Am J Surg 1992; 163: 301-4.
28. Lafferty FW. Differential diagnosis of hypercalcemia. J Bone Miner Res 1991; 6 (suppl 2): 51-9.
29. Mallette LE. The hypercalcemias. Semin Nephrol 1992; 12: 159-90.
30. Fisken RA, Heath DA, Bold AM. Hypercalcemia--a hospital survey. Q J Med 1980; 49: 405-18.
31. Mundy GR. Calcium homeostasis: Hypercalcemia and hypocalcemia. Martin Dunitz, London. 1989; 37-181.
32. Martin TJ, Suva LJ. Parathyroid hormone-related protein in hypercalcaemia of malignancy. Clin Endocrinol 1989; 31: 631-47.
33. Ratcliffe WA, Hutchesson ACJ, Bundred NJ et al. Role of assays for parathyroid-hormone-related protein in investigation of hypercalcemia. Lancet 1992; 339: 164-7.
34. Burtis WJ, Brady TG, Orloff JJ et al. Immunochemical characterization of circulating parathyroid hormone-related protein in patients with humoral hypercalcemia of cancer. N Engl J Med 1990; 322: 1106-12.
35. Nussbaum SR, Gaz RD, Arnold A. Hypercalcemia and ectopic secretion of parathyroid hormone by an ovarian carcinoma with rearrangement of the gene for parathyroid hormone. N Engl J Med 1990; 323: 1324-8.
36. Foley TP Jr, Harrison HC, Arnaud CD et al. Familial benign hypercalcaemia. J Pediatr 1972; 82: 1060-7.
37. Marx SJ, Spiegel AM, Brown EM et al. Family studies in patients with primary parathyroid hyperplasia. Am J Med 1977; 62: 698-706.
38. Marx SJ, Stock JL, Attie MG et al. Familial hypocalciuric hypercalcemia: Recognisation among patients referred after unsuccessful parathyroid exploration. Ann Intern Med 1980; 92: 351-6.
39. Marx SJ, Attie MF, Levine MA et al. The hypocalciuric or benign variant of familial hypercalcemia: clinical and biochemical features in fifteen kindreds. Medicine 1981; 60: 397-412.
40. Law WM Jr, Carney JA, Heath H III. Parathyroid glands in familial benign hypercalcemia (familial hypocalciuric hypercalcemia). Am J Med 1984; 76: 1021-6.
41. Marx SJ, Attie MF, Spiegel AM et al. An association between neonatal severe primary hyperparathyroidism and familial hypocalciuric hypercalcemia in three kindreds. N Engl J Med 1982; 306: 257-64.
42. Heath DA. Familial benign hypercalcemia.Trends Endocrinol Metab 1989; 1: 6-9.
43. Marx SJ, Spiegel AM, Brown EM et al. Divalent cation metabolism. Familial hypocalciuric hypercalcemia versus typical primary hyperparathyroidism. Am J Med 1978; 65: 235-42.
44. Heath H III. Familial benign (hypocalciuric) hypercalcemia. Endocrinol Metab Clin North Am 1989; 18: 723-40.
45. Law WM Jr, James EM, Charboneau JW et al. High-resolution parathyroid ultrasonography in familial benign hypercalcemia (familial hypocalciuric hypercalcemia). Mayo Clin Proc 1984; 59: 153-5.
46. Law WM Jr, Carney JA, Heath H III. Parathyroid glands in familial benign hypercalcemia (familial hypocalciuric hypercalcemia). Am J Med 1984; 76: 1021-6.
47. Frame B, Foroozanfar F, Patton RB. Normocalcemic primary hyperparathyroidism with osteitis fibrosa. Ann Intern Med 1970; 73: 253-7.
48. Dent CE, Jones PE, Millam DP. Masked primary (or tertiary) hyperparathyroidism. Lancet 1975; 1: 1161-4.
49. Lloyd HM. Primary hyperparathyroidism: an analysis of the role of the parathyroid tumor. Medicine 1968; 47: 53-71.
50. Mallette LE, Bilezikian JP, Heath DA et al. Primary hyperparathyroidism: clinical and

biochemical features. Medicine 1974; 53: 127-46.
51. Hayes CW, Conway WF. Hyperparathyroidism. Radiol Clin North Am 1991; 29: 85-96.
52. Palmér M, Ljunghall S, Åkerström G et al. Patients with primary hyperparathyroidism operated on over a 24-year period: temporal trends of clinical and laboratory findings. J Chronic Dis 1987; 40: 121-30.
53. Parisien M, Silverberg S, Shane E et al. The histomorphometry of bone in primary hyperparathyroidism: preservation of cancellous bone structure. J Clin Endocrinol 1990; 70: 930-8.
54. Eriksen EF, Mosekilde L, Melsen F. Trabecular bone remodelling and balance in primary hyperparathyroidism. Bone 1986; 7: 213-21.
55. Silverberg SJ, Shane E, DeLaCruz L et al. Skeletal disease in primary hyperparathyroidism. J Bone Mineral Res 1989; 4: 283-91.
56. Larsson K, Lindh E, Lind L et al. Increased fracture risk in hypercalcemia: Bone mineral content measured in hyperparathyroidism. Acta Orthop Scand 1989; 60: 268-70.
57. Martin P, Bergmann P, Gillet C et al. Long-term irreversibility of bone loss after surgery for primary hyperparathyroidism. Arch Intern Med 1990; 150: 1495-7.
58. Bilezikian JP, Silverberg SJ, Shane E et al. Characterization and evaluation of asymptomatic primary hyperparathyroidism. J Bone Mineral Res 1991; 6 (suppl 2): 85-9.
59. Rao SD, Wilson RJ, Kleerekoper M et al. Lack of biochemical progression or continuation of accelerated bone loss in mild asymptomatic primary hyperparathyroidism: evidence for biphasic disease course. J Clin Endocrinol Metab 1988; 67: 1294-8.
60. Peacock M, Horsman A, Aaron JE et al. The role of parathyroid hormone in bone loss. In: Christiansen C, Arnaud CD, Nordin BEC, eds. Osteoporosis 1. Denmark: Aalborg Stiftsbogtrykkers 1984; 463-8.
61. Peacock M. Interpretation of bone mass determination as they relate to fracture: implications for asymptomatic primary hyperparathyroidism. J Bone Mineral Res 1991; 6 (suppl 2): 77-82.
62. Wilson RJ, Rao SD, Ellis B et al. Mild asymptomatic hyperparathyroidism is not a risk factor for vertebral fractures. Ann Int Med 1988; 109: 952-62.
63. Melton LJ 3d, Atkinson EJ, O'Fallon WM et al. Risk of age-related fractures in patients with primary hyperparathyroidism. Arch Intern Med 1992; 152: 2269-73.
64. Benhamou Cl, Chappard D, Gauvain JB et al. Hyperparathyroidism in proximal femur fractures, biological and histomorphometric study in 21 patients over 75 years old. Clin Rheumatol 1991; 10: 144-50.
65. Turner G, Brown RC, Silver A et al. Renal insufficiency and secondary hyperparathyroidism in elderly patients. Ann Clin Biochem 1991; 28: 321-6.
66. Parisien M, Recker R, Silverberg SJ et al. Cancellous bone structure in postmenopausal women with primary hyperparathyroidism. In: Christiansen C, Overgaard K, eds. Third International Symposium on Osteoporosis, October 14-20, 1990. Copenhagen: Osteopress 1990; 1139-40.
67. Kleerekoper M, Villaneuva AR, Stanciu J et al. The role of three-dimensional trabecular microstructure in the pathogenesis of vertebral compression fractures. Calcif Tissue Int 1985; 37: 594-7.
68. Parisien M, Mellish RWE, Silverberg SJ et al. Maintenance of cancellous bone connectivity in primary hyperparathyroidism: trabecular strut analysis. J Bone Mineral Res 1992; 7: 913-19.
69. Broadus A. Nephrolithiasis in primary hyperparathyroidism. In: Coe F, Brennan B, Stein J. eds. Nephrolithiasis. New York: Churchill Livingstone 1980.
70. McGeown MG. Effect of parathyroidectomy on the incidence of renal calculi. Lancet 1961; 1: 586-7.
71. Lafferty FW. Primary hyperparathyroidism: changing clinical spectrum, prevalence of hypertension, and a discriminant analysis of laboratory tests. Arch Int Med 1981; 141: 1761-6
72. Silverberg SJ, Shane E, Jacobs TP et al. Nephrolithiasis and bone involvement in primary hyperparathyroidism. Am J Med 1990; 89: 327-34.

73. Parks J, Coe F, Favus M. Hyperparathyroidism in nephrolithiasis. Arch Intern Med 1980; 140: 1479-81.
74. Ljunghall S, Danielson BG, Johansson G et al. Renal stone formation in primary hyperparathyroidism. Role of tubular dysfunction. In: Smith LH, ed. Urolithiasis: Clinical and Basic Research. New York: Plenum 1981: 89-92.
75. Coe FL, Keck J, Norton ER. The natural history of calcium urolithiasis. JAMA 1977; 238: 1519-23.
76. Deaconson TF, Wilson SD, Lemann J Jr. The effect of parathyroidectomy on the recurrence of nephrolithiasis. Surgery 1987; 102: 910-2.
77. Fuss M, Pepersack T, Corvilain J et al. Infrequency of primary hyperparathyroidism in renal stone formers. Br J Urol 1988; 62: 4-6.
78. Backman U, Danielson BG, Johansson G et al. Incidence and clinical importance of renal tubular defects in recurrent renal stone formers. Nephron 1980; 25: 96-101.
79. Wells AS. Surgical therapy of patients with primary hyperparathyroidism: Long-term benefits. J Bone Mineral Res 1991; (6 suppl 2): 143-52.
80. Palmér M, Adami H-O, Bergström R et al. S. Survival and renal function in persons with untreated hypercalcaemia: a population-based cohort study with 14 years of follow-up. Lancet 1987; 1: 59-62.
81. Patten BM, Bilezikian JP, Mallette LE. Neuromuscular disease in primary hyperparathyroidism. Ann Intern Med 1974; 80: 182-93.
82. Ljunghall S, Åkerström G, Johansson G et al. Neuromuscular involvement in primary hyperparathyroidism. J Neurol 1984; 231: 263-5.
83. Delbridge LW, Marshman D, Reeve TS. Neuromuscular symptoms in elderly patients with hyperparathyroidism: Improvement with parathyroid surgery. Med J Aust 1988; 149: 74-6.
84. Wersäll-Robertson E, Hamberger B, Ehrén H et al. Increase in muscular strength following surgery for primary hyperparathyroidism. Acta Med Scand 1986; 220: 233-5.
85. Joborn C, Joborn H, Rastad J et al. Maximal isokinetic muscle strength in patients with primary hyperparathyroidism before and after parathyroid surgery. Br J Surg 1988; 75: 77-80.
86. Kristoffersson A, Bjerle P, Stjernberg N. Pre- and postoperative respiratory muscle strength in primary hyperparathyroidism. Acta Chir Scand 1988; 154: 415-8.
87. Joborn C, Rastad J, Stålberg E et al. Muscle function in patients with primary hyperparathyroidism. Muscle Nerve 1989; 12: 87-94.
88. Nielsen H. Familial occurrence, gastrointestinal symptoms and mental disturbances in hyperparathyroidism. Acta Med Scand 1955; 151: 359-66.
89. Peterson P. Psychiatric disorders in primary hyperparathyroidism. Clin Endocrinol Metab 1968; 28: 1491-5.
90. Joborn C, Hetta J, Johansson H et al. Psychiatric morbidity in primary hyperparathyroidism. World J Surg 1988; 12: 476-81.
91. Joborn C, Hetta L, Lind L et al. Self-rated psychiatric symptoms in patients with primary hyperparathyroidism and in patients with long-standing mild hypercalcemia. Surgery 1989; 105: 72-8.
92. Joborn C, Hetta J, Frisk P et al. Primary hyperparathyroidism in patients with organic brain syndrome. Acta Med Scand 1985; 219: 91-8.
93. Heath DA. Primary hyperparathyroidism: Clinical presentation and factors influencing clinical management. Endocrinol Metab Clin North Am 1989; 18: 631-46.
94. Brown GG, Preisman RC, Kleerekoper M. Neurobehavioral symptoms in mild primary hyperparathyroidism: related to hypercalcemia but not improved by parathyroidectomy. Henry Ford Med J 1987; 35: 211-5.
95. Joborn C, Hetta J, Rastad J et al. Psychiatric symptoms and cerebrospinal fluid monoamine metabolites in patients with primary hyperparathyroidism. Biol Psychiatry 1988; 23: 149-58.
96. Ljunghall S, Lithell H, Vessby B et al. Glucose and lipoprotein metabolism in primary hyperparathyroidism: Effects of parathyroidectomy. Acta Endocrinol (Kbh). 1978; 89: 580-9.

97. Ljunghall S, Palmér M, Åkerström G et al. Diabetes mellitus, glucose tolerance and insulin response to glucose in patients with primary hyperparathyroidism before and after parathyroidectomy. Eur J Clin Invest 1983; 13: 373-7.
98. Kumar S, Olukoga AO, Gordon C et al. Impaired glucose tolerance and insulin insensitivity in primary hyperparathyroidism. Clin Endocrinol 1994; 40: 47-53.
99. Ljunghall S, Åkerström G. Urate metabolism in primary hyperparathyroidism. Urol Int 1982; 37: 73-8.
100. Palmér M, Adami H-O, Bergström R et al. Mortality after operation for primary hyperparathyroidism: A follow-up of 441 patients operated on from 1956 to 1979. Surgery 1987; 102: 1-7.
101. Nainby-Luxmoore JC, Langford HG, Nelson NC et al. A case-comparison study of hypertension and hyperparathyroidism. J Clin Endocrinol Metab 1982; 55: 303-6.
102. Jones DB, Jones JH, Lloyd HJ et al. Changes in blood pressure and renal function after parathyroidectomy in primary hyperparathyroidism. Postgrad Med J 1983; 59: 350-3.
103. Bradley El III, Wells JO. Primary hyperparathyroidism and hypertension. Am Surg 1983; 49: 569-70.
104. Broulik PD, Horky K, Pacovsky V. Blood pressure in patients with primary hyperparathyroidism before and after parathyroidectomy. Exp Clin Endocrinol 1985; 86(3):346-52.
105. Diamond TW, Botha JR, Wing J et al. Parathyroid hypertension. A reversible disorder. Arch Intern Med 1986; 146: 1709-12.
106. Sancho JJ, Rouco J, Riera-Vidal R et al. A. Long-term effects of parathyroidectomy for primary hyperparathyroidism on arterial hypertension. World J Surg 1992; 16: 732-6.
107. Ronni-Sivula H. Causes of death in patients previously operated on for primary hyperparathyroidism. Ann chir Gynaecol 1985; 74: 13-8.
108. Hedbäck G, Tisell LE, Bengtsson BÅ et al. Premature death in patients operated on for primary hyperparathyroidism. World J Surg 1990; 14: 829-36.
109. Hedbäck G, Odén A, Tisell L-E. The influence of surgery on the risk of death in patients with primary hyperparathyroidism. World J Surg 1991; 15: 399-407.
110. Ostrow JD, Blanshard G, Gray SJ. Peptic ulcer in primary hyperparathyroidism. Amer J Med 1960; 29: 769-79.
111. Linos DA, vanHeerden JA, Abboud CF et al. Primary hyperparathyroidism and peptic ulcer disease. Arch Surg 1978; 113: 384-6.
112. Mixter CG jr, Keynes WM, Cope O. Further experience with pancreatitis as a diagnostic clue to hyperparathyroidism. N Engl J Med 1962; 266: 265-72.
113. Bess MA, Edis AJ, vanHeerden JA. Hyperparathyroidism and pancreatitis. Chance or a causal association? JAMA 1980; 243: 246-7.
114. Sitges-Serra A, Alonso M, de Lecea C et al. Pancreatitis and hyperparathyroidism. Br J Surg 1988; 75: 158-60.
115. Marcus R. Estrogens and progestins in the management of primary hyperparathyroidism. J Bone Mineral Res 1991; 6 (suppl 2): 125-9.
116. Shane E. Medical management of asymptomatic primary hyperparathyroidism. J Bone Mineral Res 1991; 6 (-suppl 2): 131-4.
117. Kaplan RA, Geho WB, Poindexter C et al. Metabolic effects of diphosphonate in primary hyperparathyroidism. J Clin Pharmacol 1977; 17: 410-9.
118. Shane E, Baquiran DC, Bilezikian JP. Effects of dichloromethylene diphosphonate on serum and urinary calcium in primary hyperparathyroidism. Ann Intern Med 1981; 95: 23-7.
119. Schmidli RS, Wilson I, Espiner EA et al. Aminopropylidine diphosphonate (APD) in mild primary hyperparathyroidism: effects on clinical status. Clin Endocrinol 1990; 32: 293-300.
120. Jansson S, Tisell L-E, Lindstedt G et al. Disodium pamidronate in the preoperative treatment of hypercalcemia in patients with primary hyperparathyroidism. Surgery 1991; 110: 480-6
121. Brown AJ, Ritter CR, Finch JL et al. The normocalcemic analogue of vitamin D, 22-oxacalcitriol suppresses parathyroid hormone

synthesis and secretion. J Clin Invest 1989; 84: 728-32.

122. NIH Consensus Development Conference Panel. Diagnosis and management of asymptomatic primary hyperparathyroidism: consensus development conference statement. Ann Intern Med 1991; 114: 593-7.
123. Åkerström G, Ljunghall S. Medical and radiologic evaluation and operative treatment of primary hyperparathyroidism. Curr Opinion Gen Surg 1993; 130-8.
124. Mitlak BH, Daly M, Potts JT et al. Asymptomatic primary hyperparathyroidism. J Bone Mineral Res 1991; 6 (suppl 2): 103-10.
125. Warner J, Clifton-Bligh P, Posen S et al. Longitudinal changes in forearm bone mineral content in primary hyperparathyroidism. J Bone Mineral Res 1991; 6 (suppl 2): 91-5
126. Scholtz DA, Purnell DC. Asymptomatic primary hyperparathyroidism: 10 year prospective study. Mayo Clin Proc 1981; 56: 473-8.
127. Heath DA, Heath EM. Conservative management of primary hyperparathyroidism. J Bone Mineral Res 1991; 6 (suppl 2): 117-20.
128. Parfitt AM, Rao DS, Kleerekoper M. Asymptomatic primary hyperparathyroidism discovered by multichannel biochemical screening: clinical course and considerations bearing on the need for surgical intervention. J Bone Mineral Res 1991; 6 (suppl 2): 97-101.
129. Corsello SM, Folli G, Crucitti F et al. Acute complications in the course of "mild" hyperparathyroidism. J Endocrinol Invest 1991; 14: 971-4.
130. Åkerström G, Bergström R, Grimelius L et al. Relation between changes in clinical and histopathological features of primary hyperparathyroidism. World J Surg 1986; 10: 696-702.
131. Rudberg C, Åkerström G, Palmér M et al. Late results of operation for primary hyperparathyroidism in 441 patients. Surgery 1987; 99: 643-51.
132. Satava RM, Beahrs OH, Scholz DA. Success rate of cervical exploration for hyperparathyroidism. Arch Surg 1975; 110: 625-7.
133. Cooke TJC, Boey JH, Sweeney EC et al. Parathyroidectomy: extent of resection and late results. Br J Surg 1977; 64: 153-7.
134. McGarity WC, Mathews WH, Fulenwider JT et al. The surgical management of primary hyperparathyroidism: a personal series. Ann Surg 1981; 193: 794-804.
135. Russell CF, Edis AJ. Surgery for primary hyperparathyroidism:experience with 500 consecutive cases and evaluation of the role of surgery in the asymptomatic patient. Br J Surg 1982; 69: 244-7
136. Bruining HA, van Houten H, Jettman JR et al. Results of operative treatment of 615 patients with primary hyperparathyroidism. World J Surg 1981; 5: 85-90.
137. Farnebo LO, Trigonis C, Forsgren L et al. Surgery for primary hyperparathyroidism. Experience with 400 patients during 10 years (1972-1981). Acta Chir Scand (Suppl) 1984; 520: 11-76.
138. Lafferty FW, Hubay CA. Primary hyperparathyroidism. Arch Intern Med 1989; 149: 789-96.
139. Van Heerden JA, Grant CS. Surgical treatment of primary hyperparathyroidism: An institutional perspective. World J Surg 1991; 15: 688-92.
140. Clark OH, Wilkes W, Siperstein AE et al. Diagnosis and management of asymptomatic hyperparathyroidism: Safety, efficacy and deficiencies in our knowledge. J Bone Mineral Res 1991; 6 (suppl 2): 135-42.
141. Kaplan E, Yashiro T, Salti G. Primary hyperparathyroidism in the 1990s: Choice of surgical procedures for this disease. Ann Surg 1992; 215: 300-17.
142. Malmaeus J, Granberg PO, Halvorsen J et al. Parathyroid surgery in Scandinavia. Acta Chir Scand 1988; 154: 409-13.
143. Sivula A, Ronni-Sivula H. Natural history of treated primary hyperparathyroidism. Surg Clin North Am 1987; 67: 329-41.
144. Wells SA Jr, Leight GS, Hensley M et al. Hyperparathyroidism associated with the enlargement of two or three parathyroid glands. Ann Surg 1985; 202: 533-8.
145. Wallfelt C, Ljunghall S, Bergström R et al. Clinical characteristics and surgical treatment of sporadic primary hyperparathyroidism with emphasis on chief cell hyperplasia. Surgery 1990. 107: 13-9.

146. Edis AJ, vanHeerden JA, Scholz DA. Results of subtotal parathyroidectomy for primary chief cell hyperplasia. Surgery 1979; 86: 462-9.
147. Goretzki PE, Dotzenrath C, Roeher H-D. Management of primary hyperparathyroidism caused by multiple gland disease. World J Surg 1991; 15: 693-7.
148. Saxe A, Brown E, Hamburger SW. Thyroid and parathyroid surgery performed with patient under regional anesthesia. Surgery 1988; 103: 415-20.
149. Miller DL. Pre-operative localization and interventional treatment of parathyroid tumors: when and how? World J Surg 1991; 15: 706-15.
150. Doppman JL, Miller DL. Localization of parathyroid tumors in patients with asymptomatic hyperparathyroidism and no previous surgery. J Bone Mineral Res 1991; 6 (Suppl 2): 153-8.

CHAPTER 7

Familial Hyperparathyroidism

Göran Åkerström, Britt Skogseid, Jonas Rastad

Hereditary variants of hyperparathyroidism (HPT) are difficult to treat efficiently since the underlying genetic abnormality may generate recurrence in spite of apparently adequate surgery. These entities of HPT have to be actively searched for in patients who plan to undergo parathyroid reoperation.

Hyperparathyroidism (HPT) associated with the multiple endocrine neoplasia (MEN) syndromes type 1 or 2 and other varieties of familial HPT are rather recently recognized entities of parathyroid disease. Increased awareness of their presence has revealed that these hereditary forms represent a probably underrated proportion of the patients who ultimately experience failed parathyroid surgery. Knowledge about the genetics behind these lesions, and their variable presentation and prognosis therefore commonly has to be considered especially in the context of reoperative parathyroid surgery. It is also often essential to pay attention to other endocrinopathies of the traits as a ground for adequate diagnosis and because of their influence on prognosis.

MEN-1 SYNDROME

The multiple endocrine neoplasia type I (MEN-1) syndrome is a hereditary disorder, comprising lesions within the parathyroid, the pituitary and the endocrine pancreas. Already in 1903 Erdheim reported the association between a pituitary adenoma, causing acromegaly, and four enlarged parathyroid glands in an autopsy case.[1] Several authors thereafter described similar cases, some of which also had endocrine pancreatic tumors, but these were mostly collected at autopsy and the hereditary aspects of the disease were not recognized. In 1954 Wermer emphasized the familial occurrence of MEN-1 by reporting a family where the father and four of nine siblings were affected. He proposed that the syndrome was due to inheritance of a dominant, autosomal gene with high penetrance and expression.[2] He also noted frequent occurrence of peptic ulcer in this

Current Controversy in Parathyroid Operation and Reoperation,
edited by Göran Åkerström.

kindred and regarded this as another feature of the abnormal gene.[3]

Other Endocrinopathies

It has later been appreciated that other organs besides the classical endocrinopathies could be affected as well in MEN-1.[4-6] Thus, adrenal cortical involvement was revealed in as many as 30-40% of the cases in earlier more comprehensive series.[4-6] The adrenal lesion was almost invariably symptomless, and generally reported to consist of bilateral, diffuse to micronodular or occasionally grossly nodular cortical hyperplasia or bilateral adenoma, while unilateral tumors were more rarely described.[4-8] The adrenal tumors of MEN-1 have almost invariably been benign and adrenal cortical carcinoma has been infrequently reported.[6,7,9] The presence of a Cushing's syndrome has occasionally been reported in MEN-1, and may be due to ACTH excess from a pituitary adenoma or ectopic ACTH secretion from an islet cell carcinoma. Only rarely has this syndrome been caused by an adrenal cortical tumor.[4,5,8] Skogseid et al, however, recently described a MEN-1 patient with bilateral adrenal cortical hyperplasia and rapid unilateral growth into an extensively large invasive adrenocortical carcinoma with adrenocortical hormone excess and a feminizing syndrome.[7]

It has recently been substantiated that submucosal duodenal carcinoids may be commonly revealed in MEN-1 patients. These carcinoids are generally multiple, and may vary considerably in number and size between individuals, from numerous microscopic lesions to one or a few pea-sized or larger tumors.[10] Even tiny duodenal carcinoids, however, can be clinically important as they have proved to be a common source of gastrin excess leading to a Zollinger-Ellison's syndrome in MEN-1.[10] The duodenal lesions may also stain positively for serotonin and somatostatin, but this type of hormone excess has not been associated with clinically detectable symptoms.[10] Other foregut carcinoids, with origin in the thymus, the bronchi and the gastric mucosa are also overrepresented in MEN-1. There is also claimed to be an increased incidence of thyroid adenoma, colloid goiter, differentiated thyroid carcinoma and lipoma.[4,6,8]

Genetics

In agreement with Knudson's two-mutational hit theory of hereditary neoplasms, it has recently been demonstrated that tumorogenesis in MEN-1 results from unmasking of a recessive mutation within the long arm of chromosome 11 band q13.[11-14] The first mutation is carried in the germ line, and a second somatic event thus eliminates the wild type allele of the MEN-1 locus, which is thought to involve or represent a tumor suppressor or anti-oncogene.[12] This inactivation of both alleles for the MEN-1 gene is considered as an early causal event in the tumor development and has been reported as a probable cause not only for the pancreatic endocrine neoplasia, but also for the preceding microadenomas or pancreatic cell proliferations, as well as the parathyroid lesion.[12-15] However, more pronounced growth or malignant transformation seem to occur in only a minority of the generally numerous pancreatic microadenomas within each patient. This circumstance may imply that additional chromosomal deletions or proto-oncogene activation are needed for the development of gross tumors.[16] In contrast to the pancreatic endocrinopathy, the parathyroid lesion extremely rarely becomes malignant in MEN-1.[17] Although the gene for MEN-1 still remains unidentified, genetic screening among family members is possible under certain conditions.[13] By taking advantage of restriction fragment length polymorphism (RFLP) for markers closely related to the MEN-1 locus the disease-carrying allele can be followed through generations and predisposed individuals can be identified (Fig. 7.1). Although tumor development is characteristically multifocal in MEN-1, each individual tumor is considered to represent a monoclonal lesion.[7,12,16] On the other hand it has been suggested that stimulation by a circulating mitogenic factor, re-

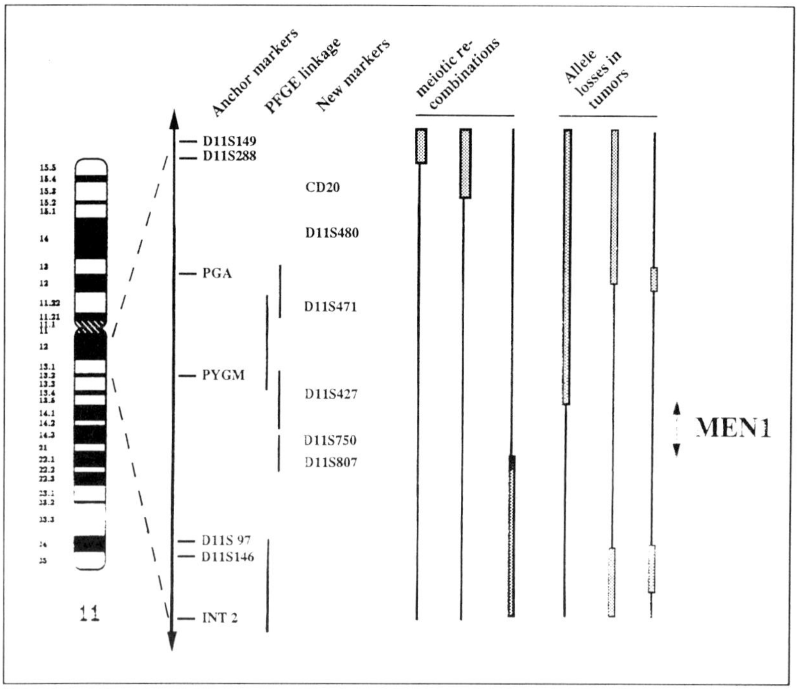

Fig. 7.1. Mapping of the MEN-1 region on chromosome 11. An enlarged map of the 11q 11-13 region shows the gene order based on combined physical mapping and linkage analysis. Anchor markers are those previously mapped in reference families. In each case the region "excluded" from analysis of recombinational events of deletion mapping is hatched. With knowledge of neighboring genes RFLP analysis can be used to detect MEN-1 gene carriers.[12,13] Reprinted with permission from Larsson C et al.[90]

sembling basic fibroblastic growth factor may cause polyclonal parathyroid hyperplasia and that this stage of proliferation precedes the secondary mutational hit.[18] However, the significance of such stimulation is controversial, since it should be expected to cause uniform and synchronous parathyroid involvement, which rarely is present in MEN-1.[18,19] The adrenocortical tumors apparently represent no primary MEN-1 lesion, but have been suggested to result from circulating growth factors or peptides, which could be produced in the environment of a more or less invariably coexisting endocrine pancreatic tumor.[7]

Diagnosis

Although MEN-1 patients represent a minority among patients with primary HPT, index cases for new kindreds are often efficiently recruited among patients with multiple parathyroid gland involvement[20,21] (Table 7.1). Thus, approximately 10-20% of the patients with multiglandular parathyroid disease will ultimately prove to have familial HPT, and apparently most often of MEN-1 origin if they are subjected to appropriate screening for the syndrome.[22-25] Even figures as high as 50% have been reported in this respect, but may indeed be overestimated, as the great tendency of the MEN-1 associated parathyroid lesion to recur after parathyroid surgery infers selection bias in most patient series.[23] Long term follow-up is often necessary in order to accurately diagnose the presence of MEN-1 among the patients with multiglandular parathyroid disease, as the individual parathyroid lesions characteristically occur asynchronously and often with considerable time-lag.[26] MEN-1 may also be diagnosed by the demonstration of hypercalcemia due to HPT in patients suffering from any of the other endocrinopathies of

Table 7.1. Biochemical screening for the MEN-1 syndrome in HPT patients (serum estimates)

chromogranin A
pancreatic polypeptide (PP)
gastrin
insulin, proinsulin/glucose
glucagon
prolactin
somatomedin C (IGF-1)
meal test with PP and gastrin analysis[16]

Screening is liberal in patients scheduled for parathyroid reoperation (where the surgical failure is not likely due to an overlooked adenoma) and is routinely performed in *younger* patients, those with *recurrent* HPT or with *multiglandular involvement.*

Only under special circumstances is a more extensive screening applied (italics), including a meal stimulation test which presently is the most sensitive for detection of concomitant endocrine pancreatic tumors.

the trait, pituitary adenoma, endocrine pancreatic tumors, or even adrenal cortical tumors or foregut carcinoids.[4,16] Thus, as many as 25% of patients with the Zollinger-Ellison's syndrome will ultimately prove to have MEN-1, while the syndrome is less prevalent and comprises only 4-10% of patients harboring insulinoma, and approximately 3% of the patients with pituitary tumors.[26-30]

Screening

The parathyroid lesion is generally claimed as the most prevalent and the earliest detected endocrinopathy of MEN-1, and HPT has thus been diagnosed in 90% or more of the patients[21] (Table 7.2). The MEN-1 associated parathyroid disease may often be evident clinically as early as during the 2nd or 3rd decades of life, and MEN-1 should be highly suspected when HPT is diagnosed in young individuals.[16,21] However, it should rarely be the cause of hypercalcemia in children before the age of 10, and under such circumstances familial hypocalciuric hypercalcemia may be a more likely diagnosis (see chapter 6). Endocrine pancreatic tumors or pituitary adenoma have in most MEN-1 kindreds not been nearly as prevalent clinically as they have been revealed at autopsy, and both these lesions have been most frequently diagnosed during the 4th decade of life.[4-6,31] However, a recent prospective screening study, utilizing sensitive biochemical markers, revealed that also the other target organs may indeed be involved in MEN-1[16] (Table 7.2). This careful screening program was found to lower the age of detection of especially the pancreatic lesion, which could frequently be demonstrated as the first presenting endocrinopathy, sometimes already in individuals 20 years or younger.[16] The prospective screening program furthermore emphasized a duration of several years from the first recognition of the presenting lesion to the development of a full scale clinical syndrome associated with the endocrine pancreatic tumor.[16] Occasionally the MEN-1 related endocrine pancreatic tumor syndromes have been clinically evident already in children, causing Zollinger-Ellison's syndrome and peptic ulcer disease, or hypoglycemic syndrome, and a hereditary trait must indeed be suspected when such young individuals are affected with any of these syndromes.[4,32] Thorough prospective screening was also found to lower the incidence of metastatic disease among the individuals with MEN-1, substantiating that the diagnosis of the individual lesions was made considerably earlier.[16] However, further studies are still needed to determine whether this type of efficient screening not only detects the individual lesions at an earlier stage, but also

Table 7.2. Frequency of different lesions among MEN-1 patients

	Screening* (%)	Autopsy** (%)
HPT	90	80-90
Pituitary tumor	19	60-70
Endocrine pancreatic tumor	75	81

* Skogseid et al[16]
** Eberle et al;[4] Ballard et al[5]

that the active screening program combined with early treatment, will really have influence on survival in MEN-1.[16] Identification of the MEN-1 gene will certainly simplify and increase the efficacy of the screening procedures in suspected MEN-1 patients, as only individuals with an identified genetic lesion will have to undergo the extensive biochemical studies.

Clinics of the MEN-1 Parathyroid Lesion

Autopsy studies as well as clinical reports substantiate that the parathyroid glands are almost invariably involved in MEN-1.[4-6,8,16,21,33] It has been claimed that screening with ionized calcium measurements is particularly valuable in MEN-1 kindreds, and that affected individuals might display only slightly raised ionized calcium, but normal total calcium measurements, and still exhibit symptoms of HPT and considerably enlarged parathyroid glands at surgery.[34,35] As such individuals are supposed to be at risk to develop further rise in serum calcium during intercurrent illness or surgery, the ionized calcium measurements have been suggested as a necessary part of the routine screening and follow-up of the MEN-1 patients.[35] In our experience the measurements of albumin corrected total serum calcium generally provide adequate basis for follow-up and treatment, and in fact we would rarely consider parathyroid surgery necessary unless there is unequivocal hypercalcemia. It has been stated that HPT in MEN-1 is generally asymptomatic and follows a mild clinical course. However, when this has been more closely evaluated there has been no significant difference in the incidence of symptoms or complications in patients with MEN-1 associated HPT as compared to those with non-familial primary HPT.[36] Symptomatic parathyroid bone disease is nowadays infrequently encountered also in MEN-1. Renal stones may be present in one-third or more of the patients, and is particularly likely to occur in younger individuals who more often exhibit a raised urinary calcium. The MEN-1 patients also frequently suffer from the common general complaints of primary HPT, characterized by more or less pronounced neuromuscular weakness or a psychiatric disability of mainly depressive character.[21,35,36]

Parathyroid Histology in MEN-1

Earlier histopathological reports of parathyroid glands in MEN-1 invariably described multiple glandular involvement with multinodular hyperplastic or adenomatous foci in individual glands.[37-39] A recent histopathological study substantiated that considerable variability within and between the individual glands was a distinct feature of the MEN-1 parathyroid lesion.[39] The glands often exhibited varying degrees of diffuse and nodular hyperplasia, areas with intermingled patterns, as well as areas of normal architecture (Fig. 7.2). Also in other series nodular changes have been present in at least two-thirds of the pathologically enlarged glands, and the largest of them have generally displayed the most markedly abnormal and nodular pattern.[39] The larger glands have often also exhibited more extensively enlarged nodules, demarcated by fibrous encapsulation or a contrasting cytoarchitecture, and often with diffusely hyperplastic or normal tissue dispersed between the nodules. Some of these glands appear adenoma-like and may even contain a characteristic peripheral rim of normal tissue. The morphological features of the MEN-1 glands are often similar to those described in patients with sporadic nodular chief cell hyperplasia, or in the patients with HPT secondary to uremia. Normal-sized glands may sometimes exhibit distinctly normal histological features, even if they coexist with a considerably enlarged gland or multiple abnormal glands in the same patient[39-41] (Fig. 7.2). The glandular enlargement may in fact be unusually marked in MEN-1 even in spite of only moderate hypercalcemia, substantiating that the lesion primarily relates to a growth regulatory disturbance of the parathyroid cells. Immunostaining for parathyroid hormone (PTH) has revealed decreased staining intensity within expanding nodules, and more intense reactivity in normal rims of parathyroid tissue, which suggests decreased capacity for storage of PTH in the abnormal cells.[39] Amyloid has been demonstrated in hyperplastic areas of MEN-1 glands and as it stains positively for PTH, it has been thought to represent abnormal cytoplasmic hormone processing.[39] Lymphoid infiltration, which is otherwise an unusual feature in pathological parathyroid glands, has been demonstrated in a proportion of the pathological glands of the MEN-1 patients.[39]

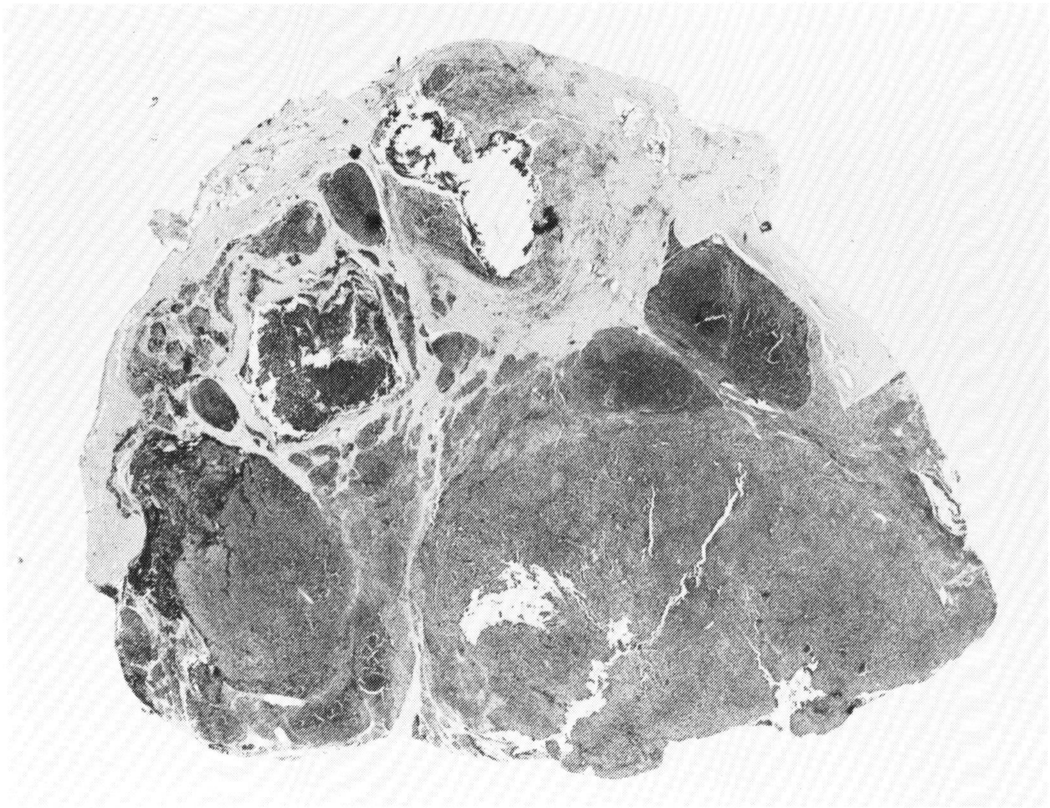

Fig. 7.2A.

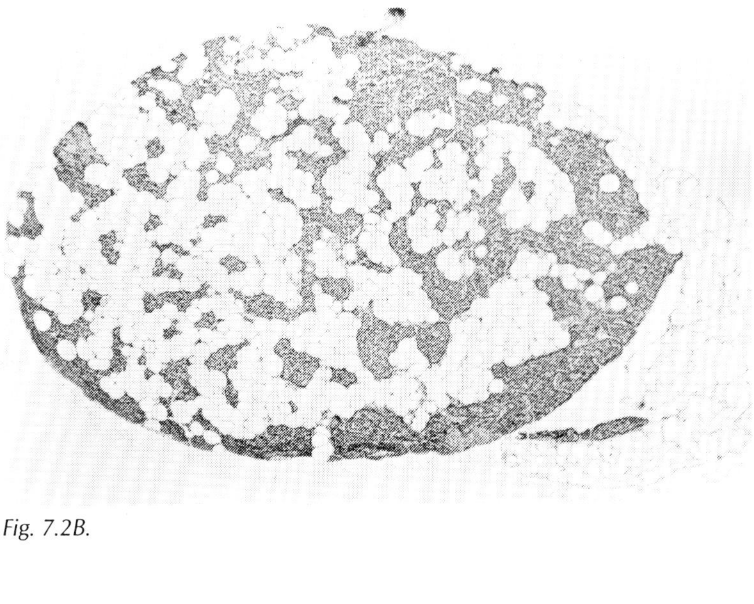

Fig. 7.2B.

Fig. 7.2. Parathyroid glands from a patient with MEN-1 associated parathyroid hyperplasia; gland (A) is markedly enlarged and exhibits nodular chief cell hyperplasia and fibrosis, while gland (B) is normal-sized and histologically normal.

Pancreatic Lesion

Pancreatic involvement has been revealed in 80% of MEN-1 necropsies, but the clinical endocrine pancreatic lesion has generally been detected with considerably lower frequency.[4-6] However, when a careful prospective screening program was adopted the pancreatic abnormalities were revealed almost as frequently as at autopsy[4,6,16] (Table 7.2). The MEN-1 pancreatic lesion characteristically consists of multiple microadenomas, together with less numerous, larger tumors, representing endocrine pancreatic adenomas or carcinomas.[4-6,42-44] The microadenomas frequently coexist with normal islets, and it has been suggested that they may originate from endocrine cell proliferations within the exocrine ducts, a feature named nesidioblastosis, rather than from islet cell hyperplasia, which indeed seems to be exceedingly rare in the MEN-1 pancreas.[43,44] The microadenomas as well as the larger lesions may display immunoreactivity for several peptides, like pancreatic polypeptide (PP), glucagon, insulin, proinsulin, somatostatin, gastrin, vasoactive intestinal peptide (VIP) and neurotensin.[43] Clinically the Zollinger-Ellison's syndrome and a peptic ulcer disease is the most prevalent of the endocrine pancreatic tumor syndromes associated with MEN-1. This syndrome may be caused by gastrin producing tumors of the pancreas, but surprisingly few of the gross pancreatic tumors have been found to stain positively for gastrin, and it has recently been emphasized that the gastrin excess in MEN-1 may often originate from one or several tiny duodenal adenomas or microadenomas.[10] The hypoglycemic syndrome is the second most common syndrome in MEN-1, while the Verner-Morrison's syndrome occurs more rarely and a glucagonoma syndrome is very unusual, although the minute microadenomas will frequently stain positively for glucagon.[42-44] Shifts between the endocrine pancreatic tumor syndromes may be experienced frequently during treatment or follow-up of the MEN-1 patients.[16] In younger MEN-1 individuals who have been recognized by biochemical screening the pancreatic endocrinopathy is almost invariably asymptomatic although the histologic lesion may comprise the full scale of proliferations from numerous microadenomas to gross tumors of appreciable size.[16] Many of the larger MEN-1 associated pancreatic tumors are clinically non-functioning and not associated with any clinically detectable tumor syndrome. These tumors are, however, equally important with respect to malignant behavior and require pancreatic surgery as the other MEN-1 pancreatic tumors, since they may also be the origin of metastases.[16,44] Surgery for the MEN-1 pancreatic lesion is thus undertaken when biochemical markers are positive, even in the absence of distinct clinical syndromes, and radiology is generally a poor indicator for the lesions.[44] Pancreatic surgery should encompass corpus and tail resection combined with enucleation of tumors in the head of the pancreas.[44] Regional lymph node or liver metastases of the pancreatic tumors may be revealed in approximately 15% of the MEN-1 patients where pancreatic involvement has been detected in the clinical routine. Metastases occur most frequently to regional lymph glands, and may also occur in association with small tumors of the pancreas or the duodenum.[42,44]

Pituitary Lesion

Pituitary tumors have been found at autopsy in approximately 60% of MEN-1 cases, while clinical screening studies of affected kindreds generally have revealed lower prevalence figures.[5,6,16,21,45] The pituitary tumors usually present with symptoms due to excessive hormone secretion or with complaints of pituitary hypofunction or local symptoms that can be related to the expanding tumor.[21,45] A majority of the MEN-1 associated pituitary tumors have been growth hormone and/or prolactin immunoreactive. At clinical evaluation prolactin-secreting lesions have been the most common, and these lesions may be the cause of amenorrhea in females as well as decreased libido and impotence in males. Occasionally pituitary lesions of

MEN-1 are associated with excessive growth hormone release leading to acromegaly. A few cases of Morbus Cushing due to corticotropin excess have also been reported, while other pituitary tumors release different combinations of hormones.[16,21,33] Two-thirds of the MEN-1 pituitary tumors are macroadenomas, and many are apparently multicentric.[30] A minority of them are non-functioning (null-cell adenomas), implying that they lack significant immunoreactivity for the pituitary hormones. The clinical diagnosis of the pituitary lesion in MEN-1 should depend on demonstration of elevated pituitary hormones and on visualization of the tumor by magnetic resonance imaging (MRI) or computed tomography (CT).

Prognosis

Complications of the peptic ulcer disease used to be the most common cause of death in untreated MEN-1 patients. Other causes of death are metastases from endocrine pancreatic carcinoma or foregut carcinoids, or complications related to a hypoglycemic syndrome.[4,5,8,45-47] Patients have also been reported to die from renal failure secondary to advanced HPT as well as from complications to pancreatic and pituitary surgery.[47] The recent improvements in medical therapy for the peptic ulcer disease, in particular omeprazole, has considerably increased survival in MEN-1, and have concomitantly also facilitated the clinical handling of these patients. Hypoglycemia is generally readily reversed by appropriate pancreatic surgery, as also the MEN-1 patients frequently harbor singular or only few insulinomas of a size that may cause symptoms. Recurrent insulinoma may be prevented by pancreatic body and tail resection.[32] At present the pancreatic malignancy exerts a major influence on survival, and in this respect some MEN-1 kindreds exhibit a more aggressive and malignant behavior of the pancreatic tumors.[16] Other kindreds tend to show a more favorable, or between kins, variable disease course.[16] Survival estimates of MEN-1 patients with endocrine pancreatic tumors have averaged 15 years from diagnosis within the clinical course.[44,48] The foregut carcinoids associated with MEN-1 may also influence survival, and although many of them run an indolent course, at least half exhibit malignant properties and may be a cause of death.[49] Also the other endocrinopathies of the trait may evolve aggressively, and knowledge of the typical pattern of development in a certain kindred may have a major influence on requirements of follow-up and treatment.[16]

Indications for Parathyroid Surgery in MEN-1

Consistent with a reported high failure rate of parathyroid operation in MEN-1, it has been advocated that surgery should be postponed until the development of marked hypercalcemia or severe HPT-related symptoms. However, this suggestion is based on retrospective analyses of patient series where the hereditary trait or even the multiglandular parathyroid involvement may not have been appreciated at the time of surgery. Our experience is that the MEN-1 patients are at similar risk of developing symptoms and complications of their parathyroid disorder as are the non-familial cases of primary HPT. We therefore subject the MEN-1 patients to surgery with virtually the same indications as applied in sporadic primary HPT, provided they exhibit unequivocal elevation of serum calcium and the diagnosis has been confirmed by inappropriately raised PTH values. The presence of a renal stone disorder or considerably increased urinary calcium excretion, as well as other symptoms of HPT, further support such decisions. The notion that elimination of the hypercalcemia may favorably influence the gastrin excess and peptic ulcer disease in an associated Zollinger-Ellison's syndrome has frequently also supported liberal indications for operation of MEN-1 associated HPT. However, such liberal indications require that the operation successfully reveals the prevailing histopathology, and furthermore that a majority of the patients rendered normocalcemic and not hypoparathyroid by surgery. Therefore less radical parathyroidectomy procedures may sometimes be performed even in MEN-1 cases if they exhibit only moderate hypercalcemia or less extensive glandular involvement.

SURGERY IN MEN-1 ASSOCIATED HPT

The MEN-1 parathyroid lesion is generally considered to represent an unusually aggressive form of hyperplastic proliferation, which has proven to be commonly associated with failed parathyroid surgery.[25,26,35,45,50-52] Although the aggressiveness of the disease may certainly vary between individuals and different MEN-1 kindreds, the reported failure rate has indeed been high, and especially so when the MEN-1 syndrome has not been recognized at the time of parathyroid surgery.[25,26,32,45,50,51] Consequently the MEN-1 cases will constitute a significant proportion of the patients who ultimately have to be considered for parathyroid reoperation.[52] Most authors therefore advocate a radical initial operation when dealing with MEN-1 associated HPT, based on the assumption that the patients invariably harbor polyclonal parathyroid hyperplasia affecting all glands.[25,26,40,52,53] Accordingly 50-80% of the MEN-1 patients have been reported to exhibit multiglandular disease at the primary exploration.[22,25,26,40,52] Since any patient undergoing operation for HPT could represent an unrecognized MEN-1 case it is essential to routinely visualize all parathyroid glands in order to recognize this pathology. However, the MEN-1 parathyroid endocrinopathy typically consists of multiple monoclonal lesions, characterized by greatly asymmetrical and asynchronous involvement. The different lesions may therefore evolve after a substantial time-lag, and some patients present initially with only one enlarged parathyroid gland and will then often be judged to harbor single adenomas. This incorrect impression may persist even after careful histopathological examination since glands excised at surgery may exhibit criteria compatible with the adenoma diagnosis, and almost half of the MEN-1 patients have at least one normal-sized gland besides the single or multiple enlarged ones.[52,54]

The time-lag for recurrence of parathyroid disease in the MEN-1 patients is unpredictable and apparently related to a highly variably growth potential within individual lesions. Decades of normocalcemia may thus be encountered after excision of one or two glands in certain MEN-1 patients, while others exhibit recurrence 3-5 years after radical subtotal three and a half gland resection.[52] In fact, superior results have been reported in patients where only singularly enlarged glands have been excised than in those with obvious multiglandular involvement subjected to a more radical surgical procedures.[54] Variation in the underlying genetic alteration, and possibly also other growth regulatory disturbances could be responsible for the variably aggressive clinical behavior of the MEN-1 parathyroid disease. Similar circumstances are possibly also reflected in the pronounced asymmetrical size and asynchronous development of the glandular pathology. The variability between individual patients and kindreds certainly have an impact on the long-term course of MEN-1 HPT, with crucial influence on the progression of hypercalcemia as well as the rate and time-lag of recurrence. However, until the MEN-1 gene has been cloned and the different constitutional mutations which correspond to different phenotypes have been identified, the optimal surgical procedure will continue to be debated, and variable outcome will possibly mainly reflect heterogeneity within different patient series.

MEN-1 parathyroid disease may be treated by classical subtotal parathyroid resection or total parathyroidectomy and immediate autotransplantation. Abundant experience indicate that either method is efficient, but they may have different applications.

Subtotal parathyroid resection remains the principle surgical procedure in parathyroid hyperplasia and so also when dealing with the MEN-1 lesion. The strategy, however, must consider the gland size and the histopathology revealed at operation. The largest parathyroid glands should always be excised at surgery, leaving remnants of the smallest, most normal-looking glands corresponding to a size of approximately 40-60 mg. Since many normal parathyroid glands are smaller, this requirement implies that in the presence of fat-cell rich, normal-sized glands a state of hypoparathyroidism may be avoided if clearly sufficient amounts of viable parathyroid tissue, i.e. up to one and a half (or even one and 3/4) of the normal sized glands are left as remnants. Remaining glands, however, need to be marked by suture for easier retrieval in case of recurrence.

Total parathyroidectomy and immediate autotransplantation appears as the preferred treatment in MEN-1 patients with four markedly enlarged glands. The procedure obviates the need to transect an enlarged and obviously diseased gland within the operative field, with its inherent risk of seeding and recurrence by implantation. Total parathyroidectomy and autotransplantation may be preferred at reoperation, since progressive adhesions will make further explorations considerably more difficult. The amount of transplanted parathyroid tissue may have to be increased to about 60-80 mg in the MEN-1 patients, in order to reduce the risk of permanent hypoparathyroidism.[41,52] The tissue selected for grafting should always originate from the patients smallest, obviously least diseased gland. This requirement is, however, not always easy to fulfill in the reoperative situation, since remaining glands may be difficult to identify.

Deficient recognition of the prevailing parathyroid pathology and inadequate excision of abnormal glands constitutes the principle causes of failed parathyroid operation in MEN-1, rather than the choice between the subtotal resection and total parathyroidectomy procedure. Considering that the most normal appearing gland(s) in each patient should be selected as residual tissue, subtotal resection may be a better choice in the presence of small, normal-sized glands, since these tiny generally fat-cell rich glands lend themselves poorly to autotransplantation. Transplant growth or recurrence may indeed have occurred when abnormal, and markedly enlarged glands, have been selected for transplantation, and this may have influenced the results of this surgery. A disadvantage of the total parathyroidectomy procedure is the extended period of postoperative hypocalcemia until the graft functions properly.

Of considerable importance for the success of parathyroid surgery in the MEN-1 patients and probably of greater importance for the outcome than the excision of normal-sized glands, is to emphasize the possible presence of *supernumerary parathyroid glands.* Careful search for such glands should always comprise an essential part of the operation. The supernumerary glands may be found in 13-15% of normal individuals and should occur with at least the same frequency in MEN-1.[55] They can be located in the fat surrounding the proper parathyroids as well as in the loose areolar fat tissue around the thyroid, or within the thymus. Even the rudiments of parathyroid tissue retrieved at these sites may become affected by the MEN-1 genetic aberration, acquire propensity for growth, and cause recurrent disease. The fat tissue around the parathyroid glands may thus be removed by dissection of the central neck compartment, and accessible parts of the thymus should always be excised via the neck incision.[55] This clearance may sometimes be more efficient in association with the total parathyroidectomy procedure. Involvement of glands in ectopic locations may also be frequently revealed in MEN-1, and the primary operation has to carefully explore even such sites. This is especially crucial in cases exhibiting marked glandular enlargement, reflecting unusual propensity for growth within the parathyroids. The supernumerary glands as well as the glands in ectopic locations may be considerably more difficult to retrieve if they are missed at the primary operation and have to be searched for at reoperation.

Persistent or recurrent HPT has been encountered after parathyroid surgery in

25-50% of the MEN-1 patients, and should be expected to occur if the surgeon was inexperienced or if less than four glands were visualized at surgery.[26,52] The failure rate is also high if the patient has been treated as if the lesion is a solitary parathyroid adenoma and is treated by unilateral exploration. We and others have encountered a histologically adenoma-like lesion to exist together with a normal associated gland ipsilaterally, and still been able to retrieve two enlarged glands on the contralateral side at reoperation. To assure that glands with the least apparent gross involvement can be left as remnants, we will refrain from removing any tissue for histology until both sides of the neck have been adequately explored. Moreover, trimming of subtotally resected glands should also preferably commence prior to excision, since it may sometimes be difficult to acquire appropriately vascularized remnants.

Considering the risks for failure when dealing with the MEN-1 parathyroid lesion, it should be important to recognize the diagnosis prior to operation. This association should indeed be suspected in all younger patients with HPT, i.e. < 40 years. These patients should be subjected to preoperative screening in order to disclose associated endocrinopathies, which may corraborate the MEN-1 diagnosis. This may include basal measurements in serum of chromogranin A, pancreatic polypeptide (PP), gastrin, insulin/proinsulin (glucose), glucagon and prolactin (Table 7.1). In cases where multiple enlargements of the parathyroid glands are unexpectedly found at operation the possible presence of MEN-1 should also be considered. Especially if the hypercalcemia is more significant, and the glands are markedly and unevenly enlarged, the surgeon should then already at the initial procedure extend the operation to include appropriate clearance of fat within the central neck compartment as well as a cervical thymectomy. Patients with recurrence after parathyroid surgery or those with diagnosed multiglandular parathyroid disease will generally also undergo screening for the MEN-1 syndrome.

MEN-2 SYNDROME

Medullary carcinoma of the thyroid was first described as a distinct clinical and pathological entity by Hazard in 1959.[56] In 1961 Sipple reported the association of medullary thyroid carcinoma and pheochromocytoma,[57] and a few years later it was determined that this combination of tumors represented a hereditary syndrome.[58,59] The multiple endocrine neoplasia (MEN) 2a syndrome has been more extensively described and reported to consist of frequently bilateral and multifocal medullary thyroid carcinoma and concomitant C-cell hyperplasia of the thyroid, together with uni-or bilateral pheocromocytoma in approximately 50% of the patients, and HPT in 10-20%.[60] The medullary thyroid carcinoma of the MEN-2a syndrome is often advanced when clinically detected, but may be revealed earlier by screening with measurements of serum calcitonin, whereby determination of pentagastrin stimulated calcitonin values may detect even minimal carcinoma or a preceding C-cell hyperplasia in young probands of a kindred.[61,62] The thyroid carcinoma should be treated by radical surgery, including clearance of neck lymph glands, and constitutes a principal cause of death in the MEN-2a syndrome.[63,64]

The MEN-2b syndrome was described in 1968, and apart from medullary thyroid carcinoma and pheocromocytoma, includes mucosal ganglioneuromatosis, but rarely parathyroid involvement.[65] MEN-2b is a rare hereditary syndrome, which, however, in 50% of the patients may be observed without a discernible family history. The syndrome may be detected in early childhood by a typical habitus, characterized by thick lips, mucosal neuroma and a Marphanoid habitus generally without associated vascular disease,[66] In this syndrome the medullary carcinoma develops earlier, has a considerably more malignant course with early metastases, and is associated with a more unfavorable prognosis than the medullary carcinoma in MEN-2a.[66,67]

Genetics

Genetic linkage studies have mapped the locus for MEN-2a, MEN-2b as well as familial medullary thyroid carcinoma to an interval on chromosome 10 q 11.2.[68] This region was shown to comprise the RET proto-oncogene, known to be involved in the tumorogenesis of papillary thyroid carcinoma, and subsequent studies were able to demonstrate germline mutations of this oncogene in MEN-2a and familial medullary thyroid carcinoma.[69] Further studies have indicated that specific mutations are related to the prevailing disease phenotype and possibly predicts the incidence of pheochromocytoma and HPT in MEN-2a.[70] The MEN-2b syndrome has however, not yet been related to any of these mutations.[70]

Parathyroid Lesion

Before the most recent discoveries of the genetics behind the MEN-2 syndrome the associated parathyroid disease was thought to be genetically determined rather than secondary to the elevated calcitonin or catecholamines. Consequently patients with sporadic medullary thyroid carcinoma or pheocromocytoma have not exhibited increased prevalence of parathyroid abnormalities. The reported incidence of morphological parathyroid changes in MEN-2a patients has, however, varied considerably in different series, and has ranged between 20 and 100%.[66,71-73] However, cases with even histologically unequivocal parathyroid gland abnormality frequently display normal or only sporadically inappropriately elevated PTH levels, and the vast majority lack hypercalcemia and other clinical signs of HPT.[74-76] The incidence of biochemically documented and clinically detectable HPT thus seems to range between 10 and 20% among MEN-2a patients. Moreover only occasional individuals exhibit obvious clinical manifestations of parathyroid disease, such as nephrolithiasis or evident neuropsychiatric disturbance.[76] Clinically important HPT thus seems to be a rare feature of the MEN-2a syndrome.

Histologically the predominant parathyroid lesion in MEN-2a is nodular chief cell hyperplasia. The hyperplasia generally affects more than one gland, but is often asymmetrical, and the enlarged hyperplastic glands often coexist with normal-sized ones. Single as well as multiple adenomas have also been described and it has been suggested that the adenomas evolve from a previous nodular hyperplasia.[66,77-79]

Treatment of MEN-2a Associated HPT

The lack of correlation of serum calcium or PTH concentrations makes slight, asymmetrical parathyroid gland enlargement most often a coincidental finding in MEN-2a. Under such circumstances only the obviously enlarged glands have to be excised.[80] In fact, the surgical management in MEN-2a associated HPT should aim to preserve parathyroid function, which indeed might be technically difficult during extensive lymph node clearance in association with total thyroidectomy for medullary carcinoma. However, all parathyroid glands need to be identified during the cervical exploration although even in patients with hypercalcemia only the grossly enlarged glands should be resected.[75,77,80,81] Subtotal parathyroidectomy is thus generally preferred rather than total parathyroidectomy with autotransplantation, and the former procedure is generally adopted even in cases where four parathyroid glands are enlarged.[77,82] Only rarely has MEN-2a been associated with recurrent parathyroid disease.[81]

NON-MEN FAMILIAL HPT

Familial HPT is known to occur also in the absence of other endocrinopathies, and apparently unassociated with MEN-1 or MEN-2a, and may then exhibit dominant or recessive inheritance.[23,24,83-86] The majority of these patients have displayed parathyroid chief cell hyperplasia, with asymmetrical involvement of the glands as in MEN-1 related HPT.[84,86] Occasionally, however, also familial occurrence of adenoma has been reported.[24] Parathyroid carcinoma has been rarely described in a familial setting as has occasional cystic adenomas.[23,87-89] These familial forms of

HPT seem to be associated with symptoms as in sporadic and MEN-1 related HPT.

REFERENCES

1. Erdheim J. Zur normalen und pathologischen histologie der glandula thyroidea, parathyroidea und hypophysis. Beitr Pathol Anat 1903; 33: 158-236.
2. Wermer P. Genetic aspects of adenomatosis of endocrine glands. Am J Med 1954; 16: 363-71.
3. Wermer P. Endocrine adenomatosis and peptic ulcer in a large kindred: inherited multiple tumors and mosaic pleitropism in man. Am J Med 1963; 35: 205-12.
4. Eberle F, Grün R. Multiple endocrine neoplasia, type 1 (MEN 1). Ergeb Inn Med Kinderheilkd 1981; 46: 75-149.
5. Ballard HS, Frame B, Hartsock RJ. Familial multiple endocrine adenoma peptic ulcer complex. Medicine (Baltimore) 1964; 43: 481-516.
6. Croisier JC, Azerad E, Lubetzki J. L'adénomatose polyendocrinienne. A propos d'une observation personelle et revenue de la litterature. Sem Hop Paris 1971; 47: 494-525.
7. Skogseid B, Larsson C, Lindgren P-G et al. Clinical and genetic features of adrenocortical lesions in multiple endocrine neoplasia type I. J Clin Endocrinol Metab 1992; 75: 76-81.
8. Lips CJM, Lamers CBHW, Vasen HFA. Multiple endocrine neoplasia syndromes. Critic Rev Oncol 1984; 2: 117-84.
9. Houdelette P, Chagnon A, Dumotier J et al. Corticosurrénalome malin dans le cadre d'un syndrome de Wermer. J Chir (Paris) 1989; 126: 385-7.
10 Pipeleers-Marichal M, Somers G, Willems G et al. Gastrinomas in the duodenums of patients with multiple endocrine neoplasia type 1 and the Zollinger-Ellison syndrome. N Engl J Med 1990; 322: 723-7.
11. Knudson AG. Mutation and cancer: Statistical study of retinoblastoma. Proc Natl Acad Sci USA 1971; 68: 820-3.
12. Larsson C, Skogseid B, Öberg K et al. Multiple endocrine neoplasia type 1 gene maps to chromosome 11 and is lost in insulinoma. Nature 1988; 332: 85-7.
13. Byström C, Larsson C, Blomberg C et al. Localization of the gene for multiple endocrine neoplasia type 1 to a small region within chromosome 11q 13 by deletion mapping in tumors. Proc Natl Acad Sci USA 1990; 87: 1968-72.
14. Thakker RV, Bouloux P, Wooding C, et al. Association of parathyroid tumors in multiple endocrine neoplasia type 1 with loss of alleles on chromosome 11. N Engl J Med 1989; 321: 218-24.
15. Friedman E, Sakaguchi K, Bale AE et al. Clonality of parathyroid tumors in familial multiple endocrine neoplasia type 1. N Engl J Med 1989; 321: 213-8.
16. Skogseid B, Eriksson B, Lundqvist G et al. Multiple endocrine neoplasia type 1—A ten year prospective screening study in four kindreds. J Clin Endocrinol Metab 1991; 73: 281-7.
17. Streeten EA, Weinstein LS, Norton JA et al. Studies in a kindred with parathyroid carcinoma. J Clin Endocrinol Metab 1992; 75: 362-6.
18. Brandi ML. Aurbach GD, Fitzpatrick LA et al. Parathyroid mitogenic activity in plasma from patients with familial multiple endocrine neoplasia type 1. N Engl J Med 1986; 314: 1287-93.
19. Brandi ML. Parathyroid tumor biology in familial multiple endocrine neoplasia type I. A model for cancer development. Henry Ford Hosp Med J 1992; 40: 181-5.
20. Muhr C, Åkerström G, Ljunghall S et al. Screening for multiple endocrine adenomatosis type I in patients with primary hyperparathyroidism. Clin Endocrinol 1984; 20: 153-62.
21. Benson L, Ljunghall S, Åkerström G et al. Hyperparathyroidism presenting as the first lesion in multiple endocrine neoplasia type 1. Am J Med 1987; 82: 731-7.
22. Boey JH, Cooke TJC, Gilbert JM et al. Occurrence of other endocrine tumors in primary hyperparathyroidism. Lancet 1975; 2: 781-4.
23. Marx SJ, Spiegel AM, Brown EM et al. Family studies in patients with primary parathyroid hyperplasia. Am J Med 1977; 62: 698-706.
24. Allo M, Thompson NW. Familial hyper-

parathyroidism caused by solitary adenomas. Surgery 1982; 92: 486-90.
25. van Heerden JA, Kent RB III, Sizemore GW et al. Primary hyperparathyroidism in patients with multiple endocrine neoplasia syndromes: Surgical experience. Arch Surg 1983; 118: 533-6.
26. Rizzoli R, Green J III, Marx SJ. Primary hyperparathyroidism in familial multiple endocrine neoplasia type I: long-term follow-up of serum calcium levels after parathyroidectomy. Am J Med 1985; 78: 467-74.
27. Lamers CGHW, Stadil F, van Torgeren JH. Prevalence of endocrine abnormalities in patients with the Zollinger-Ellison syndrome and in their families. Am J Med 1978; 64: 607-12.
28. Jensen RT, Doppmann JL, Gardner JD. Gastrinoma. In the exocrine pancreas: Biology, Pathobiology and diseases. V.L.W. Go JD, Gardner FP, Brooks E, Dimagno E, Lebenthal GS, Scheele, editor. New York, Raven Press 1986: 727-44.
29. Stefanini P, Carboni M, Patrassi N et al. Beta-islet cell tumors of the pancreas: results of a study on 1067 cases. Surgery 1974; 75: 597-609.
30. Scheithauer BW, Laws ER, Kovacs K et al. Pituitary adenomas of the multiple endocrine neoplasia type I syndrome. Semin Diagn Pathol 1987; 4: 205-11.
31. Brandi ML, Marx SJ, Aurbach GD et al. Familial multiple endocrine neoplasia type I: A new look at pathophysiology. Endocrine Reviews 1987; 8: 391-405.
32. Rasbach DA, van Heerden JA, Telander RL et al. Surgical management of hyperinsulinism in the multiple endocrine neoplasia, type 1 syndrome. Arch Surg 1985; 120: 584-9.
33. Marx SJ, Winik AI, Santen RJ et al. Multiple endocrine neoplasia type 1: Assessment of laboratory tests to screen for the gene in a large kindred. Medicine 1986; 65: 226-41.
34. Benson L, Ljunghall S, Groth T et al. Optimal discrimination of mild hyperparathyroidism with total serum calcium, ionized calcium and parathyroid hormone measurements. Ups J Med Sci 1987; 92: 147-76.
35. Shepherd JJ, Teh BT, ParameswaranV et al. Hyperparathyroidism with normal albumin-corrected total calcium in patients with multiple endocrine neoplasia type 1. Henry Ford Hosp Med J 1992; 40: 186-90.
36. Lamers CBHW, Froeling PGAM. Clinical significance of hyperparathyroidism in familial multiple endocrine adenomatosis. Am J Med 1979; 66: 422-4.
37. Underdahl LO, Woolner LB, Black BM. Multiple endocrine adenomas: report of 8 cases in which the parathyroids, pituitary and pancreatic islets were involved. J Clin Endocrinol Metab 1953; 13: 20-47.
38. Cope O, Keynes M, Roth SI et al. Primary chief-cell hyperplasia of the parathyroid glands: a new entity in the surgery of hyperparathyroidism. Ann Surg 1958; 148: 375-88.
39. Harach HR, Jasani B. Parathyroid hyperplasia in multiple endocrine neoplasia type 1: A pathological and immunohistochemical reappraisal. Histopath 1992; 20: 305-13.
40. Malmaeus J, Benson L, Johansson H et al. Parathyroid surgery in the multiple endocrine neoplasia type 1 syndrome: Choice of surgical procedure. World J Surg 1986; 10: 668-72.
41. Castleman B, Schantz A, Roth SI. Parathyroid hyperplasia in primary hyperparathyroidism. A review of 85 cases. Cancer 1976; 38: 1668-75.
42. Thompson NW, Lloyd RV, Nishiyama RH et al. MEN 1 pancreas. A histological and immunohistochemical study. World J Surg 1984; 8: 561-74.
43. Klöppel G, Willemer S, Stamm B et al. Pancreatic lesions and hormonal profile of pancreatic tumors in multiple endocrine neoplasia type 1. Cancer 1986; 57: 1824-32.
44. Grama D, Skogseid B, Wilander E et al. Pancreatic tumors in multiple endocrine neoplasia type 1: Clinical presentation and surgical treatment. World J Surg 1992; 16: 611-9.
45. Vasen HFA, Lamers CBHW, Lips CJM. Screening for the multiple endocrine neoplasia syndrome type 1. A study of 11 kindreds in the Netherlands. Arch Intern Med 1989; 149: 2717-22.
46. Lamers CB. Familial endocrine neoplasia

type 1 (Werner's syndrome). Neth J Med 1978; 21: 270-4.
47. Lips CJM, Koppeschaar HPF, Berends MJH et al. The importance of screening for the 5 MEN 1 syndrome: Diagnostic results and clinical management. Henry Ford Hosp Med J 1992; 40: 171-2.
48. Eriksson B, Skogseid B, Lundqvist G et al. Medical treatment and long-term survival in a prospective study of 84 patients with endocrine pancreatic tumors. Cancer 1990; 65: 1883-90.
49. Zeiger MA, Swartz SE, MacGillivray DC et al. Thymic carcinoid in association with MEN syndrome. Am Surg 1992; 58: 430-4.
50. Scholz DA, Purnell DC, Edis AJ et al. Primary hyperparathyroidism with multiple parathyroid gland enlargement: Review of 53 cases. Mayo Clin Proc 1978; 53: 792-7.
51. Samaan NA, Ouais S, Ordonez NG et al. Multiple endocrine syndrome type I: Clinical, laboratory findings, and management in five families. Cancer 1989; 64: 741-52.
52. Hellman P, Skogseid B, Juhlin C et al. Findings and long-term results of parathyroid surgery in multiple endocrine neoplasia type 1. World J Surg 1992; 16: 718-23.
53. Wells SA Jr, Farndon JA, Dale JK et al. Long-term evaluation of patients with primary parathyroid hyperplasia managed by total parathyroidectomy and heterotopic autotransplantation. Ann Surg 1980; 192: 451-8.
54. Kraimps JL, Duh Q-Y, Demeure M et al. Hyperparathyroidism in multiple endocrine neoplasia syndrome. Surgery 1992; 112: 1080-8.
55. Åkerström G, Malmaeus J, Bergström R. Surgical anatomy of human parathyroid glands. Surgery 1984; 95: 14-21.
56. Hazard JB, Hawk WA, Crile G Jr. Medullary solid carcinoma of the thyroid—a clinicopathologic entity. J Clin Endocrinol Metab 1959; 19: 152-61.
57. Sipple JH. The association of pheochromoytoma with carcinoma of the thyroid gland. Am J Med 1961; 31: 163-6.
58. Schimke RN, Hartmann WH. Familial amyloid-producing medullary thyroid carcinoma and pheochromocytoma. A distinct genetic entity. Ann Intern Med 1965; 63: 1027-39.
59. Williams ED. A review of 17 cases of carcinoma of the thyroid and pheochromocytoma. J Clin Path 1965; 18: 288-92.
60. Thakker RV, Ponder BAJ. Multiple endocrine neoplasia. Baillière's Clinical Metab 1988; 2: 1031-67.
61. Tashjian AH, Melvin KEW. Medullary carcinoma of the thyroid gland: studies of thyrocalcitonin in plasma and tumor extracts. N Engl J Med. 1968; 279: 279-83.
62. Hennessy JF, Wells SA, Ontjes DA et al. A comparison of pentagastrin injection and calcium infusion as provocative agents for the detection of medullary carcinoma of the thyroid. J Clin Endocrinol Metab 1974; 39: 487-95.
63. Melvin KEW, Tashjian AH, Miller HH. Studies in familial (medullary) thyroid carcinoma. Recent Progress in Hormonal Research 1972; 28: 399-470.
64. Williams ED. Thyroidectomy for genetically determined medullary carcinoma. Lancet. 1977; i: 1309-10.
65. Schimke RN, Hartmann WH, Prout TE et al. Syndrome of bilateral pheochromocytoma, medullary thyroid carcinoma, and multiple neuromas. N Engl J Med 1968; 279: 1-7.
66. Saad MF, Ordonez NG, Rashid RK et al. Medullary carcinoma of the thyroid. A study of the clinical features and prognostic factors in 161 patients. Medicine (Baltimore) 1984; 63: 319-42.
67. Norton JA, Froome LC, Farrell RE et al. Multiple endocrine neoplasia type IIb. The most aggressive form of medullary thyroid carcinoma. Surg Clin N Am 1979; 59: 109-18.
68. Gardner ED, Papi L, Easton DF et al. Genetic linkage studies map the multiple endocrine neoplasia type 2 loci to a small interval on chromosome 10q11.2. Hum Molec Genet 1993; 2: 241-6.
69. Mulligan LM, Kwok JBJ, Healey CS et al. Germ-line mutations of the RET protooncgene in multiple endocrine neoplasia type 2A. Nature 1993; 363: 458-60.
70. Mulligan LM, Eng C, Healey CS et al. Specific mutations of the RET protooncgene are related to disease phenotype in

MEN 2A and FMTC. Nature Genetics 1994; 6: 70-4.
71. Chong GC, Bearhrs OH, Sizemore GW et al. Medullary carcinoma of the thyroid gland. Cancer 1975; 35: 695-704.
72. Heath H III, Sizemore GW, Carney JA. Preoperative diagnosis of occult parathyroid hyperplasia by calcitonin infusion in patients with multiple endocrine neoplasia type 2a. J Clin Endocrinol Metab 1976; 43: 428-35.
73. Wells SA, Dilley WG, Farndon JA et al. Early diagnosis and treatment of medullary thyroid carcinoma. Arch Intern Med 1985; 145: 1248-52.
74. Steiner Al, Goodman AD, Powers SR. Study of a kindred with pheochromocytoma, medullary thyroid carcinoma, hyperparathyroidism and Cushing's disease: multiple endocrine neoplasia, type 2. Medicine (Baltimore) 1968; 47: 371-409.
75. Block MA, Jackson CE, Tashjian AH. Management of parathyroid glands in surgery for medullary thyroid carcinoma. Arch Surg 1975; 110: 617-24.
76. Block MA. Surgical treatment of medullary carcinoma of the thyroid. Otolaryngol Clin North Am 1990; 23: 453-73.
77. Brunt LM, Wells S. Advances in the diagnosis and treatment of medullary thyroid carcinoma. Surg Clin North Am 1987; 67: 263-79.
78. Sarosi G, Doe RP. Familial occurrence of parathyroid adenomas, pheochromocytoma, and medullary carcinoma of the thyroid with amyloid stroma (Sipple's syndrome). Arch Intern Med 1968; 68: 1305-9.
79. Padberg BC, Holl K, Schröder S. Pathology of multiple endocrine neoplasias 2a and 2b: A review. Horm Res 1992; 38 (suppl 2): 24-30.
80. Dralle H, Scheumann GFW, Kotzerke J et al. Surgical management of MEN-2. Rec Res Cancer Res 1992; 125: 167-95.
81. Block MA, Jackson CE, Greenwald KA et al. Clinical characteristics distinguishing hereditary from sporadic medullary thyroid carcinoma, treatment implications. Arch Surg 1980; 115: 142-8.
82. O'Riordain DS, O'Brien T, Grant CS et al. Surgical management of primary hyperparathyroidism in multiple endocrine neoplasia types 1 and 2. Surgery 1993; 114: 1031-9.
83. Jackson CE. Hereditary hyperparathyroidism associated with recurrent pancreatitis. Ann Intern Med 1958; 49: 829-36.
84. Goldsmith RE, Sizemore GW, Chen I-Wen younger et al. Familial hyperparathyroidism Ann Intern Med 1976; 84: 36-43.
85. Sandler LM, Moncrief MW. Familial hyperparathyroidism. Arch Dis Child 1980; 55: 146-7.
86. Law WH Jr, Hodgson SF, Heath H III. Autosomal recessive inheritance of familial hyperparathyroidism. N Engl J Med 1983; 309: 650-3.
87. Mallette LE, Bilezikian JP, Ketcham AS et al. Parathyroid carcinoma in familial hyperparathyroidism. Am J Med 1974; 57: 642-8.
88. Dinnen JS, Greenwood RH, Jones JH et al. Parathyroid carcinoma in familial hyperparathyroidism. J Clin Path 1977; 30: 966-75.
89. Mallette LE, Malini S, Rappaport MP et al. Familial cystic parathyroid adenomatosis. Ann Intern Med 1987; 107: 54-60.
90. Larsson C, Weber G, Jansson M. Sublocalization of the multiple endocrine neoplasia type 1 gene. Henry Ford Hosp Med J 1992; 40: 159-61.

CHAPTER 8

Reoperation in Primary Hyperparathyroidism

Göran Åkerström, Claes Juhlin

"The ultimate success in the management of patients with continuing hyperparathyroidism depends on the surgeon, for he alone must recognize where the mistake lies and how to correct it" (Wang[1]).

The success rate of cervical exploration in primary hyperparathyroidism (HPT) has improved during recent decades, and up to 95-98% of the patients can now expect cure by the initial surgery.[1-17] This is due to increased knowledge of the pathology and the variable anatomy of the parathyroids together with a considerably increased experience among surgeons devoted to this surgery.[1-3,8,15-17] Along with more efficient diagnosis of HPT, the primary surgical treatment has been undertaken also in individuals with only moderate hypercalcemia and generally less impressive glandular enlargement.[8,18-24] The operation is nowadays commonly performed also outside the larger centers, sometimes by surgeons who have achieved less extensive training.[22,23] Under such circumstances parathyroid surgery may be difficult, associated with a higher failure rate than has been reported from the experienced referral centers.[22,23]

Disease remaining after neck exploration has ever since the first days of parathyroid surgery been beset with problems.[1] Reoperation in HPT has thus been regarded as a surgical challenge associated with a considerably lower rate of success than the primary operation, and the repeated surgery has often been afflicted with a higher rate of complications, some of them severe.[1,3-5,25-29] Due to accumulated experience with these difficult cases the success rate of reoperation has also increased, however, and may indeed at specialized centers now approach that of the primary operation.[1,3,4,8,11,17,23,30-39] Since the complication rate has decreased concomitantly also, this surgery may now be offered with confidence a favorable chance of success and safety.

Current Controversy in Parathyroid Operation and Reoperation, edited by Göran Åkerström.

DIAGNOSIS

Facing a parathyroid reoperation it is essential to *reconfirm the diagnosis* by repeating the measurements of serum calcium and intact parathyroid hormone (PTH).[34-37]

Until recently a substantial proportion of the patients who remained hypercalcemic after surgery were subsequently found to have raised serum calcium values for reasons other than HPT.[7,8,16,21,38] In particular this was common in patients with severe hypercalcemia, where the neck exploration was sometimes part of the diagnostic procedure. The risk of this error is now minimal, since a diagnosis of HPT can be firmly established by inappropriately raised values of intact PTH.[40] It is also possible to temporarily ameliorate severe hypercalcemia by medical treatment, so that parathyroid surgery can be postponed until the diagnosis is definitive.[41] Occasionally HPT can coexist with another disease such as sarcoidosis or malignancy, causing persistently elevated serum calcium values after apparently adequate surgery. A dual reason for the hypercalcemia may then be revealed by demonstration of low or normal PTH values after surgery.

An important diagnosis to exclude in patients with hypercalcemia persisting after neck exploration is *familial hypocalciuric hypercalcemia (FHH)*, which has been claimed to be present in up to 10% of patients evaluated for reoperation.[11,35,36,42,43] FHH should especially be suspected in younger individuals with mild, asymptomatic hypercalcemia, possibly prone to be referred for reoperative surgery because of their age. The presence of a *family history* of mild and uncomplicated hypercalcemia and previous unsuccessful parathyroid surgery supports a diagnosis of FHH. These patients are thus identified by careful examinationof the family history and determination of the urinary calcium excretion; whereby a 24h urinary calcium/creatinine quotient of less than 0.01 supports a diagnosis of FHH. However, the discrimination is not always easy, since patients with HPT may also exhibit mildly elevated serum calcium and low urinary calcium excretion. A definitive diagnosis may therefore require serum calcium screening of family members.[35,42,43]

Examination of both the patient and the family history also serves to recognize the presence of a multiple endocrine neoplasia (MEN) syndrome or other varieties of familial HPT in patients evaluated for reoperation. The MEN-2 syndrome is unusual in this context, but the MEN-1 syndrome occurs frequently among patients requiring repeat parathyroid surgery.[11,23,30,34-39,44-49] Efforts should therefore be made to reveal a history of other endocrinopathies, affecting the pituitary, the endocrine pancreas or the adrenals, in the patient or the relatives. The concomitant presence of HPT and peptic ulcer disease is highly suggestive of MEN-1 but may sometimes have been unnoticed by a treating physician. In addition laboratory screening for MEN-1 should liberally be undertaken in younger patients, those with recurrent HPT as well as any patient with expected or proven multiglandular involvement. (For details concerning this screening and the MEN-1 syndrome see chapter 7). Since the MEN-1 lesions occur asynchronously the patients may have had a single gland enlarged at the previous operation, even with adenoma criteria.[4,49] It is essential to identify the patients with MEN-1 or familial HPT, prior to reoperation, since their variety of multiglandular disease requires special consideration.[49]

The patient history may also provide information of previous neck irradiation, since an adenoma on the irradiated side might be the expected lesion.[36,50,51]

REVIEW OF OPERATIVE NOTES, PATHOLOGY AND PATIENT RECORDS

Careful review of reports from the previous neck surgery, as well as reexamination of histopathology specimens and scrutiny of patient records constitute important parts of the evaluation prior to reoperation.[11,31,36,38] Unfortunately the operative notes will often be inadequate when they are most eagerly needed after difficult primary operations or when surgery was performed by less experienced surgeons.[52] Such notes frequently lack sufficient details and fail to describe the size and location of identified glands or excised specimens.[31] Sketches of the operative anatomy are also often missing. Inadequate operative reports may suggest surgical inexperience and may indicate that a remaining gland can be easily retrieved from a normal position.[52]

Whether *routine biopsy of normal parathyroid glands* should be performed in conjunction with primary parathyroid surgery has been a matter of controversy.[5,17,19,31,33,36,53,54] In the context of reoperative parathyroid surgery such biopsies have often been especially required; in their absence during the primary operation glandular identification cannot be taken for granted.[36] However, even if such biopsies help plan reoperation, the normal glands will be considerably more difficult to identify at the subsequent surgery, if they still remain. It is common that sequential sampling of normal parathyroid glands may easily result in hypocalcemia when an enlarged and diseased gland is subsequently removed at reoperation.[23] In fact, the number of excised normal parathyroid glands or necessary biopsies from them tend to decrease with increasing surgical experience, and many surgeons will refrain from them completely unless they are really needed. More valuable for reoperation would be to have the normal-sized parathyroids marked by suture and a carefully drawn map describing their location. Moreover, when reviewing the operative notes questions may arise whether an identified parathyroid gland is superior or an inferior; it has been strongly emphasized that this distinction is difficult unless two ipsilateral glands have been visualized.[36]

The histopathology specimens should be evaluated with regard to the size of the excised glands as well as their histology. A common error is that a histologically normal gland has been judged as abnormal because the weight has not been determined or it is enveloped in a fat pad and thereby falsely interpreted as enlarged. Unfortunately, an inexperienced pathologist may contribute to this mistake. Occasionally the histopathological reexamination will identify characteristics highly suggestive of nodular chief cell hyperplasia in a gland previously interpreted to represent an adenoma. If the previous operative reports and reexamination of the histology specimens indicate that only normal tissue was removed at the primary operation a missed adenoma is the likely cause of persistent disease, while remaining hypercalcemia after previous removal of abnormal tissue suggests multiglandular involvement.[1,52]

The patient records may reveal further details concerning the patient and the family history, as well as symptoms and complications of the disease, which may constitute important grounds for decisions about surgery. The records may also provide information about the course of hypercalcemia before or after the previous operation. Limited decrease in serum calcium may have occurred even without removal of pathological tissue due to ischemia in a pathological gland.[10]

INDICATIONS FOR REOPERATION

It has been said that the second most difficult decision in surgery is when to operate, but the most difficult decision is when to reoperate.[15,31,39] When the diagnosis of HPT has been firmly established it is necessary to reevaluate whether the severity of the disease, with respect to metabolic disturbances, complications and symptoms, justifies repeat surgery.[1,34-36] This decision should depend largely on the options for cure as well as on expected effects on symptoms in relation to the risks of the operation. Earlier studies suggested that reoperative surgery was associated with considerable risk and even mortality.[28] More recent experience, however, indicates increased efficacy and safety and combined with new methods for localization of parathyroid glands prior to surgery the expected outcome may be nearly as favorable as for the primary parathyroid operation.[1,19,23,31,32,34-39]

Most surgeons will defer reoperation in patients with mildly hypercalcemic, asymptomatic and uncomplicated HPT, and in general terms consider reoperative surgery indicated in patients with symptoms, complications or more markedly elevated serum calcium values.[1,11,34-39] The symptoms that are generally considered are previous or present episodes of *renal stones* (demonstrated by the patient history or radiology), nephrocalcinosis or marked hypercalciuria; *bone disease* (reflected in even minor radiological changes typical for osteitis fibrosa, diminished bone density or elevated alkaline phosphatases); *renal function impairment* (raised serum creatinine or impaired creatinine clearance). Indications for reoperation generally also includes the neuromuscular weakness and psychiatric disability commonly associated with HPT, e.g. being weakness and fatigue, lack of initiative, depression, decreased ability to concentrate, memory loss or confusion.[35,55-60] Most series of reoperative patients have reported the presence of more advanced symptoms than in the general patient with primary HPT, and commonly 50% of the patients have exhibited renal stones, up to 10% have had some evidence of renal function impairment or renal failure, while signs of bone disease or the more vague neurobehavioral disturbance have been present in roughly 25%.[20,23,32-35] Many patients have concomitantly displayed several of these symptoms.[32,35,36]

Consistent with other authors our indications for reoperation are principally the same as those for primary operation, with the exception that either more marked elevation of serum calcium or more evident symptoms are generally required.[35] In our experience decisions to postpone surgery have generally involved patients with serum calcium values lower than 2.70-2.80 mmol/l. However, even such moderate serum calcium elevation has not been a hindrance in patients with renal stones who can be cured by reoperation. Our indications may be considered liberal but are apparently shared by others.[35] However, it needs to be strongly emphasized that the parathyroid tumor or the eventual multiple tumors in patients with mild hypercalcemia will be considerably smaller in size than commonly reported in reoperative series.[36] Our considerations with respect to these indications have made increase the cuation with which we perform the reoperation rather than to refuse surgery when we consider it needed. Decisions about surgery, however, also depend to a great extent on the adequacy of the primary operation, the age of the patient as well as the results of radiological localization studies. In patients previously operated upon by an inexperienced surgeon the indications are liberal, since the reoperation may be considered merely as a completion of the operative procedure. In contrast, in moderately hypercalcemic patients with previously extensive or already repeated parathyroid operations, including possibly previous mediastinal exploration, we will often try to postpone surgery and await positive localization, knowing that access to the cervical area relates to time elapsed from the primary surgical event. However, a significant rise in serum calcium will often be experienced during follow-up of these patients, thereby favoring operation even in the absence of positive localization. In elderly patients or in patients with complicating illness it should be more crucial to evaluate whether the expected improvement justifies the increased surgical risk. Elderly persons who essentially only feel poorly may represent difficult decisions in this respect and more marked hypercalcemia, i.e. > 2.8 mmol/l or higher, may be required. However, the experience is that when reoperation is undertaken it is more or less uneventful even in these individuals.

Patients with MEN-1 or Familial HPT

Patients with MEN-1 and familial HPT present special problems after failed exploration or recurrent disease. Many of these patients have primarily been operated upon without knowledge of the hereditary aspects of the disorder and the multiglandular involvement has often not been recognized at the time of surgery.[24,29,44,49,61] If the primary operation has been incomplete and hypercalcemia persists, these patients will generally undergo reoperation and subjected to either a classical subtotal parathyroid gland resection or, in the presence of marked four-gland enlargement, to total parathyroidectomy and autotransplantation. Either of these operations will be combined with removal of the thymus and clearance of fat within the central neck compartment. The symptoms and complications are essentially the same as in patients with sporadic primary HPT, and therefore also the indications for surgery.[62] Many of the patients are young and tend to have a high urinary calcium excretion and may therefore be prone to develop renal stones. Moreover, if a patient concomitantly suffers from Zollinger Ellison syndrome, elimination of the hypercalcemia is generally considered important for amelioration of the peptic ulcer disease. Once the MEN-1 patient has been subjected to a complete parathyroid operation, implying either subtotal or the total parathyroidectomy, recurrent disease is likely to be due to ectopic or supernumerary glands.[39] A new exploration will then be more difficult and sometimes should await positive localization unless the hypercalcemia is more marked.[39] (For further details see chapter 7).

TIMING OF REOPERATION

Experience with reoperative parathyroid surgery has demonstrated that timing is essential for safe performance and optimal results. If failure occurs in a patient with severe hypercalcemia and the need to obtain a cure is urgent the patient be referred and evaluated promptly for a second operation. The operation has to be undertaken within a week of the initial surgery since thereafter marked fibrotic adhesions will increase the difficulties of the exploration.[21,35] If more than one week has passed it is generally wise to postpone surgery at least 3 months until the inflammatory reaction after the previous surgery has subsided. If the patient has moderate hypercalcemia, surgery may preferably and without risk be postponed even longer, up to 6 and even 12 months, and during this time the patient can undergo localization studies.

When the indications are clear, surgery can be postponed but not entirely omitted. Thus, patients with mild hypercalcemia without symptoms or with previously extensive or already repeated surgery may be followed for a few years, but in our experience the serum calcium values will generally subsequently rise and establish more urgently the indications for reoperation.

PERSISTENT VS RECURRENT DISEASE

In patients subjected to reoperative parathyroid surgery it is customary to try to determine whether the disease is persistent or recurrent.[23,29-36,39,63-67] The more commonly applied definition of *persistent hypercalcemia* implies that the serum calcium levels have never returned to normal after the neck exploration or that they have risen to abnormally high values already within 6 months after the operation.[4,23,30,34-36,67] Accordingly *recurrent hypercalcemia* indicates reappearance of abnormally elevated serum calcium values after more than 6 months of postoperative normocalcemia. Recurrence should in a stricter sense be consistent with subsequent development of abnormal hyperfunction in gland or glands which were normal at the time of the initial operation.[63] However, development of hypercalcemia should require considerably longer than 6 months, and it is certainly intriguing that surgically caused ischemia of an abnormal gland has resulted in temporary normalization of the serum calcium value and recurrent hypercalcemia.[10] It is moreover not always easy to distinguish between persistence or recurrence when patients have not been followed closely after surgery. Thus, the definitions may often be theoretically insufficient but are still considered of value by allowing comparison between different patient series. Persistent hypercalcemia is generally the result of surgical failure, due to inability to identify the prevailing parathyroid abnormality or to deal with it accurately at surgery. Most commonly an adenoma has been overlooked and more occasionally hyperplasia has not been recognized or has not been adequatelyresected.[1,19,23,61] Persistent hypercalcemia has generally comprised 80-90% of patients undergoing parathyroid reoperation.[11,19,23] Recurrent hypercalcemia has been a more rare cause of such operation, but the incidence may be considerably higher if many MEN-1 patients are included in the series, and may then amount to 10-20% of the reoperations.[10,23,30,39]

CAUSES OF FAILED PRIMARY OPERATIONS

The most common cause of *persistent hypercalcemia* is surgical inability to visualize the parathyroid glands at the initial neck exploration.[1,3-12,19-21,23,31-39,52,54,63-66] The majority of missed adenomas has subsequently been retrieved from normal locations and fewer have been ectopic. The inability to recognize and adequately resect hyperplastic glands has generally also been related to inadequate glandular visualization. These failures thus commonly result from surgical inexperience, and ensuing reoperations have often revealed that the areas where normal or ectopic glands should be searched for have not been explored.[19,20,23,32,54] Misleading or absent histopathology have sometimes contributed to the error.[12,21,23,32] Occasionally incomplete excision of an abnormal gland has been the cause of persistent hypercalcemia.[21,23]

Recurrent hypercalcemia has been most commonly associated with multiglandular disease.[1,3-5,10,11,20,21,23,24,30,34-39,44,63-67] This has been related to the inability to visualize four parathyroid glands at surgery, whereby hyperplasia may not have been detected and adequately resected. Misleading or absent histopathology may have contributed also to this error.[23] Many recurrences, however, originate in glands which were normal at the time of the initial surgery and some have been caused by development of an abnormality in a supernumerary gland.[8,52,63] Recurrent hypercalcemia most frequently occurs in patients with MEN-1 syndrome, either early or with a delay of several years after the primary operation.[11,23,30,39] Recurrence in patients previously operated on for true adenomas is more rare, but has occasionally occurred due to growth of a new adenoma generally with considerable delay after the primary operation.[8,10,23] Occasionally recurrent HPT has been related to remnant hypertrophy in a patient subjected to subtotal parathyroid resection, or hyperfunction in autotransplanted parathyroid tissue.[38,67,68] Rare instances of recurrent disease have resulted from violation of a tumor capsule during a primary operation, with resulting spillage and implantation of parathyroid cells.[23]

RADIOLOGICAL LOCALIZATION STUDIES

It was previously a more or less unanimous experience that radiological localization studies frequently failed to correctly identify the abnormal gland or glands prior to reoperation and the majority of patients therefore had to undergo surgery without positive localization.[1,3,4,9-12,20,23,25-28,33,35,38,39,66] Under such circumstances previous operative notes and the imaginativeness of the surgeon executing the secondary operation can sometimes direct the search to the appropriate areas, but generally a meticulous and complete exploration of the neck and sometimes also the mediastinum is required in order to identify and conclusively deal with the lesion.[1] Recently the efficacy of particularly noninvasive radiological localization studies has increased considerably and consequently such studies have been extensively utilized in patients scheduled for reoperative parathyroid surgery.[69,70] (Review of these methods and additional references are provided in chapter 5).

Most surgeons utilize a combination of noninvasive methods prior to reoperation and perform invasive studies only when the other methods fail. Presently the more efficient of the noninvasive methods are percutanous ultrasonography (US), computed tomography (CT), tallium/technetium scintigraphy and more recently also positron-emission tomography (PET).[69-71] Since the results of the noninvasive studies are additive it should be important to use them in combination. The accuracy of both US and CT has increased in our experience and these methods will reveal approximately 50% of the abnormal glands prior to reoperation. It is crucial that the radiological studies include also the sites where ectopic parathyroid glands may be located. Thus, both CT and US examinations should scan the submandibular region and the area around the carotid artery bifurcation, where unusual undescended glands may hide. The examinations should also include the vascular sheath and the surrounding areas all the way down to the clavicle. CT is particularly valuable for visualization of mediastinal glands and the examination should encompass the middle mediastinum where rare glands may reside. Tallium/technetium scintigraphy has generally been the least awarding of these methods, but may reveal additional glands in the most unusual, ectopic locations. Both CT and US will also provide an image of the anatomy of the neck region, so that thyroid abnormalities, which may be important to be aware of at surgery can be identified. Magnetic resonance tomography (MRT) will also provide an image of the neck region and mediastinum and since it can detect additional glands its use should be considered if the other investigations are negative. More recently in our experience PET investigations have the highest sensitivity when compared with the other methods.[71] Development of PET may be promising for the future, but the method must be combined with CT for imaging of anatomy. If glandular localization remains equivocal after the noninvasive studies selective venous catheterization and sampling for determination of the PTH concentration in vein effluents of the area will be performed. This investigation may provide correct localization of the side of lesion, but is associated with false positive results since the venous drainage especially of the lower neck may occasionally pass over to the contralateral side. Our experience with arteriography has even in the hands of specially trained radiologists been unrewarding.

If localization studies are negative but firm indications for reoperation still exist surgery will be undertaken in any case. However, in patients subjected to several previous operations positive radiological localization may be considered more crucial; surgery may be postponed and new attempts of glandular imaging may be undertaken after a period follow-up.

SURGICAL ANATOMY

The anatomical distribution of abnormal glands in patients subjected to parathyroid reoperation could be expected to differ from glands recovered during primary cervical explorations, since surgical failure is more likely to occur with glands in abnormal locations. Variation in this respect is, however, essentially related to the number of cases referred after previous explorations by more or less inexperienced surgeons.[1,3-5,10,23,32,33,35-39,65] Unusual anatomical locations have been more common in cases with recurrent than in those with persistent disease, as well as in patients with multiglandular involvement and familial, MEN-1 related HPT.[39] The reported distribution of abnormal glands may also reflect the efficacy of radiological localization methods, since patients with positive localization are more likely to be accepted for repeat surgery. Nevertheless, the overwhelming experience from reoperative parathyroid surgery is that even under these circumstances a majority of abnormal glands will be retrieved from normal locations or from the most common ectopic positions. Thus, around 40-50% of tumors originating in *superior parathyroid* glands have been found to occupy a normal position, attached to the dorsal aspects of the superior thyroid pole or situated slightly behind the thyroid, enveloped in layers of pretracheal fascia[1,3-5,10,23,33,35-39,65,74] (Fig. 8.1). Superior glands may also be located on the medial surface of the upper thyroid lobe, but few have been found medial to the superior thyroid artery. Reflecting a suggested displacement of the enlarged, superior parathyroid around 20% of such tumors have been retrieved at reoperation from the tracheoesophageal groove or the retropharyngeal/retroesophageal space and as many as 40% from the posterior superior mediastinum.[1,3-5,10,23,33,35-39,65,72-74] Altogether these locations have generally comprised up to 50-70% of the superior abnormal glands retrieved at reoperation (Figs. 8.1 and 8.2).

Consistent with the greater variation in distribution of normal inferior glands, the location of *inferior parathyroid* tumors has been variable also in reoperative series.[1,3-5,10,23,33,35-39,65,74] Unusual locations of abnormal inferior glands are often described in such series, but probably represent selection of difficult cases rather than in vivo displacement of the enlarged inferior gland.[1,73] The majority, comprising around 40% of the abnormal inferior glands have been found close to the inferior thyroid pole or within the thyreothymic ligament, while approximately 20% have been in the cervical thymus and nearly 30% deeper in the anterior mediastinum and then generally in the thymus[1,3,23,35-39,65,74-78] (Figs. 8.1 and 8.2). Even in reoperative series only few inferior abnormal glands have been in intrathyroidal or undescended positions or within the mediastinum outside the thymus.[74-89] Only occasionally have either superior or inferior parathyroids been located within the carotid sheath.[35-39,72,73] They have also been located around the large vessels in the mediastinum, whereas inferior ones have been located around the origin of these vessels from the aorta, while rare superior tumors have been retrieved from the middle mediastinum.[72-78,85-89]

Tumors originating in *supernumerary glands* have been overrepresented in reoperative series, and have been commonly found in the thymus and sometimes in the mediastinal part of this gland.[1,4,10,35,38,39,90-93] Occasional supernumerary lesions have occurred in the neck in a position between the normal locations of the superior and inferior glands.

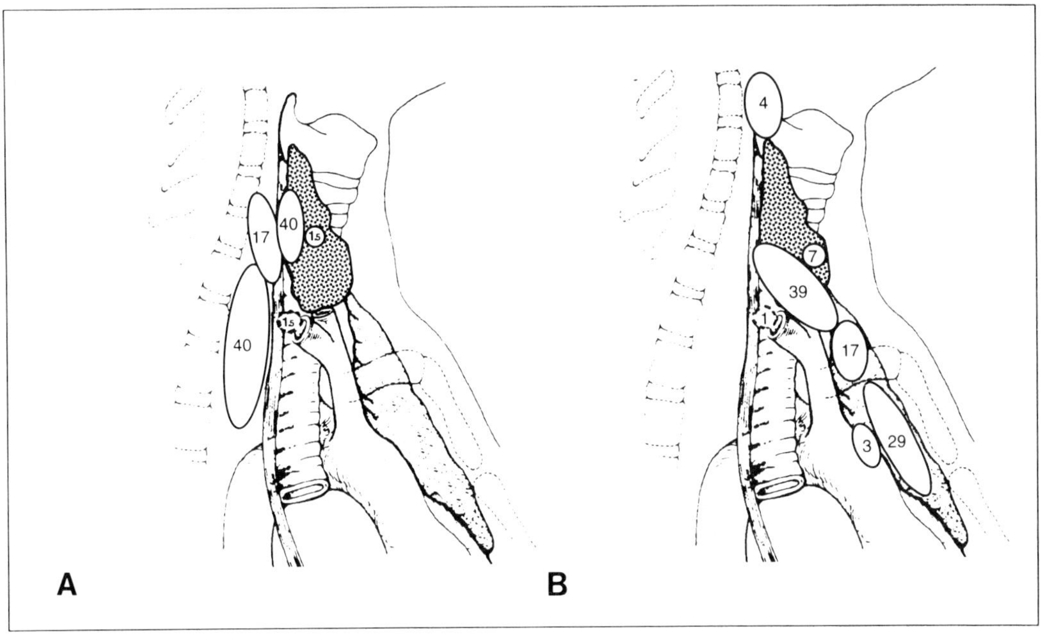

Fig. 8.1. Anatomic distribution (per cent) of abnormal parathyroid glands retrieved at reoperation for primary HPT by pooling and approximation of data from Wang,[1] Edis et al,[3] McCarity et al,[33] Grant et al,[35] Cheung et al,[38] Levin et al,[39] Rothmund et al,[65] Åkerström et al.[23] (A) Superior glands: Normal position 40, retroesophageal or tracheoesophageal groove 17, posterior superior mediastinum 40, intrathyroidal 1,5, carotid sheath 1,5. (B) Inferior glands: Normal position around inferior thyroid pole or within thyreothymic ligament 39, cervical thymus 17, mediastinal thymus 29, mediastinal outside thymus 3, intrathyroidal 7, undescended 4, carotid sheath 1.

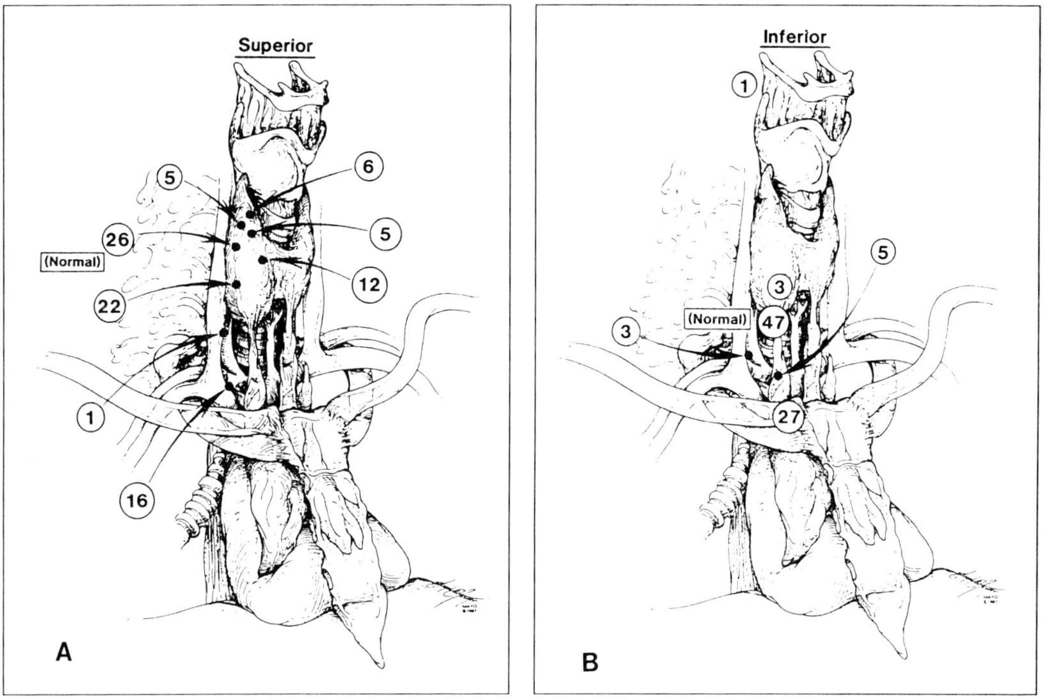

Fig. 8.2. Location and number of abnormal parathyroid glands excised at reoperation. (A) Superior glands: 26 normal position, 22 tracheoesophageal groove, 16 posterior superior mediastinum, 12 retroesophageal, 6 medial to upper pole of thyroid, 1 in carotid sheath, 5 under thyroid capsule, 5 intrathyroidal. (B) Inferior glands: 47 normal, 5 cervical thymus, 27 mediastinal thymus, 3 within carotid sheath, 3 intrathyroidal, 1 undescended. Reprinted with permission from Grant C et al.[74]

Other unusual glandular abnormalities, such as *bilobated, multilobated or divided glands* have also been the cause of operative failures, but have been described infrequently.[23]

MEDIASTINAL PARATHYROID GLANDS

Dissection studies have demonstrated that parathyroid glands occur commonly in the thymus, but deeply within the mediastinal thymus in only 2% of normal individuals.[94-96] Such studies have also revealed that proper supernumerary glands with a size equivalent to a normal gland as well as dispersed rudiments of parathyroid tissue may reside within the thymus. In particular, patients with parathyroid hyperplasia might be expected to have a high incidence of mediastinal parathyroid lesions.[96]

The first reported median sternotomy for removal of an abnormal parathyroid gland was performed by Drs. E. Churchill and O. Cope in 1932.[97] Subsequently several authors reported retrieval of parathyroid tumors from the medistinal thymus in patients with HPT.[1,4,23,28,72-78,85-89,98-103] However, the majority of the mediastinal parathyroid lesions has later proven to be accessible from the neck at the initial cervical exploration if careful dissection of the retrosternal anterior superior mediastinum has been undertaken.[1,3,28,34-39,72-78,85-89,98-103] Reports from primary operations in patients with HPT have revealed parathyroid tumors with deep mediastinal location in no more than 1-2% of cases, which compares well with the location of glands in normal individuals.[72,73,87] In reoperative series, however, mediastinotomy has been needed in 10-20% of patients and this overrepresentation probably has been due to selection of difficult cases for the repeat surgery.[1,3,4,19,29,30,33,35,36,75,76,99] Wang has proposed that some of the tumors which required mediastinotomy for removal could initially have been reached in the thoracic inlet, but due to operative division of thymic attachments to the thyroid during the primary operation they slipped deeper into the mediastinum.[1] The majority, comprising 80-90% of reported medistinal parathyroid tumors have been adenomas.[1,75-78,85-89,98-103] There may, however, have been an underrated prevalence in patients with hyperplasia and the possibility to retrieve hyperplastic glands this location should be higher especially if MEN-1 cases are included in the series.[34-39,72,73,75-78,104] Most of the mediastinal lesions have their origin in inferior parathyroid glands and occur in the anterior mediastinum.[1,73,75-78,85-89,98-103] Approximately 80% of these glands will be located within thymic tissue, most often in the vicinity of the innominate vein.[1,75-78,89] A minority, 20%, are located outside the thymic capsule, generally behind it, anterior to or around the aortic arch or the origin of the large vessels, and such lesions may be situated to the left of the aortic arch[73,75-78,89] (Figs. 8.3 and 8.4). Some mediastinal tumors have occurred on the pleural surfaces, near the hili of the lungs, anterior to the pulmonary arteries or on the pericardial surface, occasionally with proximity to the left auricle.[1,23,72-78,85,89] Very rarely have they been reported within the pericardium.[72,73,85]

The vascular supply to mediastinal parathyroid tumors may originate from the inferior thyroid artery, whereby a large vascular pedicle may be seen entering the anterior superior mediastinum.[77] More commonly these are lesions supplied by mediastinal vessels originating from the internal mammary artery.[77]

Approximate+ scintigraphy or even angiography, but occasionally technetium thymic cysts or lymph nodes technetium been reported to provide false positive images.[76,77,102] In cases with reliable preoperative localization to the mediastinum the surgeon may perform an immediate median sternotomy. However, since the majority of abnormal parathyroid glands occur within the neck it is more common to postpone the mediastinotomy until a new complete neck exploration has been performed and then undertake a combined cervical and mediastinal exploration.[72,78,98] The combined approach also has the advantage of providing excellent exposure of the anatomic recesses behind the clavicles at the level of the thoracic inlet.[77]

MIDDLE MEDIASTINAL PARATHYROID GLANDS

Recent reports have emphasized the possibility that abnormal parathyroid glands may occasionally be located within the middle mediastinum.[86-88] This compartment contains the heart, the ascending aorta, the lower half of the superior vena cava, the pulmonary artery and veins, the azygos vein and the phrenic nerves. Parathyroid tumors have been found in the aortopulmonary window, or in sites posterior to the aorta or the pulmonary arteries and ventral to the tracheal carina or one of the bronchi[23,86-88,105-107] (Fig. 8.5). Parathyroid tumors in the aortopulmonary window may be readily exposed but they may be easily confused with pigment loaded lymph glands which are prevalent in this area.[88] A parathyroid lesion usually stands out and may be distinguished from these lymph glands by its characteristic brown color, glistening surface and loose attachments to the surrounding fat.[88] The area behind the aortic arch and the pulmonary artery would supposedly not be explored unless preoperative localization has clearly visualized a suspect tumor with this location.[88] Access to this area requires retraction of the great vessels and eventually also ligation and division of the innomminate vein.[88]

UNDESCENDED PARATHYROID GLANDS

In 1979 Edis et al emphasized the significance of an undescended parathyroid adenoma as a possible cause of primary HPT.[83] The authors clarified that due to a defect in embryological development an inferior gland could remain undescended high up in the neck at the level of the angle of the mandibule or the hyoid bone. Concomitantly the thymus or parts of it

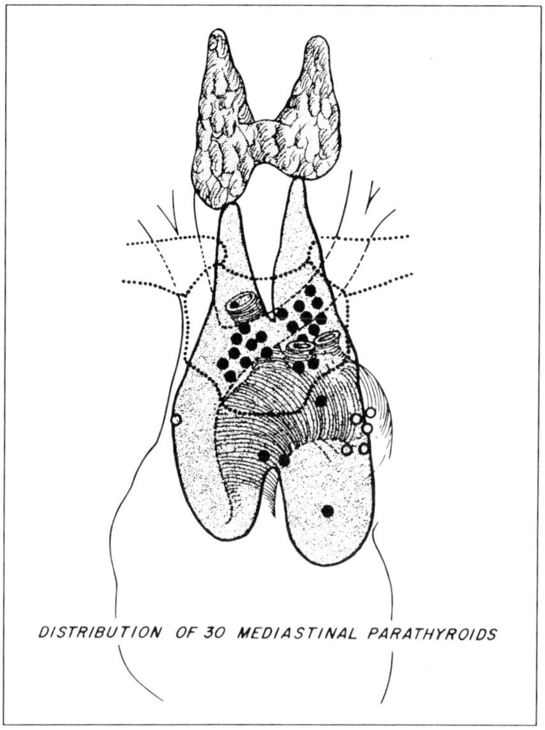

Fig. 8.3. Schematic representation of sites of 30 mediastinal parathyroid glands (both primary operation and reoperation). Solid dots indicate glands enclosed in thymus; open dots, those behind thymus. Reprinted with permission from Wang CA.[1]

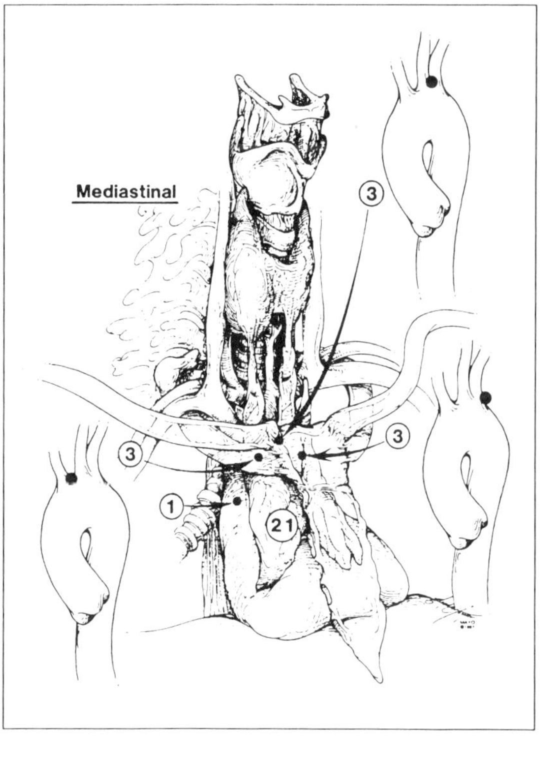

would generally fail to descend normally in which case the parathyroid tumor would be surrounded by a variable amount of thymic tissue and parathymic fat. Such an undescended parathyroid gland has often been named a parathymus because of its developmental association with the thymus.[83,108,109] Most undescended glands have been located medial to the carotid artery and the jugular vein, usually adjacent to, but sometimes also included within the carotid sheath. Undescended parathyroids have been uncommon in autopsy series of normal subjects,[94-96] and they have also been unusual in primary explorations for HPT, with an estimated prevalence of probably less than 1%.[21,33,39,73,83,84] However, due to referral selection such glands have been considerably more common in some reoperative series and have sometimes comprised up to 7-9% of inferior parathyroid tumors.[1,3,5,35,36,83,84,109-111]

The presence of an undescended parathyroid gland is important to emphasize in reoperative patients and particularly the possibility of imaging these glands by preoperative localization procedures.[84] Noninvasive studies such as US and CT, and to some extent also thallium/technetium scintigraphy, are often additive in this respect, and may together accurately identify 60-70% of the undescended glands if images are obtained up to the level of the mandibule.[84] The glands may also be identified by arteriography if the superior thyroid artery is cannulated.[84] Most undescended glands reported this far have been parathyroid adenomas, but certainly enlarged hyperplastic glands can be retrieved from the same position[1,3,5,35,36,83,84,109,111] (own unpublished observation). If a parathyroid tumor is preoperatively localized in an undescended position it may be best to

Fig. 8.4. Location and number of mediastinal parathyroid glands requiring sternotomy for excision at reoperation: 21 mediastinal thymus, 3 at origin of each of the aortic arch vessels, 1 at tracheal carina. Reprinted with permission from Grant C et al.[74]

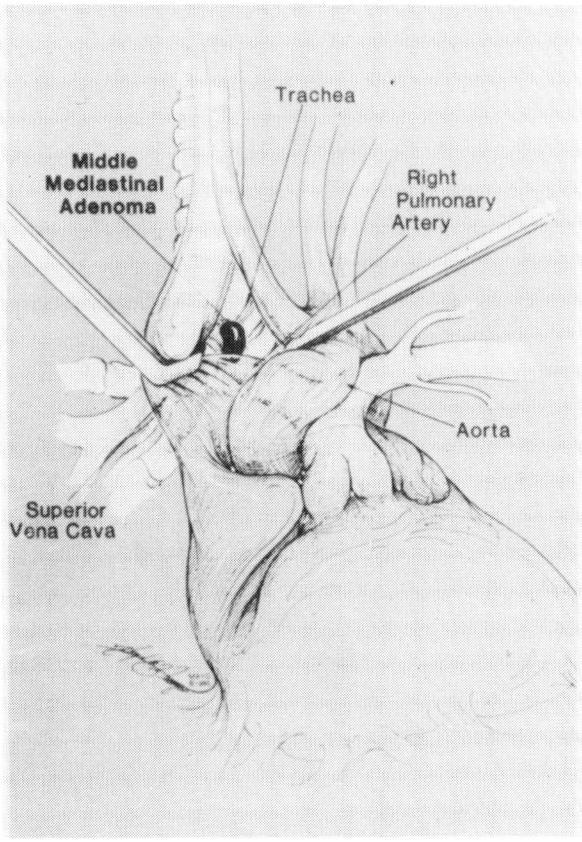

Fig. 8.5. Middle mediastinal parathyroid gland, anterior to the right main bronchus and posterior to the right pulmonary artery. Reprinted with permission from Curley IR et al.[88]

avoid a complete reexploration of the neck and instead try to deliver the gland via a more direct approach.[36,84]

INTRATHYROIDAL PARATHYROID GLANDS

A close association between the thyroid and the parathyroid glands during embryological development implies that the parathyroids often remain in intimate contact with the surface of the thyroid gland in adult life.[94-96] Such parathyroids are often concealed within the pretracheal fasciae layers and may be separated from the thyroid first when the external fascia layer has been detached and occasionally not until the surgical thyroid capsulae is cut open.[96] The parathyroids may also often be hidden in crevices of the thyroid and especially in connection with a nodular goiter may they be partially engulfed within protuberant thyroid tissue.[96] Fibrosis occurring after neck exploration may also contribute to the entrapment of a parathyroid.[82] Glands concealed in this way are generally not considered to truly intrathyroidal, but it may certainly be difficult to distinguish between the varieties. True intrathyroidal glands have been rare in autopsy series obviously because of difficulties associated with the demonstration of normal-sized glands in this location.[94-96]

The incidence of intrathyroidal glands in patients undergoing primary parathyroid surgery has varied, between 0.5 to 3% or more, but they should be uncommon since comprehensive patient series have often failed to report their presence.[72,73,80] Among patients subjected to reoperation the incidence of such glands has been even more variable, with figures commonly around 5% but occasionally also higher.[1,3,21,33,35,36,38,39] Most intrathyroidal glands reported this far have been adenomas,[79-82,112-118] but the incidence may be even higher in hyperplasia.[39,104] An unusual MEN-1 patient has been described where the thyroid lobe on one side contained two intrathyroidal pathological lesions.[80] Other reports have described the presence of bilateral or supernumerary intrathyroidal glands as well as an occasional case of intrathyroidal parathyroid carcinoma.[80,81,117] There has been considerable controversy whether the superior or the inferior parathyroids will most commonly be found in an intrathyroidal location, but apparently this may occur with either.[23,35,79,80,82] Wang reported superior parathyroids in intrathyroidal positions and suggested that during embryological development a superior parathyroid could be entrapped and incorporated into the thyroid.[79,85] Most other authors have suggested that inferior parathyroid glands were more likely to occupy an intrathyroidal position.[17,73,80] Consistent with the latter proposal intrathyroidal glands are most commonly found within the lower parts of the thyroid, from the middle of this gland to its inferior pole.[80]

During investigations prior to reoperative parathyroid surgery an intrathyroidal parathyroid gland may sometimes be detected by percutaneous US or CT and may then be subjected to guided fine needle biopsy for PTH determination in the aspirate or cytological examination.[69,70,119,120] An intrathyroidal gland may sometimes also be palpated intraoperatively and may mimic a thyroid nodule, but it might be nonpalpable and may then be demonstrated by intraoperative US, or by incisions into the thyroid parenchyma.[73,80] An intrathyroidal parathyroid a characteristic smooth, yellow-brownish, glistening surface, in clear contrast to the hard, irregular, and reddish thyroid tissue. Incisions have to be performed cautiously, since penetration of the parathyroid tumor capsule may result in implantation.[80] The intrathyroidal parathyroid may be dissected free or removed by resection of the lower thyroid pole.[80]

Histological diagnosis of an intrathyroidal tumor may present difficulties, especially if the gland consists of parenchymal cells arranged in a follicular pattern, whereby it may mimic a follicular thyroid tumor.[80,81] Immunostaining for thyroglobulin and PTH may aid in this diagnosis, but the PTH stainings have sometimes been difficult, and specific monoclonal antiparathyroid antibodies may be superior for the discrimination.[80,81,121,122] The differential diagnosis may also include medullary thyroid carcinoma, since parathyroid adenomas may contain amyloid.[81] Staining for calcitonin and carcinoembryonic antigen (CEA) may solve this problem, since either or both of these markers will be positive in medullary carcinoma.[81]

UNUSUAL ECTOPIC LOCATIONS

The presence of parathyroid glands within the *carotid sheath* should be rare, since Gilmour found this location to comprise only 0.25% of superior glands, whereas inferior ones were never seen in this position.[94] Norris first drew attention to this site as a possibly location for abnormal parathyroid glands, and subsequently several authors have reported similar findings.[19,35,39,73,123-126] The origin of parathyroid tumors within the carotid sheath is not always clear, and Grant et al recognized both superior and inferior glands in this location.[35] Levin and Clark suggested that parathyroid tumors within the sheath should represent inferior ones, while those posterior to it were denoted superior glands.[39]

Parathyroid tumors located in the *lateral cervical triangle* of the neck, i.e. lateral to the carotid sheath, have been described occasionally.[72,73,126,127] These glands should be exceedingly rare since only one such case was encountered in 1400 operations for primary HPT.[72] Udekwu et al described two such tumors retrieved from reoperative patients; both involved supernumerary glands and were thought to represent superior ones.[126,127]

SUPERNUMERARY PARATHYROID GLANDS

The accurate number of supernumerary parathyroid glands in normal individuals still remains somewhat uncertain, and the significance of such glands in patients with HPT is even more difficult to assess. Dissection studies have revealed supernumerary glands in up to 13% of normal individuals.[94-96] These consisted of proper supernumerary glands as well as split or rudimentary ones, and the majority of them were concealed within the thymus, but also occurred in the typical fat pad surrounding the normal parathyroids as well as occasionally between the normal locations of superior and inferior glands.[96] It is likely that dissection studies will underestimate this incidence and there are indeed embryological prerequisites for more frequent occurrence, particularly likely to be of clinical significance in patients with hyperplasia.[96,104,128-130] Most commonly an additional fifth gland is present, but occasional individuals have had six glands or more, and up to 17 glands have been asynchronously removed in a patient with MEN-1.[49,96,129] It is obvious that the presence of supernumerary glands in patients with HPT is not always detected or of significance if pathology involves only glands in normal location.

Several authors have drawn attention to the presence of parathyroid tumors affecting a fifth supernumerary gland in patients with primary HPT, and have demonstrated that many of these glands were located within the mediastinal thymus. Subsequent series verified such tumors as an important entity in HPT.[85,89-93,131-133] Abnormal supernumerary parathyroid glands have been revealed in patients subjected to reoperative parathyroid surgery, but with variable incidence, which in some series has amounted to 3-10%.[3,10,34-39] The majority of these supernumerary parathyroid tumors have been diagnosed as adenomas and have been retrieved from the mediastinum, but some of them have occurred in normal or other ectopic positions.[34-39] In sporadic primary parathyroid hyperplasia supernumerary glands have been demonstrated in up to 13%, and have been emphasized as an important cause of both persistent and recurrent disease.[45,72,73,130] Levin and Clark demonstrated hyperfunctioning supernumerary glands in 20% of their reoperative patients, and many of the tumors caused recurrent disease in patients with MEN-1 associated parathyroid hyperplasia.[39] Inability to identify supernumerary glands may thus be a very significant cause of operative failure when dealing with the parathyroid lesion of the MEN-1 syndrome.[23,39,49,104] The high incidence of supernumerary glands implies strongly that the neck exploration in HPT should not be terminated in patients with hyperplasia until four glands have been identified and also all possible sites of ectopic glands have been adequately explored. This is particularly important in the MEN-1 patients and emphasizes that excision of the thymus and clearance of fat in the neck compartment is necessary part of both primary and reoperative procedures in these patients. Patients with secondary HPT may harbor supernumerary parathyroids in up to 15-40%, emphasizing further that the embryological parathyroid remnants may be stimulated to grow to clinically significant lesions.[129,132,133]

PREOPERATIVE SEEDING/ IMPLANTATION OF PARATHYROID TISSUE

In 1943 Burk autotransplanted a piece of a parathyroid adenoma into the cervical strap muscles, and the patient 2 years later returned with recurrence due to growth of the implanted glandular specimen.[134] This observation demonstrated that small pieces of benign parathyroid tissue had an unusual ability to survive in a muscle bed. A subsequent report by Black and Ackerman in 1959 described recurrent hypercalcemia due to cell seeding from a ruptured parathyroid adenoma and growth of multiple brown nodules at the site of the original lesion.[135] Several authors have reported similar cases among reoperative patients with both primary and secondary HPT.[136-142] Sokol reviewed the literature and found 11 such patients, and the present authors have reported three cases and recently experienced another.[138,143] The majority have been associated with recurrent disease and only few with persistence.[23,138,143] The implantation has been caused by violation of the tumor capsule and glandular rupture or deliberate transection of a parathyroid gland during surgery.[135-143] The recurrent disease has occurred 1-23, mean 9 years after the initial operation, and the patients have represented difficult reoperative cases since the lesions have invariably been impossible to localize preoperatively.[143] Implantation has typically resulted in multiple, a few millimeter large brownish or occasionally slightly grayish nodules, which often have been surrounded by prominent fibrosis.[135-143] The case we recently encountered lacked these typical demarcated nodules and instead revealed vaguely visible large islets of parathyroid tissue with a slight brown tinge but otherwise extremely difficult to distinguish grossly from the surrounding fat of the neck. Histologically the lesions have generally lacked encapsulation, but have exhibited a tendency to invade fat or muscle bundles and have generally been surrounded by pronounced fibrosis.[143] These features have sometimes made discrimination from parathyroid carcinoma difficult, but the implanted benign tissue has typically lacked mitoses, clear signs of invasion and has not been associated with metastases.[138,143] The characteristic, proliferating parenchymal cell nodules lacking fat cells and the surrounding fibrosis serve to distinguish the implanted abnormal tissue from the condition where ectopic foci of normal parathyroid rudiments are embryologically dispersed within the thymus or the fat of the neck.[130,136,138,143] The implantation and subsequent growth of implanted lesions seem to be particularly prone to occur in association with larger parathyroid tumors and may thus represent an inherent aggressiveness of the primary lesion.[144] Several of the reported cases have occurred in association with rupture of parathyroid cysts.[137,143]

Reoperation is generally very difficult in cases with implantation.[138,143] It has been suggested that they should receive more or less the same treatment as parathyroid carcinoma, implying that the area of implantation is cleared of all suspect nodules and that the surrounding fibrosis and fat are removed concomitant with hemithyroidectomy.[143] It has also been claimed that the recurrent laryngeal nerve may need to be sacrificed during these dissections but in the cases we encountered the nerve could be dissected and preserved.[138,143] When seeding has occurred in wound or strap, muscles complete excision of these structures has been required.[144] Provided that clearance of the appropriate area has been efficiently executed, the patients may have a relatively favorable likelihood of cure by surgery.[138] This is in contrast to cases where similar implants have occurred in association with parathyroid carcinoma, where recurrence should invariably occur and generally within a shorter time period.[138]

Recognition of the risks associated with incautious removal of parathyroid lesions suggests that extreme care be taken to avoid capsule rupture or crushing of the tissue in association with surgery. Parathyroid tumors must be gently handled by their pedicle and all dissection should always diligently follow capsular surfaces of the lesions. Whether routine biopsy of abnormal parathyroid glands could result in this type of implantation has not been demonstrated but caution is appropriate. Growth of spilled normal tissue probably does not occur since this would require growth stimulation or presence of genetic abnormality.

LOCALLY RECURRENT PARATHYROID TUMORS

Growth of Autografted Tissue

Wells and other authors have developed and refined the technique of parathyroid autotransplantation and demonstrated that both normal and abnormal tissue will survive and function appropriately when grafted to an appropriate site.[145] The technique of autotransplantation has therefore been combined with total parathyroidectomy in primary as well as reoperative treatment of parathyroid hyperplasia, but also more generally in association with reoperative surgery when an excised parathyroid tumor is likely to represent a patient's last remaining gland.[11,36,146-148] It has subsequently been demonstrated that proliferation within the autografted parathyroid tissue, and concomitant functional disturbance may cause recurrent hypercalcemia in up to 33% of patients who have received such transplants.[149] Occasionally growth has been remarkable within the autografted tissues, originating from either adenoma or hyperplastic glands.[144,150-153] Removal of the autografts from implantation sites in muscles have sometimes been associated with considerable difficulties and occasionally this has required extensive muscle resection of, for instance, the sternocleidoid muscle.[144] It appears unlikely that the excessive growth is related to the transplantation per se, but rather that rapidly proliferating tissue has been selected for the graft. The sternocleidoid muscle may thus be used for implantation of normal parathyroids which have been devascularized in association with thyroid surgery, but appears unsuitable for implantation of abnormal parathyroid tissue. The forearm muscle should be more appropriate, but it is also possible that sites other than muscle may be advantageous because of easier retrieval of the implant.[154] However, careful selection of tissue for implantation, implying that the smallest gland in each patient is utilized seems to reduce or possibly eliminate the risk of this complication.[155] More commonly the growth of such autografts is less impressive and it may in fact be a difficult clinical problem to determine whether the recurrent hypercalcemia is graft dependent or caused by residual parathyroid tissue within the neck. US and thallium/technetium scintigraphy may be used to identify expanding nodules or activity within the transplanted tissue and a recently described arm occlusion test may help to verify that this is the source of the increased PTH secretion.[156] If the transplant is the likely cause of hypercalcemia it can be excised, whereby the presence of nodular growth at the site, as well as histological verification of proliferating parathyroid tissue substantiate that the operation will probably normalize the hypercalcemia. Lack of effect is common and suggests that remaining hyperfunctioning parathyroid tissue prevails in the neck. (See chapter 9)

Incomplete Tumor Excision

Another type of failure which may result in locally recurrent tumor is incomplete excision of the original parathyroid tumor.[23,110,137,144] This may occur when a parathyroid tumor is bi-, or multilobated or unusually elongated (Fig. 8.6). In other cases a more or less impressive tumor remnant may have been inadvertently left behind because it lies within or under the thyroid gland, between vessels or under the recurrent laryngeal nerve. A remnant may also have been left when bleeding obscured the field during surgery. This may result in persistent as well as recurrent hypercalcemia, since even tiny glandular remnants may grow to clinically significant lesions after years of observation.[23] We have sometimes encountered such glandular remnants adjacent to the laryngeal entrance of the recurrent laryngeal nerve where the surgeon may have been particularly cautious with the dissection. Such glandular remnants may be difficult to recover during reoperation, but it may be recommendable to approach the tumor remnant from a side opposite to the nerve and preserve nerve function by dissection close to the tumor capsule. Some of these tumor remnants have elicited considerable fibrosis and since they sometimes appear hard and white-gray they can be difficult to distinguish from parathyroid carcinoma. Histology will frequently reveal fibrosis and lack of encapsulation, but in other aspects the lesions will generally exhibit clearly benign features.

Remnant Recurrence

Remnant recurrence has been reported to cause either persistent or recurrent hypercalcemia in up to 14% of patients subjected to subtotal parathyroidectomy for primary parathyroid hyperplasia.[38,157] Although occasionally such remnants have exhibited remarkable growth potential this is probably rare and persistent or recurrent hypercalcemia in these patients are more likely to result from previously unidentified or supernumerary glands. Consequently this type of operative failure has been infrequently reported in series of reoperative patients with HPT.[38] The likelihood of remnant growth should be higher in pa-

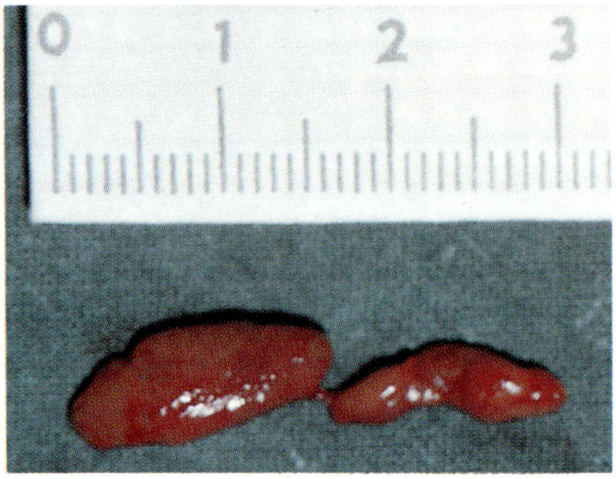

Fig. 8.6. Bilobated parathyroid adenoma, part of which may easily be left behind.

tients with the MEN-1 syndrome. As more marked propensity for growth is reflected in more or less impressive glandular enlargement, the risk for remnant recurrence should be markedly reduced if apparently normal-sized parathyroids were routinely selected as the residual tissue in conjunction with the subtotal parathyroid resection. If considerable growth of the remnant is identified at reoperation—and this is likely to represent the patient's last remaining tissue—it seems advisable to excise the remnant and use part of it for immediate or delayed autotransplantation (see below).[148]

HISTOPATHOLOGY

In recent series 80-90% of the patients with primary HPT have had single parathyroid adenomas as the cause of the disease. It is consequently likely that persistent HPT due to failure to appropriately visualize the glands at surgery also commonly involves an overlooked single adenoma. In contrast, the most likely cause of disease in the minority of patients who have recurrent HPT has been hyperplasia or multiple gland disease. A summary of a few selected, more or less comprehensive series of patients undergoing reoperation have denoted the following causes for *persistent HPT:*[21,23,34,39]

- missed adenomas 60-70%
- inadequately resected hyperplasia 20-30%
- double adenomas 10-20%
- carcinoma 1-2%.

Utilizing the same sources the causes for recurrent HPT have encompassed:

- inadequately resected hyperplasia 70-80%
- incomplete adenoma excision 5-10%
- recurrent (asynchronous) adenoma 5-10%
- seeding (or carcinoma) 2-5%.

Many authors report increasing incidence of hyperplasia or multiple adenomas in patients subjected to reoperation and these different entities of multiple gland disease have in some series involved up to 30-40% of reoperations.[10,11,21,23,30,32,34-39] This has especially been common if MEN-1 patients have been overrepresented in the series.[11,23,39] (For details concerning parathyroid carcinoma see chapter 10).

REOPERATION

The description below particularly emphasizes technical aspects of parathyroid reoperations, details of which have been previously provided by other authors.[1,5,10,11,17,19,21,35,36,61,66,110,147,148,158,159] Prior to reoperative surgery the *vocal cord function* always needs to be carefully investigated by indirect laryngoscopy. Review of the patient history and medical records is undertaken with the particular purpose of revealing a possible transient vocal cord paralysis in association with the previous surgery, since this may indicate that a laryngeal nerve may be especially vulnerable during the subsequent surgery. Finally, by examining once again the notes from previous operations, reports on histopathology and the results of localization studies the surgeon sets out a plan for the forthcoming operation. Decisions about the most convenient approach in reoperative cases often requires careful consideration together with imaginativeness and intuition, but may be most awarding in directing the search towards the appropriate sites. The patient is prepared for the exploration and obtains adequate information about the planned operation. Appropriate prophylaxis against thrombosis is provided as well as liberal preoperative antibiotics, if the procedure is expected to be long or involves mediastinotomy. Thus, even if a direct approach to an expected lesion is attempted the surgeon should always be prepared to undertake an extensive exploration of the cervical area as well as a complete mediastinal dissection. With increasingly effective parathyroid imaging, and more reliable localization, reoperation in HPT may sometimes be unexpectedly expeditious and occasionally even shorter than the primary exploration.

In the operating room care is taken to position the patient with maximal neck extension and shoulder support. The skin is cleaned from the jaw to the umbilicus to allow concomitant cervical exploration and mediastinotomy. The neck is entered via the previous skin incision, which is excised if unattractive. Not unusually the incision is too short or placed too high in the neck and may need widening. Dissection of superior and inferior platysma/skin flaps is performed by electrocautery with the tissue under traction and with extension from above the thyroid cartilage to the sternal notch. Additional exploration depends on whether a direct approach can be undertaken to deliver a previously localized lesion or if complete exploration of the neck is needed.

Frozen section verification of excised tumors is an integral part of any of these procedures (see chapter 3 for details of pathology).

Direct Approach

Attempts at a direct approach are utilized if one suspects an overlooked adenoma remains after previous surgery and has been localized by radiology prior to operation. This approach may be used to deliver both *superior* and *inferior* parathyroid tumors in their most common, *normal* as well as *ectopic* locations, and it may be particularly suitable for retrieval of inferior glands in their more unusual, *undescended* position. By directing the exploration straight towards the site of a localized lesion these operations may often expediently deliver the tumor without the extensive and sometimes hazardous dissections within the scar tissue resulting from the previous exploration.

A commonly utilized *lateral approach* via the vascular sheath avoids general adhesions in the midline, but also serves to identify and save major vessels from injury during the subsequent exploration.[160] The vascular sheath is approached via dissection between the medial border of the sternocleidoid muscle and the strap muscles, as the carotid artery and the jugular vein are easily identified. Mobilization of the carotid artery and the jugular vein is undertaken, and in the presence of harsh fibrotic adhesions this may be easier to initiate in virgin areas high and low in the neck. Dissection and division of the tendinous part of the omohyoid muscle helps to identify the appropriate layer of dissection in the sheath. When the large vessels have been identified without injury from the thyroid, dissection along them continues generally all the way down to the clavicle, after which the pretracheal fascia is divided to allow medial mobilization of the thyroid and exploration of its dorsal and lateral surfaces.

In our experience a *superior parathyroid tumor* has most often been preoperatively localized dorsal to the thyroid, and occasionally is it easily delivered from an untouched space between the layers of the pretracheal fascia. More commonly the gland resides in a previously dissected area at the latero-posterior surface of the superior thyroid lobe. It may then be necessary to find a cleavage plane under the strap muscles to be able to entirely expose the dorsal aspects of the upper thyroid all the way between the superior and inferior thyroid arteries. Many overlooked superior parathyroid tumors have in our experience resided directly on the thyroid, just behind its posterior edge, some of them medially, and these glands are easily delivered after medial rotation of the thyroid and meticulous exploration of its surface.

The common ectopic positions for overlooked superior parathyroid tumors are the areas lateral or posterior to the pharynx or the esophagus. By traction applied to the thyroid and division of the fascial layer the retroesophageal space is easily explored by blunt dissection and a finger may be inserted directly onto the prevertebral fascia to explore the posterior space all the way down to the superior posterior mediastinum (see chapter 4). Subsequently this space is opened up totally by division of the lateral attachments of the pretracheal fascia to the vascular sheath down to the clavicle. Caudally this division is kept close to the sheath whereby the *recurrent laryngeal nerve* is preserved and allowed to fall medially. Occasionally the nerve is identified early during these dissections and may also be followed along its course, but generally it is not dissected if encased in scar tissue. The dissection should be lateral, away from the pertinent areas of the nerve, especially on the right side where the nerve has an oblique course, and a non-recurrent nerve even may be present higher in the neck. If a parathyroid tumor has descended towards the tracheoesophageal groove or the posterior superior mediastinum the nerve can be on either side, but most commonly medially and anteriorly and is preserved by dissection close to the tumor capsule.

A *direct approach to an inferior parathyroid gland* located in its most common position near the inferior thyroid pole or the cervical thymus implies that the area under the strap muscles must be explored. Only rarely is this efficiently achieved by medial retraction of these muscles. Suggested alternatives to overcome this problem utilize midline separation of the muscles, or their transection or removal below the thyroid. In our hands a semilateral approach longitudinally through the strap muscles will often facilitate their dissection from the thyroid surface and allow lateral retraction, whereby the inferior thyroid pole and the most common sites for inferior glands are well exposed.[23] If no gland is retrieved immediately the cervical thymus is diligently dissected and accessible parts of the thymus are delivered from the superior anterior mediastinum. Since an inferior gland is occasionally laterally positioned below the thyroid, the tissues around and medial to the tracheoesophageal groove require dissection. An inferior parathyroid tumor is generally medial and anterior to the recurrent laryngeal nerve, but may occasionally be under it. If the inferior gland is still not readily identified, dissection progresses from medial to lateral on the surface of the inferior thyroid pole and cranially along its lateral border, allowing fibrotic tissue to slip posteriorly from its surface. This dissection continues up to the purported nerve-artery intersection. *Palpation* is important in the context of parathyroid reoperation and may identify a parathyroid tumor as a well circumscribed soft lesion within or adjacent to the inferior thyroid pole. If the parathyroid tumor is suspected to be within the thyroid substance there is generally remarkably little bleeding if the thyroid is cut by one or several transverse incisions, which may be closed subsequently by suture. More often, an intraoperative US examination will be done at this stage to identify a possible intrathyroidal gland. Although partial thyroid resection may be undertaken, *hemithyroidectomy* is rarely considered in these situations since the yield of pathological glands tends to be remarkably low and normal parathyroids will often be removed concomitantly. This procedure will also seriously complicate any subsequent surgery and may interfere with localization studies.

A particularly direct route of exploration can be utilized if an *undescended inferior parathyroid tumor* has been localized prior to surgery.[36,84] A high, short transverse incision at the level of the carotid artery bifurcation or along the anterior border of the sternocleidomastoid muscle may be utilized, followed by dissection of the vascular sheath, after which the tumor is often easily delivered from a site generally medial to the carotid artery. (Fig. 8.7)

Complete Cervical Exploration

Unfortunately many patients have to undergo reoperation without identification of a tumor prior to surgery. Moreover, false positive localization occurs with any of the localization methods, whereby a suspected parathyroid tumor may not uncommonly be revealed at reoperation as a thyroid lesion. Although exploration in the absence of positive localization may sometimes be terminated if an overlooked adenoma is identified, many of these patients have to undergo complete, bilateral neck exploration, and this is also frequently required in the presence of hyperplasia or associated MEN-1 syndrome.

The *complete cervical exploration* will generally utilize lateral approaches according to the same principles as outlined for the direct approach, comprising one side at a time. Dissection of the vascular sheath is performed; entry is generally semilaterally via the strap muscles or these muscles are simply removed below the thyroid. Thereafter, the exploration ensues with visualization first of the *normal sites* for superior and inferior glands and thereafter the *ectopic* locations. The dissection ultimately follows the lateral surface of the thyroid, first from its uppermost part down to the nerve-artery intersection and then from the inferior pole, laterally and cranially to the same point.

The area at the level of the nerve-artery intersection, or the middle of the thyroid, often remains the most difficult site to explore. In order to approach this area safely the recurrent laryngeal nerve may have to be identified within the generally virgin tissue caudally in the neck and followed cephalad, whereby the inferior thyroid artery branches may be dissected concomitantly.

Intraoperative US may be utilized early during these dissections and may identify intrathyroidal and undescended parathyroid tumors as well as those in juxtathyroidal glands around the middle of the thyroid lobe.[36,161-164] This investigation may also disclose the safest approach for delivery of tumors, which for glands at the level of the nerve-artery intersection may occasionally be from the medial aspects of the thyroid rather than via the lateral, harsh scar tissue.

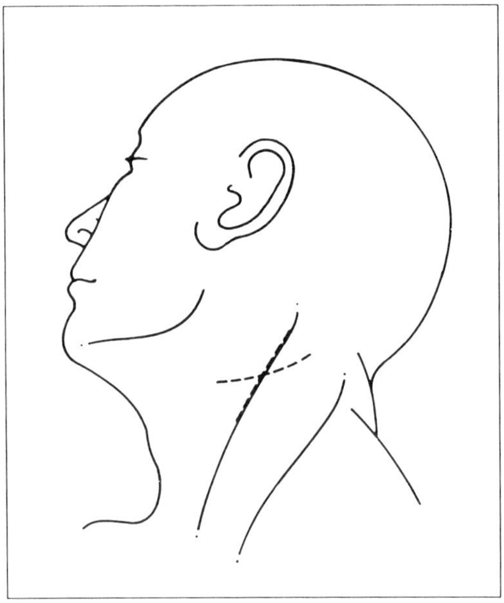

Fig. 8.7. Sketch of the neck, showing placement of the skin incision for direct approach to an undescended parathyroid gland. Reprinted with permission from Fraker et al.[84]

Finally the exploration includes the areas around and within the vascular sheath from above the carotid artery bifurcation to the clavicle and has extended medially to the mid line. Subsequent to exploration of one side the same procedure is repeated contralaterally, but requires that the recurrent laryngeal nerve ipsilaterally definitely is preserved.

Identification of normal parathyroid glands is often warranted during these dissections and frequently possible unless they have been previously biopsied. Occasionally we have encountered clips marked normal glandular remnants of adenoma, having been erroneously mistaken for normal glands during the previous surgery because major parts of the tumors have been concealed by the thyroid tubercle or the nerve-artery intersection.

We have also experienced *incompletely excised parathyroid tumors* in difficult locations in relation to the nerve and apparently the surgeon at the previous operation has been hesitant to dissect such glands. Reoperation has retrieved overlooked parathyroid tumors occupying most of the inferior thyroid lobe or unusually outstretched and thin lesions have been mistaken for the esophageal wall.

MEDIASTINAL EXPLORATION

The majority of mediastinal parathyroid tumors may be retrieved from the neck incision, either by transcervical thymectomy for inferior derived glands or by the delivery of ectopic superior glands in the posterior mediastinum.[1,3,4,8,10-12,17,20,21,23,34-39,72-78,85,89,98-103] Mediastinal exploration is therefore generally not performed in association with reoperation unless the neck has been once again completely explored. *Direct mediastinomy* may be undertaken exceptionally in cases with positive tumor localization in positions not accesible from the neck.[75-78,85,89,99-103] If, however, no suspect lesion is identified during extensive cervical exploration, immediate mediastinotomy will provide the most satisfactory exposure of both the neck and the mediastinum.[77] This allows identification of both recurrent laryngeal nerves close to their origin and efficient exposure of the large vessels.[23] When tumors occupy the upper mediastinum or the patient has an unusually osteoporotic sternum, a partial sternal split may be undertaken.[148] For the vast majority a complete sternal split provides better exposure, and gives minimal discomfort even in elderly individuals. Most mediastinal tumors are located within the thymus, at the level of and around the innominate vein, and it may be rewarding to follow venous branches which may lead to a tumor. Some tumors are not detected until the surgeon has completely removed and dissected the thymic specimen, or they may even be discovered by the pathologist.[76] Approximately 10-15% of mediastinal glands occur outside the thymus, most of them on the anterior aspects of the aortic root or arch, or around the origin of the large vessels in the superior mediastinum[74-78,85,89,99-103] (Figs. 8.3 and 8.4). The lateral areas under the clavicles should receive special attention as tumors at these sites have a tendency to be concealed within fibrosis and attached anteriorly. Parathyroid tumors may also be located laterally on the pleural surfaces so special care should be taken to avoid injury to the phrenic nerves.[75-78,89] More rarely a parathyroid tumor may intrude within the aortopulmonary window and may then require diligent dissection from the left recurrent laryngeal nerve where it passes around the aortic arch.[86-88] A difficult area to explore is the site to the left and lateral to the aortic arch, where occasional glands have been located.[35,76] The area of the middle mediastinum posterior to the aortic arch and the pulmonary arteries, and in front of the trachea may be approached via sternotomy, but generally requires that the innominate vein is divided. Such dissections are not attempted without positive localization.[86-88]

Re-sternotomy may sometimes be undertaken in patients with primary HPT if appropriate indications are present. Since the innominate vein may attach to the posterior sternal surface, fatal bleeding may ensue unless great caution is undertaken when opening the mediastinum. Generally this is performed by saw through the ventral bone layer and with scissors from the xiphoid in upwards direction through the posterior layer of the bone. Overlooked lesions in the mediastinum may be encountered particularly after a previous partial sternal split.

RESECTION OF SELECT MEDIASTINAL ADENOMAS VIA ANTERIOR MEDIASTINOTOMY

Schlinkert et al recently described a technique to remove parathyroid tumors, which preoperatively had been accurately localized to the mediastinum, via a simple anterior mediastinotomy[165] (Fig. 8.8). This approach has previously been utilized for sampling of lymph nodes prior to pulmonary surgery, as well as for removal of the thymus in patients with myasthenia gravis.[166] Access to the medistinum is obtained via incision over and removal of the second costal cartilage, and entry through its bed. Parathyroid tumors located in or near the caudal parts of the thymus can be expediently retrieved by this maneuver, but the exposure is insufficient for glands located deeper in the mediastinum.[165] The described technique has been unusually convenient for the patients and suggested to be particularly suitable for older individuals or those with intercurrent disease who might have difficulties following an ordinary mediastinal exploration.[165] Although it has previously been suggested that mediastinal parathyroid tumors may be removed by mediastinoscopy, caution has to be urged against this approach since the mediastinoscope has to be inserted into the anterior mediastinum with its major vascular components rather than into the avascular plane anterior to the trachea.[165,167]

CLOSED MEDIASTINAL EXPLORATION

Wells et al recently described a method for complete delivery of the entire thymic gland through a cervical incision by the use of a special retractor for elevation of the sternum.[168] This technique has also been used in patients with myasthenia gravis.[168,169] The neck is first explored after which the strap muscles are split down to the sternal notch, the cleido-cleido ligament is divided vertically and the cervical extensions of the thymus are carefully dissected. Thereafter the anterior surface of the thymus is dissected from the sternum and by simultaneous traction, first the right and then the left posterior parts of the thymus are loosened until the gland is completely delivered. Veins entering the thymus from the innominate vein have to be ligated during this procedure and occasionally some adhesions to the pleura or the pericardium have to be cut. At present few other surgeons have experience with this delivery, which certainly appears attractive since it may apparently obviate the need for sternotomy in many patients with mediastinal lesions.[168]

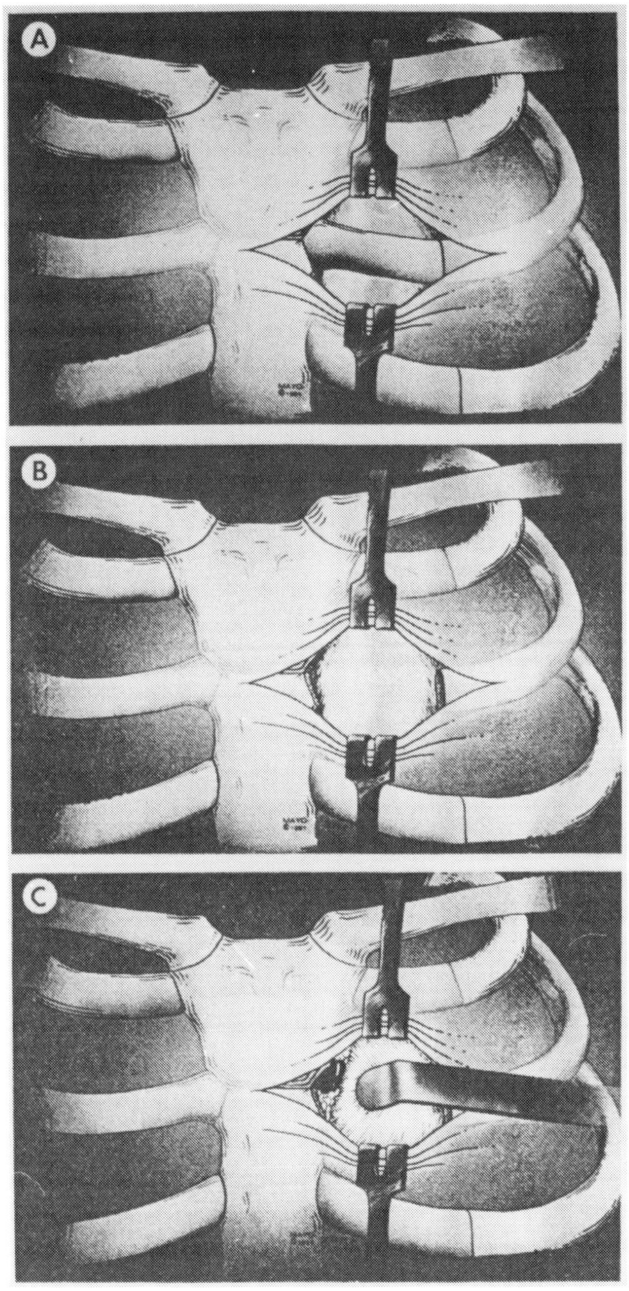

Fig. 8.8. Diagrams depicting technique of anterior mediastinotomy. (A) Incision over costal cartilage. (B) Costal cartilage resected to expose pleura. (C) Pleura reflected to expose parathyroid adenoma. Reprinted with permission from Schlinkert RC et al.[165]

INTRAOPERATIVE ULTRASOUND

Intraoperative US was recently demonstrated as a new important means to improve glandular localization in association with parathyroid reoperation, and it was demonstrated to significantly reduce the time required for these operations.[36,161-164] Intraoperative US may have the capacity to detect up to 80% of all enlarged glands encountered during reoperation and is therefore more sensitive than any other imaging technique.[163,164] It may provide particularly good visualization of intrathyroidal glands; in so doing it may more or less obviate the need for blind thyroid lobectomy and also facilitate safe enucleation or partial lobectomy for delivery of these lesions.[163,164] The intraoperative US investigation can frequently also demonstrate undescended glands.[163,164] This far the size of presently available probes has limited their efficacy in visualizing glands posterior to the thyroid or in the posterior superior mediastinum, and one-third of superior glands may therefore remain undetected with this method. The construction of smaller probes is expected to overcome this problem.[163,164] The sensitivity of the method for detection of glands within the cervical operation field may be used to indicate immediate progress to median sternotomy if abnormal gland is discovered by US examination in the neck.[163,164]

Occasional false positives may occur with this method and in particular lymph nodes or thyroid adenoma have been mistaken for parathyroid lesions.[163,164] The intraoperative US can occasionally be recommended for use during primary parathyroid surgery, if a fourth gland is not found, and may then reveal such glands especially if they occupy intrathyroidal or undescended positions. The method may also guide the surgeon towards the most appropriate and safe approach for delivery of an entrapped in scar tissue from previous surgery.

URINARY cAMP AND SERUM PTH DETERMINATION GUIDING PARATHYROID SURGERY

Urinary cAMP determinations have been used to decide when to terminate a reoperative parathyroid procedure.[36,170] The cAMP levels have been found to drop significantly from a baseline value within 1-2 hours following removal of abnormal parathyroid tissue.[36] Recent methods have utilized a rapid assay for determination of intact PTH, whereby decrease in PTH levels may be recognized shortly after removal of a parathyroid tumor or multiple lesions.[171-178] Including the time for the PTH determination, evaluation of the operative outcome may thus be provided in one hour or less. Such methods have been suggested to predict with considerable confidence the presence of residual abnormal glands in patients with parathyroid hyperplasia. The intraoperative measurements of PTH appear preferable in this context and could certainly have advantages in selected reoperative cases where extensive scar tissue precludes adequate dissection although it has to be appreciated that false results may be encountered.[175] In fact, asymmetrical and asynchronous glandular involvement in hyperplasia reduces the possibility to safely exclude multiglandular disease with these methods and limits the unquestionable value to minorities of reoperative patients. It is unlikely that the measures can compete with the assessment of glandular pathology which is obtained at an adequate exploration by a trained parathyroid surgeon.

PARATHYROID OPERATION AFTER PREVIOUS THYROID SURGERY

The concomitant presence of HPT and thyroid abnormalities, mainly colloid goiter (30%) but also thyroid carcinoma, implies that up to 5% of patients with HPT will have to undergo surgery after previous thyroid operations.[131,179-182] Kadowaki et al have emphasized that parathyroid surgery under such circumstances may be associated with difficulties similar to those encountered during a parathyroid reoperation.[182] A proportion of these patients may have acquired recurrent laryngeal nerve injury at the previous surgery, which together with scarring and fibrosis may considerably complicate the parathyroid operation.[182] If a long time has elapsed after the previous thyroid operation the fibrosis may have subsided, the exploration may be a lot easier than expected. It is nevertheless recommended that noninvasive radiological methods are utilized to localize a parathyroid tumor as this may obviate the need of bilateral exploration. At surgery a lateral approach is often utilized if exploration has to be made on the previously operated side.[182] Exploration is most difficult after previous hemithyroidectomy in which case caudal identification of the recurrent laryngeal nerve in virgin tissue may be required.[182] The risk of hypocalcemia after removal of a parathyroid tumor is often increased since it is always uncertain whether the normal parathyroid glands remain viable after the previous surgery.[182] The exploration may, under these circumstances, be terminated after unilateral exploration if a suspected adenoma is retrieved.[182]

RESULTS OF REOPERATIVE PARATHYROID SURGERY

A few decades ago reports on limited series of patients undergoing reoperation for primary HPT revealed a success rate with respect to resolution of hypercalcemia amounting to 60-70%.[25,27-29] Improvement in this respect has been considerable during recent years and especially at larger centers the development of methods for radiological localization of abnormal parathyroid glands and accumulated experience have raised the efficacy of treatment.[1,3,4,6-8,14,19,20,30-39,65,66,69-71] Thus, recent more comprehensive patient series have revealed a cure rate after parathyroid surgery reoperation of 85-95% (Table 8.1).[1,3,6,8,23,35-39] The success rate depends also on criteria for selection of the patients undergoing this surgery, their levels of serum calcium and the size of the retrieved tumors as well as the number of patients who have previously undergone primary surgery at an institution other than the referral center. The outcome is thus generally better if the previous parathyroid surgery was performed by less experienced surgeons than if the failures were encountered at the reoperating surgeons own institution. Results of radiological localization studies should also have considerable influence, and the outcome overall has been considerably better for cervical as compared to mediastinal explorations.[1,11]

At our institution preoperative localization studies have been increasingly successful, as a result of close collaboration between the radiologists and the surgeons. In sharp contrast to what was routine a few years ago it is now common that the parathyroid lesion is localized prior to reoperation. Difficulties with reoperation are, however, considerably increased in patients with MEN-1 related HPT, who are particularly prone to recurrent hypercalcemia due to involvement of ectopic and supernumerary glands.[11,23,39]

A problem of increasing significance is that referring physicians may have tried to correct their mistakes by performing yet another parathyroid operation before submitting the patient to the larger center for appropriate investigations and thereby possibly *rerepeated parathyroid surgery*. This will considerably increase the difficulties of the reoperation, especially if the primary procedures have been associated with liberal excision of tissues, including parts of or entire normal parathyroids or a thyroid lobe, or if it has resulted in recurrent laryngeal nerve paralysis. It is increasingly important that surgeons without adequate training for reoperative parathyroid surgery be dissuaded from attempting this difficult procedure, otherwise the mistakes leading to higher incidence of failed primary operations will be repeated.

COMPLICATIONS

In earlier series of reoperative parathyroid surgery, complications were common and severe: tetany, bilateral recurrent laryngeal nerve paralysis and even deaths due to injury of large vessels.[26,28] In more recent series the mortality has been exceedingly low, and when occurring it has been associated with operations on debilitated patients, many with severe hypercalcemic crises.[23,29,35-39] Bilateral recurrent laryngeal nerve paralysis requiring tracheostomy has been extremely rare and generally transient among reoperative patients.[11,20,28,183] Still, however, unilateral recurrent laryngeal nerve paralysis has occurred with a frequency generally around 3-6%, and temporary paralysis has been even more common.[1,4,11,19-21,33-39,52,65] In a prospective study by Patow et al on 163 patients subjected to parathyroidectomy, the incidence of recurrent laryngeal nerve paralysis was 6%, 8 patients experienced unilateral and 2 bilateral involvement, despite intraoperative visualization of both nerves.[183] Other series have, however, reported nerve complications more uncommonly, although tran-

Table 8.1. Results of reoperation

Author, year, reference	No. of patients	Successful reoperations %
Hellström, 1957[25]	20	70
Romanus et al, 1973[27]	11	73
Beazley et al, 1975[28]	35	74
Livesay et al, 1976[29]	20	63
Wang, 1972[1]	112	91
Edis et al, 1978[3]	51	84
Bruining et al, 1981[6]	53	81
Granberg et al, 1982[8]	53	83
Brennan et al, 1985[37]	175	90
Grant et al, 1986[35]	157	89
Cheung et al, 1989[38]	83*	86
Levin et al, 1989[39]	81	86
Carty et al, 1991[36]	206	96
Åkerström et al, 1992[23]	69	90

The figures in this table are not mutually comparable, because of variable patient selection. However, the depicted information reveals increased efficacy of parathyroid reoperation during recent years.
* *Includes also six patients with secondary HPT*

sient paresis should be expected to occur with some frequency in the more difficult cases.[23,35,184] The right recurrent laryngeal nerve is twice as often injured during this surgery due to a more oblique course in the lower neck and a less constant relation to the trachea as compared to the left nerve which generally remains well hidden in the tracheoesophageal groove.[183] Occasionally a non-recurrent right laryngeal nerve, being present in 0.2-0.4%, may be mistaken for a branch of the thyroid artery and can be divided[185] (Fig. 8.9). Contrary to the experiences in thyroid surgery, the recurrent laryngeal nerve may not require dissection in association with parathyroid surgery and it may in fact at reoperation be more or less impossible to deliver the nerve without damage if it is severely encased in scar tissue after the previous surgery. It may be more awarding to use common landmarks in order to appreciate the course of the nerve and approach the pertinent areas with caution[185] (Fig. 8.10). The laryngeal entrance of the nerve is identified as the palpable inferior cornu of the thyroid cartilage, but most superior glands will reside dorsal and lateral to this point.[186] When dissections require identification of the recurrent laryngeal nerve this is generally most easily accomplished in virgin tissues within the lower neck whereafter it may be traced cranially, appreciating that it may divide into two major functional branches.[187]

The recurrent laryngeal nerve may also be injured in dissections of the mediastinum, and it is especially vulnerable where it passes around the aortic arch or the brachiocephalic trunk.[87] The *phrenic nerve* may rarely be injured in deep dissections of the neck, but more easily in conjunction with mediastinal explorations by lateral dissection towards the pleural surfaces.[76] Many authors have reported injury to the sympathetic trunk with a resulting Horner's syndrome when dissections have been performed towards the vertebral space in the neck.[11,23,35] A sympathetic ganglion may have been excised under such circumstances; it may represent parathyroid tumor. Some authors have reported injury to the carotid artery which may indeed be friable because of adventitial adhesions after previous surgery.[11,19,32,35] Injury to this artery as well as the jugular vein may generally be easily repaired by suture but have occasionally been reported to require prosthetic replacement. The morbidity after reoperative surgery includes also hematoma, wound infections and occasional episodes of pulmonary embolism. The risk of complications is generally reported to be higher in association with mediastinotomy due to increased risk of lung complications, sternal dehiscence and infection, as well as injury to the first rib or brachial plexus.[89,110,165] Many of these complications may be prevented by careful technique, preoperative antibiotics as well as liberal drainage of the neck wound and the mediastinal space after sternotomy. In our experience the problems associated with sternotomy have been few and the inconveniences have been limited even in elderly individuals.

The most common complication of reoperative parathyroid surgery and the one that has been most difficult to prevent is postoperative *hypoparathyroidism*, being encountered with an incidence of 15 to 25% after parathyroid reoperation.[1,3,8,11,23,34-39] It has frequently occurred subsequent to sequential excision of normal parathyroid glands prior to identification of an adenoma but has also resulted from excessive removal of hyperplastic parathyroid tissue.[23] The risk is increased after previous thyroid surgery or if thyroid and parathyroid procedures have been performed concomitantly.[182] The incidence of postoperative hypoparathyroidism may be reduced if surgeons in general refrain from biopsy or excision of parathyroid glands until exploration on both sides allows reasonable assessment of the underlying pathology.

CRYOPRESERVATION AND AUTOLOGOUS TRANSPLANTATION OF PARATHYROID TISSUE

Since patients undergoing reoperative surgery for primary HPT are afflicted with a high incidence of postoperative hypoparathyroidism, several authors have advocated routine cryopreservation of the excised parathyroid tissue to be used for delayed autografting if needed.[34,36,147-149,188] Frequently as a result of sequential excision of glands during previous surgery a residual pathological gland may sometimes constitute the patient's only remaining parathyroid tissue. If this is obvious at the time of reoperation immediate autografting is advocated. However, especially in patients with MEN-1 associated hyperplasia (as well as secondary parathyroid hyperplasia) at least one-third of the patients may not require such transplantation because of functioning supernumerary parathyroid tissue.[147,148] Since cryopreserved tissues have functioned less efficiently when grafted, as compared to the immediately performed graft, it may sometimes be a delicate task to decide whether to transplant immediately or to cryopreserve.[3,34,36] Recent improvements with cryopreservation have reported an increased success rate of up to 80%, and it is possible that when this method is more commonly adopted it may considerably reduce the risks of hypoparathyroidism in association with parathyroid reoperation.[34,36]

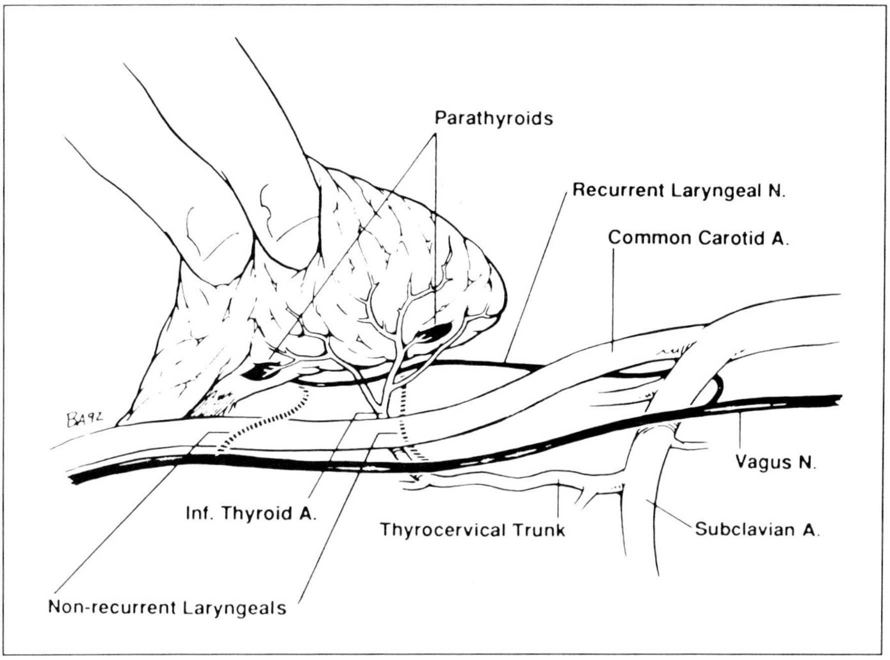

Fig. 8.9. Anatomy of the recurrent laryngeal nerve. Potential sites for a nonrecurrent laryngeal nerve are indicated by the dashed lines. This anatomic variant occurs almost exclusively on the right side. Reprinted with permission from Kahky HP et al.[185]

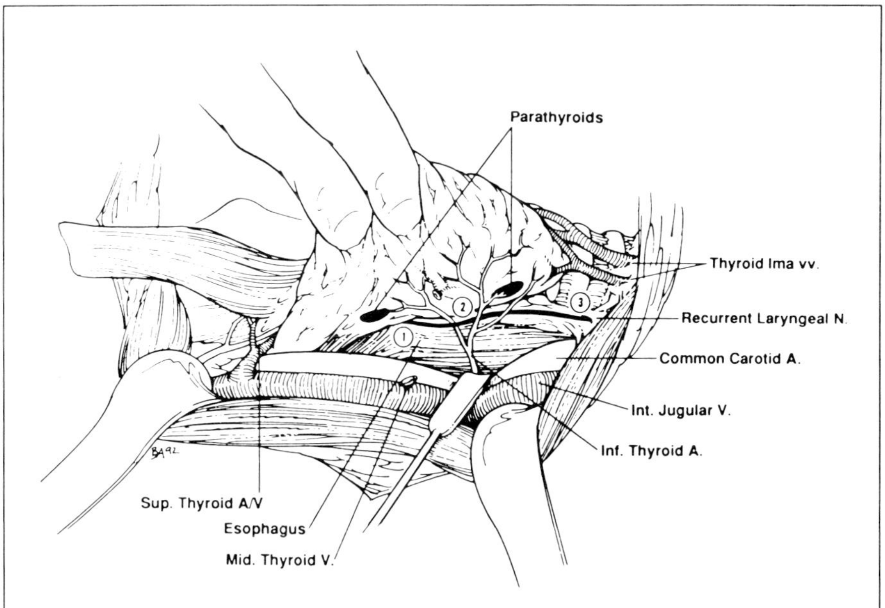

Fig. 8.10. During thyroidectomy, the recurrent laryngeal nerve is at greatest risk for injury (1) at the ligament of Berry, (2) during ligation of branches of the inferior thyroid artery, and (3) at the thoracic inlet. Reprinted with permission from Kahky HP et al.[185]

References

1. Wang CA. Parathyroid re-exploration. A clinical and pathological study of 112 cases. Ann Surg 1977; 186: 140-5.
2. Satava RM, Beahrs OH, Scholz DA. Success rate of cervical exploration for hyperparathyroidism. Arch Surg 1975; 110: 625-8.
3. Edis AJ, Sheedy PF, Beahrs OH et al. Results of reoperation for hyperparathyroidism, with evaluation of preoperative localization studies. Surgery 1978; 84: 384-93.
4. Brennan MF, Doppman JL, Marx SJ et al. Reoperative parathyroid surgery for persistent hyperparathyroidism. Surgery 1978; 83: 669-76.
5. Martin JK, van Heerden JA, Edis AJ et al. Persistent postoperative hyperparathyroidism. Surg Gynecol Obstet 1980; 151: 764-8.
6. Bruining HA, van Houten H, Juttman JR et al. Results of operative treatment of 615 patients with primary hyperparathyroidism. World J Surg 1981; 5: 85-90.
7. Russel CF, Edis AJ, Purnell DC. The reasons for persistent hypercalcaemia after cervical exploration for presumed primary hyperparathyroidism. Br J Surg 1983; 70: 198-201.
8. Granberg P-O, Johansson G, Lindvall N et al. Reoperation for primary hyperparathyroidism. Am J Surg 1982; 113: 296-300.
9. Katz AD, Hopp D. Parathyroidectomy. Review of 338 consecutive cases for histology, location, and reoperation. Am J Surg 1982; 144: 411-5.
10. Palmer JA, Rosen IB. Reoperative surgery for hyperparathyroidism. Am J Surg 1982; 144: 406-10.
11. Brennan MF, Wells SA. Reoperation for suspected hyperparathyroidism. In: IDA Johnston, NW Thompson, eds. Endocrine Surgery. London: Butterworth, 1983: 41-52.
12. Katz AD, Formichella D. Fifty-three reoperations for hyperparathyroidism. Am J Surg 1989; 158: 385-7.
13. Wells AS. Surgical therapy of patients with primary hyperparathyroidism: Long-term benefits. J Bone Mineral Res 1991; 6 (suppl 2): 143-52.
14. McGarity WC, Mathews WH, Fulenwider JT et al. The surgical management of primary hyperparathyroidism: a personal series. Ann Surg 1981; 193: 794-804.
15. van Heerden JA, Grant CS. Surgical treatment of primary hyperparathyroidism: An institutional perspective. World J Surg 1991; 15: 688-92.
16. Clark OH, Wilkes W, Siperstein AE et al. Diagnosis and management of asymptomatic hyperparathyroidism: Safety, efficacy and deficiencies in our knowledge. J Bone Mineral Res 1991; 6 (suppl 2): 135-42.
17. Kaplan E, Yashiro T, Salti G. Primary Hyperparathyroidism in the 1990s: Choice of surgical procedures for this disease. Ann Surg 1992; 215: 300-17.
18. Attie JN, Kahfif RA. Surgical exploration in asymptomatic hypercalcaemia. Am J Surg 1976; 132: 449-52.
19. van Vroonhoven TJ, Muller H. Causes of failure in the surgical treatment of primary hyperparathyroidism: lessons from 51 successful reoperations. Br J Surg 1978; 65: 297-300.
20. Prinz RA, Gamvros OI, Allison DJ et al. Reoperations for hyperparathyroidism. Surg Gynecol Obstet 1981; 152: 760-4.
21. Billings PJ, Milroy EJG. Reoperative parathyroid surgery. Br J Surg 1983; 70: 542-6.
22. Malmaeus J, Granberg P-O, Halvorsen J et al. Parathyroid surgery in Scandinavia. Acta Chir Scand 1988; 154: 409-13.
23. Åkerström G, Rudberg C, Grimelius L et al. Causes of failed primary exploration and technical aspects of re-operation in primary hyperparathyroidism. World J Surg 1992; 16: 562-9.
24. Haff RC, Ballinger WF. Causes of recurrent hypercalcemia after parathyroidectomy for primary hyperparathyroidism. Ann Surg 1971; 173: 884-91.
25. Hellström J. The causes of unsuccessful or inadequate parathyroidectomy in hyperparathyroidism. Acta Chir Scand 1957; 112: 79-91.
26. Clark OH, Taylor S. Persistent and recurrent hyperparathyroidism. Br J Surg. 1972; 59: 555-8.
27. Romanus R, Heimann P, Nilsson O et al. Surgical treatment of hyperparathyroidism. Prog Surg 1973; 12: 22-76.
28. Beazley RM, Costa K, Ketcham AS. Reoperative parathyroid surgery. Am J Surg

1975; 130: 427-9.
29. Livesay JJ, Mulder DG. Recurrent hyperparathyroidism. Arch Surg 1976; 111: 688-91.
30. Clark OH, Way LW, Hunt TK. Recurrent hyperparathyroidism. Ann Surg 1976; 184: 391-402.
31. Organ CH Jr, Albano WA. Surgical management of recurrent and persistent hyperparathyroidism. Surg Gynecol Obstet 1980; 151: 237-40.
32. Roslyn JJ, Mulder DG, Gordon HE. Persistent and recurrent hyperparathyroidism. Am J Surg 1981; 142: 21-5.
33. McGarity WC, Goldman AL. Reoperation for primary hyperparathyroidism. Ann Surg 1981; 194: 134-9.
34. Brennan MF, Marx SJ, Doppman J et al. Results of reoperation for persistent and recurrent hyperparathyroidism. Ann Surg 1981; 194: 671-6.
35. Grant CS, van Heerden JA, Charboneau JW et al. Clinical management of persistent and/or recurrent primary hyperparathyroidism. World J Surg 1986; 10: 555-65.
36. Carty SE, Norton JA. Management of patients with persistent or recurrent primary hyperparathyroidism. World J Surg 1991; 15: 716-23.
37. Brennan MF, Norton JA. Reoperation for persistent and recurrent hyperparathyroidism. Ann Surg 1985; 201: 40-44.
38. Cheung PSY, Borgström A, Thompson NW. Strategy in reoperative surgery for hyperparathyroidism. Arch Surg 1989; 124: 676-80.
39. Levin KE, Clark OH. The reasons for failure in parathyroid operations. Arch Surg 1989; 124: 911-15.
40. Nussbaum SR, Zahradnik R, Lavigne J et al. Highly sensitive two-site immunoradiometric assay for parathyrin and its clinical utility in evaluating patients with hypercalcemia. Clin Chem 1987; 33: 1364-7.
41. Jansson S, Tisell L-E, Lindstedt G et al. Disodium pamidronate in the preoperative treatment of hypercalcemia in patients with primary hyperparathyroidism. Surgery 1991; 110: 480-6.
42. Marx SJ, Stock JL, Attie MG et al. Familial hypocalciuric hypercalcaemia: recognition among patients referred after unsuccessful parathyroid exploration. Ann Intern Med 1980; 92: 351-6.
43. Robinsson PJ, Corrall RJM. The importance of distinguishing familial hypocalciuric hypercalcaemia from asymptomatic primary hyperparathyroidism prior to neck exploration. Clin Otolaryngol 1990; 15: 141-6.
44. Marshden P, Day JL. Hyperparathyroidism: The risk of recurrence. Clin Endocrinol 1973; 2: 9-13.
45. Edis AJ, van Heerden JA, Scholz DA. Results of subtotal parathyroidectomy for primary chief cell hyperplasia. Surgery 1979; 86: 462-9.
46. Prinz RA, Gamvros OI, Sellu D et al. Subtotal parathyroidectomy for primary chief cell hyperplasia of the multiple endocrine neoplasia type I syndrome. Ann Surg 1981; 193: 26-9.
47. van Heerden JA, Kent RB, Sizemore GW et al. Primary hyperparathyroidism in patients with multiple endocrine neoplasia syndromes. Arch Surg 1983; 118: 533-5.
48. Rizzoli R, Green J, Marx SJ. Primary hyperparathyroidism in familial multiple endocrine neoplasia type 1: Long-term follow-up of serum calcium levels after parathyroidectomy. Am J Med 1985; 78: 467-74.
49. Kraimps JL, Duh Q-Y, Demeure M et al. Hyperparathyroidism in multiple endocrine neoplasia syndrome. Surgery 1992; 112: 1080-8.
50. Tisell L-E, Carlsson S, Lindberg S et al. Autonomous hyperparathyroidism, a possible late complication of neck radiotherapy. Acta Chir Scand 1976; 142: 367-73.
51. Prinz RA, Paloyan E, Lawrence AM et al. Radiation-associated hyperparathyroidism: A new syndrome? Surgery 1977; 82: 296-302.
52. Silver CE, Velez FJ. Parathyroid re-exploration. Am J Surg 1992; 164: 606-9.
53. Wells SA, Leight GF, Ross AJ. Primary hyperparathyroidism. Curr Probl Surg 1980; 17: 398-463
54. Stoffer SS, Szpunar WE, Hamburger SW et al. Unsuccessful parathyroid surgery. Keeping the risk of failure minimal. Postgrad Med 1982; 72: 80-2.

55. Peterson P. Psychiatric disorders in primary hyperparathyroidism. Clin Endocrinol Metab 1968; 28: 1491-5.
56. Numann PJ, Torppa AJ, Blumetti AE. Neuropsychologic deficits associated with primary hyperparathyroidism. Surgery 1984; 96: 1119-23.
57. Joborn C, Hetta J, Johansson H et al. Psychiatric morbidity in primary hyperparathyroidism. World J Surg 1988; 476-81.
58. Joborn C, Hetta J, Frisk P et al. Primary hyperparathyroidism in patients with organic brain syndrome. Acta Med Scand 1985; 219: 91-8.
59. Joborn C, Rastad J, Stålberg E et al. Muscle function in patients with primary hyperparathyroidism. Muscle Nerve 1989; 12: 87-94.
60. Åkerström G, Ljunghall S. Medical and radiologic evaluation and operative treatment of primary hyperparathyroidism. Curr Opinion Gen Surg; 1993; 130-8.
61. Edis AJ, Beahrs OH, Sheedy PF II: Reoperation for hyperparathyroidism. World J Surg 1977; 1: 731-8.
62. Lamers C, Froeling PGAM. Clinical significance of hyperparathyroidism in familial multiple endocrine adenomatosis (MEA 1). Am J Med 1979; 66: 422-4.
63. Muller H. True recurrence of hyperparathyroidism: proposed criteria of recurrence. Br J Surg 1975; 62: 556-9.
64. Carter WB, Carter DL, Cohn HE. Cause and current management of reoperative hyperparathyroidism. Am Surg 1993; 59: 120-4.
65. Rothmund M, Wagner PK, Seesko H et al. Lehren aus re-operationen bei 55 patienten mit primären hyperparathyreoidismus. Dtsch Med Wochenscr 1990; 115: 1579-85.
66. Auguste L-J, Attie JN, Schnaap D. Initial failure of surgical exploration in patients with primary hyperparathyroidism. Am J Surg 1990; 160: 333-6.
67. Block MA, Frame B, Kleerekoper M et al. Surgical management of persistence or recurrence after subtotal parathyroidectomy for primary hyperparathyroidism. Am J Surg 1979; 138: 561-6.
68. Mallette LE, Blevins T, Jordan PH et al. Autogenous parathyroid grafts for generalized primary parathyroid hyperplasia: Contrasting outcome in sporadic hyperplasia versus multiple endocrine neoplasia type I. Surgery 1987; 101: 738-45.
69. Miller DL. Pre-operative localization and interventional treatment of parathyroid tumors: When and how? World J Surg 1991; 15: 706-15.
70. Doppman JL, Miller DL. Localization of parathyroid tumors in patients with asymptomatic hyperparathyroidism and no previous surgery. J Bone Mineral Res 1991; 1991: 6 (Suppl 2): 153-8.
71. Hellman P, Sundin A, Bergström M et al. Positron emission tomography with ^{11}C-methionine in hyperparathyroidism. Surgery, in press.
72. Thompson NW, Eckhauser FE, Harness JK. The anatomy of primary hyperparathyroidism. Surgery 1982; 92: 814-21.
73. Thompson NW. Surgical anatomy of hyperparathyroidism. Prog Surg 1986; 18: 59-79.
74. Grant CS, Charboneau JW, James EM et al. Reoperative parathyroid surgery. Wien Klin Wochenschr 1988; 100: 360-3.
75. Roslyn JJ, Gordon HE, Mulder DG. Mediastinal parathyroid adenomas. A cause of persistent hyperparathyroidism. Am Surg 1983; 49: 523-7.
76. Norton JA, Schneider PD, Brennan MF. Median sternotomy in reoperations for primary hyperparathyroidism. World J Surg 1985; 9: 807-13.
77. Wang C-A, Gaz RD, Moncure AC. Mediastinal parathyroid exploration: A clinical and pathologic study of 47 cases. World J Surg 1986; 10: 687-95.
78. Conn JM, Goncalves MA, Mansour KA et al. The mediastinal parathyroid. Am Surg 1991; 57: 62-6.
79. Wang C-A. Hyperfunctioning intrathyroid parathyroid gland: A potential cause of failure in parathyroid surgery. J. R. Soc. Med 1981; 74: 49-52.
80. Wheeler MH, Williams ED, Path FRC et al. The hyperfunctioning intrathyroidal parathyroid gland: A potential pitfall in parathyroid surgery. World J Surg 1987; 11: 110-4.

81. Sawady J, Mendelsohn G, Sirota RL et al. The intrathyroidal hyperfunctioning parathyroid gland. Mod Pathol 1989; 6: 652-7.
82. Feliciano DV. Parathyroid pathology in an intrathyroidal position. Am J Surg 1992; 164: 496-500.
83. Edis AJ, Purnell DC, van Heerden JA. The undescended "parathymus". An occasional cause of failed neck exploration for hyperparathyroidism. Ann Surg 1979; 190: 64-8.
84. Fraker DL, Doppman JL, Shawker TH et al. Undescended parathyroid adenoma: An important etiology for failed operations for primary hyperparathyroidism. World J Surg 1990; 14: 342-8.
85. Scholz DA, Purnell DC, Woolner LB et al. Mediastinal hyperfunctioning parathyroid tumors: Review of 14 cases. Ann Surg 1973; 178: 173-8.
86. Stocks AE, Hartley LCJ. Hypercalcaemia. The case of the missing adenoma. Med J Austr 1986; 145: 92-4.
87. McHenry C, Walsh M, Jarosz H et al. Resection of parathyroid tumor in the aorticopulmonary window without prior neck exploration. Surgery 1988; 104: 1090-4.
88. Curley IR, Wheeler MH, Thompson NW et al. The challenge of the middle mediastinal parathyroid. World J Surg 1988; 12: 818-24.
89. Russel CF, Edis AJ, Scholz DA et al. Mediastinal parathyroid tumors: Experience with 38 tumors requiring mediastinotomy for removal. Ann Surg 1981; 193: 805-9.
90. Monchik JM, Nelson TG, Powell DA. Adenoma in a fifth parathyroid gland: The role of selective venous catheterization. Surgery 1973; 73: 782-5.
91. Palmer JA, Sutton FR. Importance of a fifth parathyroid gland in the surgical treatment of hyperparathyroidism. Can J Surg 1978; 21: 350-1.
92. Wang C-A, Mahaffey JE, Axelrod L et al. Hyperfunctioning supernumerary parathyroid glands. Surg Gynecol Obstet 1979; 148: 711-4.
93. Russell CF, Grant CS, van Heerden JA. Hyperfunctioning supernumerary parathyroid glands. An occasional cause of hyperparathyroidism. Mayo Clin Proc 1982; 57: 121-4.
94. Gilmour JR. The gross anatomy of the parathyroid glands. J Pathol 1938; 46: 133-49.
95. Wang CA. The anatomic basis of parathyroid surgery. Ann Surg 1976; 183: 271-5.
96. Åkerström G, Malmaeus J, Bergström R. Surgical anatomy of human parathyroid glands. Surgery 1984; 95: 14-21.
97. Cope O. The story of hyperparathyroidism at the Massachusetts General Hospital. N Engl J Med 1966; 274: 1174-82.
98. Cope O. The occurrence of parathyroids in the anterior mediastinum and the division of the operation into two stages. Ann Surg 1941; 114: 706-33.
99. Nathaniels EK, Nathaniels AM, Wang C-A. Mediastinal parathyroid tumors: a clinical and pathological study of 84 cases. Ann Surg 1970; 171: 165-70.
100. Freeman JB, Sherman BM, Mason EE. Transcervical thymectomy. An integral part of neck exploration for hyperparathyroidism. Arch Surg 1976; 111: 359-64.
101. Rothmund M, Diethelm L, Brünner F et al. Diagnosis and surgical treatment of mediastinal parathyroid tumors. Am Surg 1976; 183: 139-45
102. Nudelman IL, Deutsch AA, Reiss R. Primary hyperparathyroidism due to mediastinal parathyroid adenoma. Int Surg 1987; 72: 104-8.
103. Clark OH. Mediastinal parathyroid tumors. Arch Surg 1988; 123: 1096-9.
104. Liechty RD, Weil III R. Parathyroid anatomy in hyperplasia. Arch Surg 1992; 127: 813-6.
105. Deleplanque G, Kraimps JL, Coste G et al. Une observation d'adénome parthyroidien localisé dans le médiastin moyen. Ann Chir 1989; 43: 393-6.
106. Proye C, Lefebvre J, Bourdelle-Hego MF et al. Adenome parathyroidien mediastinal moyen de la fenetre aorto-pulmonaire. 2 observations. Chirurgie 1988; 114: 166-73.
107. Obara T, Fujimoto Y, Tanaka R et al. Mid-mediastinal parathyroid lesions: Preoperative localization and surgical approach in two cases. Jpn J Surg 1990; 20: 481-6.
108. Weller GL. Development of the thyroid, parathyroid and thymus glands in man.

Carneg. Inst. Washington, Publ No 443, Contrib Embryol 1933; 141: 93-139.
109. Gaz RD, Doubler PB, Wang C-A. The management of 50 unusual hyperfunctioning parathyroid glands. Surgery 1987; 102: 949-57.
110. Cohn KH, Silen A. Lessons of parathyroid reoperations. Am J Surg 1982; 144: 511-7.
111. Levin KE, Gooding GAW, Okerlund M et al. Localizing studies in patients with persistent or recurrent hyperparathyroidism. Surgery 1987; 102: 917-25.
112. Tolstedt GE, Cammock EE, Bell JW. Hyperparathyroidism associated with intrathyroid parathyroid glands. Amer J Surg 1960; 100: 757-60
113. Buchanan LC. Hidden parathyroid adenoma. Am Surg 1952; 18: 439-42.
114. Attie JN, Estrin J, Khafif RA et al. Parathyroid adenomas discovered incidentally during explorations of the thyroid. Am J Surg 1967; 114: 538-42.
115. Spiegel AM, Marx SJ, Doppman JL et al. Intrathyroidal parathyroid adenoma or hyperplasia. An occasionally overlooked cause of surgical failure in primary hyperparathyroidism. JAMA 1975; 234: 1029-33.
116. Bainbridge ET, Barnes AD. Primary hyperparathyroidism due to overactive intrathyroid parathyroid glands: A potential cause of failed exploration. Br J Surg 1982; 69: 200-2.
117. Davis O, Scanlon EF, Pollak ER et al. Bilateral intrathyroidal hyperplastic parathyroid glands. J Surg Oncol 1984; 27: 271-4.
118. Billings PJ, Milroy EJG. Overactive intrathyroid parathyroid glands. Br J Surg 1982; 69: 498.
119. Clark OH, Gooding GAW, Ljung BM. Locating a parathyroid adenoma by ultrasonography and aspiration biopsy cytology. West J Med 1981; 135: 154-8.
120. Rastad J, Johansson H, Lindgren PG et al. Ultrasonic localization and cytologic identification of parathyroid tumors. World J Surg 1984; 8: 501-8.
121. Juhlin C, Rastad J, Klareskog L et al. Parathyroid histology and cytology with monoclonal antibodies recognizing a calcium sensor of parathyroid cells. Am J Pathol 1989; 135: 321-328.
122. Bjerneroth G, Juhlin C, Grimelius L et al. Improvement in histological diagnosis of primary hyperparathyroidism with a monoclonal antiparathyroid antibody. Endocr Pathol 1992; 3: 83-92.
123. Norris EH. The parathyroid glands and the lateral thyroid in man: Their morphogenesis, histogenesis, topographic anatomy and perinatal growth. Carneg. Inst. Washington Publ No 479, Contrib Embryol 1937; 479: 247-94.
124. Kurtay M, Crile G Jr. Aberrant parathyroid gland in relationship to the thymus. Am J Surg 1969; 117: 705-8.
125. Summers G. Parathyroid exploration. A review of 125 cases. Arch Otolaryngol Head Neck Surg 1991; 117: 1237-41.
126. Salti G, Fedorak I, Yashiro T et al. Continuing evolution in the operative management of primary hyperparathyroidism. Arch Surg 1992; 127: 831-7.
127. Udekwu AO, Kaplan EL, Wu T-C et al. Ectopic parathyroid adenoma of the lateral triangle of the neck: Report of two cases. Surgery 1987; 101: 114-8.
128. Gilmour JR. The embryology of the parathyroid glands, the thymus and certain associated rudiments. J Pathol Bacteriol 1937; 45: 507-22.
129. Nobori M, Saiki S, Tanaka N et al. Blood supply of the parathyroid gland from the superior thyroid artery. Surgery 115; 417-23.
130. Reddick RL, Costa JC, Marx SJ. Parathyroid hyperplasia and parathyromatosis. Lancet 1977; 1: 549.
131. Hooghe L, Kinnaert P, Van Geertruyden J. Surgical anatomy of hyperparathyroidism. Acta Chir Belg 1992; 92: 1-9.
132. Edis AJ, Levitt MD. Supernumerary parathyroid glands: Implication for the surgical treatment of secondary hyperparathyroidism. World J Surg 1987; 11: 398-401.
133. Wells SA, Stirman JA Jr, Bolman RM III. Parathyroid transplantation. World J Surg 1977; 1: 747-56.
134. Burk LB. Recurrent parathyroid adenoma. A case report. Surgery 1947; 21: 95-101.
135. Black BK, Ackerman LV. Tumors of the parathyroid: A review of 23 cases. Cancer

1950; 3: 415-44.
136. Palmer JA, Brown WA, Kerr WH et al. The surgical aspects of hyperparathyroidism. Arch Surg 1975; 110: 1004-6.
137. Rattner DW, Marrone GC, Kasdon E et al. Recurrent hyperparathyroidism due to implantation of parathyroid tissue. Am J Surg 1985; 149: 745-8.
138. Åkerström G, Rudberg C, Grimelius L et al. Recurrent hyperparathyroidism due to peroperative seeding of neoplastic or hyperplastic parathyroid tissue. A case report. Acta Chir Scand 1988; 154: 549-52.
139. Fitko R, Roth SI, Hines JR et al. Parathyromatosis in hyperparathyroidism. Hum Pathol 1990; 21: 234-7.
140. Kessler M, Avila JM, Renoult E et al. Reoperation for secondary hyperparathyroidism in chronic renal failure. Nephrol Dial Transplant 1991; 6: 176-9.
141. Fulmer DH, Rothschild EO, Myers WPL. Recurrent parathyroid adenoma. Arch Intern Med 1969; 124: 495-501.
142. Penington A, Ihle B, Billson V et al. Recurrent secondary hyperparathyroidism due to implanted parathyroid tissue: A case report. Austr N Z J Surg 1990; 60: 821-3.
143. Sokol M, Kavolius J, Schaaf M et al. Recurrent hyperparathyroidism from benign neoplastic seeding: A review with recommendations for management. Surgery 1993; 113: 456-61.
144. Fraker DL, Travis WD, Merendino JJ. Locally recurrent parathyroid neoplasms as a cause for recurrent and persistent primary hyperparathyroidism. Ann Surg 1991; 213: 58-65.
145. Wells SA, Ellis GJ, Gunnells JC et al. Parathyroid autotransplantation in primary parathyroid hyperplasia. N Engl J Med 1976; 295: 57-62.
146. Saxe AW. Parathyroid transplantation: A review. Surgery 1984; 95: 507-26.
147. Saxe AW, Brennan MF. Reoperative parathyroid surgery for primary hyperparathyroidism caused by multiple-gland disease: Total parathyroidectomy and autotransplantation with cryopreserved tissue. Surgery 1982; 91: 616-21.
148. Saxe AW, Brennan MF. Strategy and technique of reoperative parathyroid surgery. Surgery 1981; 89: 417-23.
149. Wells SA, Farndon JR, Dale JK et al. Long-term evaluation of patients with primary parathyroid hyperplasia managed by total parathyroidectomy and heterotopic autotransplantation. Ann Surg 1980; 192: 451-8.
150. Klempa I, Steinau U, Frei U et al. Morphologische aspekte der parathyroideatransplantation. Beitrag zur klinischen relevanz des induzierten, invasiven gewebswachstums. Chirurg 1978; 49: 704-10.
151. Brennan MF, Brown EM, Marx SJ et al. Recurrent hyperparathyroidism from an autotransplanted parathyroid adenoma. N Engl J Med 1978; 299: 1057-9.
152. Frei U, Klempa I, Schneider M et al. Tumour-like growth of parathyroid autografts in uraemic patients. Proc Eur Dial Transpl 1981; 18: 548-55.
153. Coulon G, Mantion G, Saint-Hillier Y et al. Récidive d'un hyperparathyroidisme sur autogreffe parathyroidienne. Hyperplasia ou carcinome? Ann Pathol 1986; 6: 340-4.
154. Jansson S, Tisell L-E. Autotransplantation of diseased parathyroid glands into subcutaneous abdominal adipose tissue. Surgery 1987; 101: 549-56.
155. Malmaeus J, Benson L, Johansson H et al. Parathyroid surgery in the multiple endocrine neoplasia type I syndrome. Choice of surgical procedure. World J Surg 1986; 10: 668-72.
156. Casanova D, Sarfiti E, De Francisco A et al. Secondary hyperparathyroidism: Diagnosis of site of recurrence. World J Surg 1991; 15: 546-50.
157. Block MA, Frame B, Kleerekoper M. Surgical management of persistence or recurrence after subtotal parathyroidectomy for primary hyperparathyroidism. Am J Surg 1979; 138: 561-6.
158. Thompson NW. The techniques of initial parathyroid exploration and reoperative parathyroidectomy. In: Thompson NW, Vinik AI, eds. Endocrine Surgery Update. Grune & Stratton 1983; 365-83.
159. Norton JA. Reoperative parathyroid surgery: indication, intraoperative decision-making and results. In: Rothmund M, Wells SA Jr, eds. Parathyroid surgery. Prog Surg (Karger,

Basel) 1986; 18: 133-45.
160. Feind CR. Re-exploration for parathyroid adenoma. Am J Surg 1964; 108: 543-6.
161. Sigel B, Kraft AR, Nyhus LM et al. Identification of a parathyroid adenoma by operative ultrasonography. Arch Surg 1981; 116: 234-5.
162. Charboneau JW, Grant CS, James EM et al. High-resolution ultrasound-guided percutaneous needle biopsy and intraoperative ultrasonography of a cervical parathyroid adenoma in a patient with persistent hyperparathyroidism. Mayo Clin Proc 1983; 58: 497-500.
163. Norton JA, Shawker TH, Jones BL et al. Intraoperative ultrasound and reoperative parathyroid surgery: An initial evaluation. World J Surg 1986; 10: 631-9.
164. Kern KA, Shawker TH, Doppman JL et al. The use of high-resolution ultrasound to locate parathyroid tumors during reoperations for primary hyperparathyroidism. World J Surg 1987; 11: 579-85.
165. Schlinkert RT, Whitaker MD, Argueta R. Resection of select mediastinal parathyroid adenomas through an anterior mediastinotomy. Mayo Clin Proc 1991; 66: 1110-3.
166. McNeill TM, Chamberlain JM. Diagnostic anterior mediastinotomy. Ann Thorac Surg 1966; 2: 532-9.
167. Adinolfi M, Browder W, Wallin JD et al. Excision of mediastinal parathyroid gland by mediastinoscopy. South Med J 1983; 76: 1496-7.
168. Wells SA, Cooper JD. Closed mediastinal exploration in patients with persistent hyperparathyroidism. Ann Surg 1991; 214: 555-61.
169. Cooper JD, Al-Jilaihawa AN, Pearson FG et al. An improved technique to facilitate transcervical thymectomy for myasthenia gravis. Ann Thorac Surg 1988; 45: 242-7.
170. Norton JA, Brennan MF, Saxe AW et al. Intraoperative urinary cyclic adenosine monophosphate as a guide to successful reoperative parathyroidectomy. Ann Surg 1984; 200: 389-95.
171. Nussbaum SR, Thompson AR, Hutcheson KA et al. Intraoperative measurement of parathyroid hormone in the surgical management of hyperparathyroidism. Surgery 1988; 104: 1121-7.
172. Brasier AR, Wang CA, Nussbaum SR. Recovery of parathyroid hormone secretion after parathyroid adenomectomy. J Clin Endocrinol Metab 1988; 66: 495-500.
173. McHenry CR, Pollard A, Walfish PG et al. Intraoperative parathormone level measurement in the management of hyperparathyroidism. Surgery 1990; 108: 801-8.
174. Davies C, Demeure MJ, St John A et al. Study of intact (1-84) parathyroid hormone secretion in patients undergoing parathyroidectomy. World J Surg 1990; 14: 355-60.
175. Proye CAG, Goropoulos A, Franz C et al. Usefulness and limits of quick intraoperative measurements of intact (1-84) parathyroid hormone in the surgical management of hyperparathyroidism: Sequential measurements in patients with multiglandular disease. Surgery 1991; 110: 1035-42.
176. Ryan MF, Jones SR, Barnes AD. Clinical evaluation of a rapid parathyroid hormone assay. Ann Clin Biochem 1992; 29: 48-51.
177. Robertson GSM, Iqbal SJ, Bolia A et al. Intraoperative parathyroid hormone estimation: a valuable adjunct to parathyroid surgery. Ann Roy Coll Surg Engl 1992; 74: 19-22.
178. Irvin GL, Dembrow VD, Prudhomme DL et al. Clinical usefulness of an intraoperative "quick parathyroid hormone" assay. Surgery 1993; 114: 1019-23.
179. Ellenberg AH, Goldman L, Gordon GS et al. Thyroid carcinoma in patients with hyperparathyroidism. Surgery 1962; 51: 708-17.
180. Liang VO, Frame B, Block MA. Associated primary hyperparathyroidism and thyroid lesions: surgical considerations. Arch Surg 1969; 98: 709-12.
181. Lever EG, Refetoff S, Strauss FH II et al. Coexisting thyroid and parathyroid disease: are they related? Surgery 1983; 94: 893-900.
182. Kadowaki MH, Fulton N, Schark C et al. Difficulties of parathyroidectomy after previous thyroidectomy. Surgery 1989; 106: 1018-24.
183. Patow CA, Norton JA, Brennan MF. Vocal cord paralysis and reoperative parathyroidectomy. Ann Surg 1986; 203: 282-5.

184. van Heerden JA, Beahrs OH, Woolner JB. The pathology and surgical management of primary hyperparathyroidism. Surg Clin North Am 1977; 57: 557-63.
185. Kahky MP, Weber RS. Complications of surgery of the thyroid and parathyroid glands. Surg Clin North Am 1993; 73: 307-21.
186. Wang C. The use of the inferior cornu of the thyroid cartilage in identifying the recurrent laryngeal nerve. Surg Gynecol Obstet 1975; 140: 91-4.
187. Nemiroff PM, Katz AD. Extralaryngeal divisions of the recurrent laryngeal nerve. Surgical and clinical significance. Am J Surg 1982; 144: 466-9.
188. Romanus ME, Farndon JR, Wells SA] Jr. Transplantation of the parathyroid glands. In: IDA Johnston, NW Thompson, eds. Endocrine Surgery. London: Butterworth, 1983: 25-40.

CHAPTER 9

Secondary Hyperparathyroidism

Jonas Rastad, Göran Åkerström

Secondary hyperparathyroidism is an inevitable consequence of mainly chronic renal insufficiency, and may add considerable morbidity to patients already suffering from this severe disorder. Parathyroid surgery usually is rewarding in these patients, although objective evaluation of even short-term surgical outcome is complicated. Yet, persistent renal insufficiency leads to inevitable relapse, in which case parathyroid reoperation might be unusually complicated. In such instances primary and secondary parathyroid surgery should be regarded as one of the possible, and perhaps underrated, options in the continuous struggle to limit the potentially severe complications of renal failure.

Secondary hyperparathyroidism (HPT) requiring parathyroid surgery virtually only relates to progressive kidney diseases and less commonly to long-term lithium therapy, although this condition also may arise from gastrointestinal absorption defects, dietary vitamin D deficiency, liver diseases and pseudohypoparathyroidism. The term tertiary HPT has been used to define secondary HPT accompanied by spontaneous hypercalcemia, clinically persistent HPT after renal transplantation and concurrence of parathyroid adenoma and hyperplasia.[1-3] This ambiguity as well as the quantitative rather than qualitative differences in parathyroid gland dysfunction within these conditions suggest that the denomination tertiary HPT should be abandoned.[4,5] The main purpose of the current chapter is to describe some aspects on pathophysiology, diagnosis, clinical findings, and medical therapy to provide a background for the section on parathyroid reoperation in uremic HPT.

UREMIC HYPERPARATHYROIDISM

HPT is an inevitable consequence of disturbances in renal function, and it should be expected to occur in all patients with chronic renal insufficiency. Moreover the biochemical and morphological evidences of parathyroid involvement generally increase with the increased severity

Current Controversy in Parathyroid Operation and Reoperation, edited by Göran Åkerström.

and duration of the functional renal impairment and seems to occur independent of the cause of this disturbance.[6-12] The principal clinical problem in these patients thus rarely relates to the diagnosis of secondary HPT per se, but rather to the extent of complications and symptoms of the disease as well as their optimal mode of management. Although new concepts for medical prophylaxis and therapy of secondary HPT have been widely accepted and might the diminish role of parathyroid surgery,[13-16] it has been demonstrated that such surgery still might be required in up to 40% of European patients undergoing truly long-term dialysis.[17]

Pathogenesis of HPT

The development of HPT in uremia has attracted considerable interest and the sequence of pathophysiologically important events has been extensively reviewed recently.[17-21] Briefly the original "trade-off" hypothesis emphasizes the importance of phosphate retention from imbalance in dietary phosphate intake and renal excretion during progressive nephron loss.[22,23] The resulting hyperphosphatemia at least transiently lowers serum calcium mainly by physicochemical complexing and thereby enhances parathyroid gland activity. Such hypocalcemia, however, constitutes no requisite for the development of uremic HPT upon experimental analysis and seems to occur in only fractions of patients developing secondary HPT.[24] The resulting excess of parathyroid hormone (PTH) stimulates phosphaturia, and participates in maintaining phosphate homeostasis until the glomerular filtration rate approaches about 30% of normal. This control, however, requires continuous parathyroid gland perturbation, which might contribute to the development of secretory dysregulation and glandular enlargement.

Experimental studies supporting the relevance of phosphate accumulation relate to the demonstration of stimulated serum PTH values and parathyroid tissue mass during exposure to phosphate enriched diets, as well as partial amelioration of these derangements by restricted phosphate intake in uremia.[17,20,23] However hyperphosphatemia is not readily demonstrable during an oral phosphate load, and phosphate restriction has not been consistently associated with decreased parathyroid gland secretion in incipient renal failure. Although the pathogenic importance of serum phosphate may be equivocal in uremic HPT, restriction of phosphate intake and maintenance of acceptable serum phosphate levels comprise the cornerstone in the medical therapy of renal insufficiency.[14,25] Moreover the acidosis of uremia and furosemide treatment may enhance circulating PTH values and perhaps contribute to the progression of secondary HPT.[26,27]

Calcitriol ($1,25(OH)_2D_3$) participates in a feedback control system exerting profound regulation on the parathyroid gland.[28-30] In addition calcitriol stimulates intestinal calcium and phosphate absorption, influences bone modeling, and exerts widespread endocrine and paracrine actions on cell proliferation, differentiation, secretion, and immune activity.[31,32] Calcitriol is synthesized mainly in the proximal kidney tubule, where activity of 1-α-hydroxylase is stimulated by PTH and inhibited by calcium as well as calcitriol. The enzyme also seems sensitive to phosphate, whereby successful phosphate restriction in some but not other studies has tended to normalize decreased serum calcitriol values in patients with moderately severe renal failure.[18,33,34] Established uremia invariably should be expected to be accompanied by a severe shortage of calcitriol due mainly to the nephron loss per se and the generally modest capacity of extrarenal calcitriol production.[35] This deficiency might be aggravated by subnormal levels of $25(OH)D_3$ from reduced sun exposure, medications and nephrotic proteinuria, since 1-α-hydroxylase activity becomes substrate dependent in uremia.[36,37]

The extent of renal impairment causing calcitriol deficiency is controversial. Low serum values have been registered in at least some patients exhibiting glomerular filtration rates of 60-80 ml/min.[36,38-42]

Mild renal insufficiency might be accompanied by maintained calcium absorption and numerically normal levels of circulating calcitriol, but this circumstance possibly relates, at least partially, to the concomitantly elevated serum PTH value. Moreover total serum calcitriol values may comprise an unsatisfactory estimate on its cellular availability due mainly to extensive serum protein binding and reduced metabolic clearance in renal disease. Free serum calcitriol values nevertheless have been positively correlated to the glomerular filtration rate.[43] The dependency of calcitriol production on PTH and calcium, and the importance of calcitriol in regulating parathyroid cell secretion and proliferation suggest that this aspect of the calcium homeostasis must also be evaluated in terms of hormonal feedback control.[31,44] The classical sequence of calcitriol deficiency leading to intestinal calcium malabsorption and secondary HPT thus is much more complex than initially anticipated. This relationship is further complicated by the occurrence of target organ resistance to the calcemic actions of PTH even in moderate renal impairment, which is a poorly understood phenomenon and possibly relates mainly to phosphate retention, calcitriol deficiency, and PTH excess itself.[40,45,46] Some light into this intriguing circumstance has recently been obtained by demonstration of down-regulation of the PTH receptor in experimental uremia.[47]

Parathyroid Cell Secretory Regulation

Parathyroid secretory stimulation in renal insufficiency possibly is multifactorial. Frank or relative hypocalcemia naturally comprise a prominent secretogogue and hypercalcemia conversely may decrease the secretion, although attenuated calcium sensitivity is a conspicuous feature of the PTH release in uremic HPT.[4,5,48,49] Calcitriol has been found to suppress parathyroid cell secretion by enhancing its calcium sensitivity and by reducing PTH gene transcription independent of any direct action on the extracellular calcium concentration.[13,28,29,50] These circumstances are consistent with the decreased serum PTH level and the enhanced calcium sensitivity of its secretion usually obtained with vitamin D treatment especially in slight to moderate renal failure, although rise in the serum calcium concentration might be frequent in certain subgroups of uremic HPT.[20,51-55] There seems to be resistance to the regulatory actions of calcitriol, however, since decreased and markedly heterogeneous expression of its receptor has been substantiated in the pathological parathyroid tissue of human and experimental HPT due to renal insufficiency.[56-59] Moreover vitamin D treatment in patients with established uremia commonly induces only limited reduction of an excessively increased PTH level, which may be accompanied by the induction of frank hypercalcemia of potentially adverse significance.

A prominent net effect of HPT and perhaps hitherto unexplored dysfunctions in uremics includes a rise in the intact serum PTH value. This rise occurs even at clearly subclinical levels of renal disturbance, increases with the extent and duration of this impairment, and demonstrates maintained but attenuated dependence on the ionized plasma calcium concentration.[12,43,60] Although the amplitude of intact PTH excess may be impressive in established uremia, considerable interindividual variation occurs. Normal levels may rarely be encountered even after longer-term hemodialysis and especially in individuals with low bone turnover. Apart from interacting with expected functions in kidney and bone, the substantial PTH excess has been causally coupled to increased cytoplasmic calcium levels facilitating nephrocalcinosis and participating in disturbances in neuronal transmitter release, pancreatic islet functions, as well as granulocytic, T-cell, and platelet actions.[21,61]

Clinical evidence and rare studies in vitro support that aluminum may accumulate in the parathyroid tissue and inhibit PTH release.[62,63] Moreover all patients with HPT should be evaluated for magnesium deficiency, since wasting of this cation by e.g. magnesuria may induce suppressed PTH secretion, hypocalcemia and skeletal disease being largely reversible upon supplementation.[64] Chromogranin constitutes a tissues-unspecific marker of neuroendocrine tissues, which is co-stored with native hormones in secretory granules and co-released upon stimulation. This protein is accumulated in the circulation of uremics and possibly participates in autoregulation of PTH release.[65,66]

Parathyroid Cell Proliferation

Indirect evidence supports coupling of the dedifferentiated calcium regulation of PTH secretion to the enhanced parathyroid cell proliferation in HPT.[67-69] A consequence of this relationship includes a correlation of serum PTH values and total glandular weight in normo- and hypercalcemic individuals with uremic HPT.[8,10,11] Moreover total gland and parenchymal cell weights, as serum PTH, tend to increase with duration and severity of both clinical and subclinical renal diseases, which also seems to encompass the tendency for nodule formations as well as the oxyphil cell content of these glands.[8,9,70] Such parenchymal nodules display greater disturbances in secretion and indices of parenchymal proliferation in subtotal parathyroid resection and parathyroid autotransplantation.[59,71-73] Furthermore hypocalcemia has been demonstrated experimentally to enhance parathyroid cell proliferation,[74] and calcitriol seems to decrease parenchymal growth by interaction with proto-oncogene products.[28,30,75,76] Provided these mechanisms comprise the most significant stimulators of proliferation, it is intriguing that the glandular enlargement characteristically is asymmetrical in uremic HPT associated with normal or elevated serum calcium values.[9,11] However substantially enlarged parathyroid glands of uremic HPT have displayed loss of a tumor suppressor gene on chromosome 11q13, which has been considered to cause neuroendocrine cell proliferation in multiple endocrine neoplasia type 1.[77] Endothelin comprises another factor which is accumulated in renal diseases and seems to interact in parathyroid cell secretion and proliferation.[78,79]

Renal Osteodystrophy

Uremic bone involvement comprises a virtually obligatory finding in chronic renal insufficiency, but the time of onset, extent and type of skeletal derangement differ between the patients.[42,80] Several factors including prominence of vitamin D deficiency in the population, aluminum exposure, and type, duration and intensity of the kidney disease, diabetes mellitus, as well as medications including corticosteroids and calcium salts might contribute to this variability. Diagnosis and differentiation between the heterogeneous and often mixed abnormalities collectively described as renal osteodystrophy require bone biopsy. This diagnostic tool should be utilized liberally especially prior to parathyroid surgery, since overt normoparathyroidism postoperatively is potentially harmful to patients suffering from states of reduced bone turnover.

Osteitis fibrosa constitutes the most prevalent form of bone involvement in secondary HPT.[49,80,81] Briefly this classical disorder of high bone turnover is characterized by signs of profound hyperparathyroid activity with a plethora of osteoblasts, osteoclasts and osteocytes, predominance of abnormal woven bone formation, fibroblast proliferation with bone marrow fibrosis, and irregular mineralization. Clinically these patients may demonstrate subperiostal resorption upon radiography, preferentially of the digital phalanxes, clavicular head, proximal tibia and humerus, and rare bone cysts or even "brown tumor" formations. Vertebral trabecular bone may display central osteosclerosis upon computed tomography.[83] An excess of intact serum PTH characteristically is present in these patients, who rather frequently display elevated levels of serum alkaline phosphatases and osteocalcin as well as a relatively moderate tendency for hypercalcemia upon treatment with vitamin D and calcium salts.

Patients with low bone turnover of uremia may suffer from osteomalacia and adynamic skeletal involvement. Osteomalacia principally comprises defective mineralization considered to relate to aluminum accumulation and perhaps also vitamin D deficiency and acidosis. The affected bone characteristically displays marked increases in lamellar osteoid, decreased osteoblasts and osteoclasts, as well as reduced formation and resorption surfaces in addition to sparse woven bone, absence of marrow fibrosis, and a high aluminum content.[49,84-86] Clinically these patients frequently show modestly elevated serum PTH, normal osteocalcin and alkaline phosphatase values, as well as radiographic signs of generalized osteopenia. The currently rare but severely affected patients may display stress or pseudofractures and Looser's zones in the ribs, scapula and femoral neck. The frequent use of vitamin D and phosphate binders with restricted aluminum content suggest temporal decay in the incidence of uremic osteomalacia.

Adynamic or aplastic osteodystrophy constitutes a rather recently recognized condition of increasing prevalence, which is characterized by decreased matrix formation and sparse bone cells without evidence of defective mineralization.[42,49,87,88] The severely decreased bone modeling of these patients increases the risk of mechanical failure. Also this disorder has been associated with aluminum accumulation in many of the currently prevailing patients, but increasing patient age, diabetes mellitus, iron overload, corticosteroid therapy and peritoneal dialysis may become of increasing pathogenic significance. Patients with hypoparathyroidism either by medical suppression or surgery exhibit increased risk for the development of osteomalacia and adynamic osteodystrophy, and excess PTH may participate in maintaining skeletal mineralization during aluminum accumulation.[89,90] Patients with adynamic osteodystrophy characteristically demonstrate normal serum PTH, alkaline phosphatase and osteocalcin levels, and the tendency for development of hypercalcemia upon vitamin D treatment may be marked especially in relation to the prevailing level of intact serum PTH.

Biochemistry of Surgical Relevance in Uremic HPT

The biochemical alterations of HPT is less readily evaluated in nephropathies compared to primary HPT. Most patients with uremia display a normal serum calcium concentration despite the presence of biochemically unequivocal HPT.[38] Total serum calcium with or without correction for serum albumin, however, may be less reliable in uremia.[91] This index of calcium homeostasis should be evaluated by measurement of the ionized plasma calcium level, since dysionization mainly seems to participate in generating clinically less relevant elevations in total serum calcium level. The serum calcium concentration should be compared to concomitant serum phosphate determinations, since elevations in either or both of these ions comprise a common failure of medical uremia treatment and influence considerations for parathyroid operation. Intact serum PTH values increase early in renal dysfunction and correlates inversely to GFR.[12,43,60] This elevated PTH is a manifestation of the defective calcium regulation of parathyroid cell secretion even in the presence of frank hypocalcemia. Dynamic testing by citrate/calcium infusion or low/high calcium dialysis accurately assesses the derangement in calcium regulated PTH secretion, but this measure rarely is necessary in the clinical follow-up. Borderline HPT in patients with mild renal dysfunction and in those with meager elevation of intact serum PTH despite established uremia rarely should be considered for parathyroid operation. In contrast to carboxyterminal or midregional serum PTH, rises in intact PTH should be regarded as accurately reflecting the parathyroid secretory stimulation. Although defective metabolism of even intact PTH may occur in renal dysfunction, the serum levels largely have been found to correlate with histomorphometric indices of bone turnover.[19,60,92] Intact serum PTH thus comprises an important means of establishing the degree of uremic HPT as well as the risk of osteitis fibrosa, and may in itself strengthen the indication for parathyroid operation. Corrections of decreased plasma bicarbonate, $1,25(OH)_2D_3$ and magnesium levels may participate in reducing or increasing the PTH concentration, respectively, but these derangements rarely seem to exert any greater impact on decisions concerning parathyroid surgery.

Evaluation of the bone involvement in uremic HPT is mandatory prior to parathyroid operation. Although individuals with excessive elevations in intact serum PTH and gradually increasing alkaline phosphatase and osteocalcin levels possibly harbor hyperparathyroid bone disease, mixed skeletal involvement with risks of postoperatively dominant osteomalacia cannot be adequately assessed in the absence of bone biopsy. This line of reasoning actually seems to apply even in the presence of radiologically demonstrable osteitis fibrosa.[93] Determination of aluminum accumulation is important not only with respect to bone biopsy stainings, whereby serum levels of this trivalent cation may be measured and perhaps deferoxamine tests and treatment may become necessary.[94,95] The establishment of vitamin D deficiency with low $1,25(OH)_2D_3$ values may increase the risk of low turnover bone disease and consequently this would be interesting to assess especially upon suspicion of insufficiently explored vitamin D_3 therapy.

Clinical Manifestations of Surgical Relevance in Uremic HPT

Symptoms of skeletal involvement generally are more prominent and common in osteomalacia than in patients with even advanced osteitis fibrosa. This distinction may relate to the increased risk of fracture particularly to the axial skeleton, painful pseudofractures, and deformity classically including kyphoscoliosis, acetabular protrusion, and femoral malpositioning. Bone pain usually is dull, insidious in onset, and aggravated by movements and weight bearing. It characteristically affects the lumbar region, hips, ankles, wrists and shoulders, and the skeleton may be tender upon palpation. Acute bone pain should increase the suspicion of fracture, which may be due to even moderate trauma, rare brown tumors and bone cysts, as well as repetitive strain. Osteomyelitis, skeletal amyloidosis, myeloma and metastases should also be considered. Epiphysiolysis as well as aseptic necrosis of especially the femoral head may cause severe disability and preferentially occur in children, patients with corticosteroid treatment and those with diabetes mellitus. Myopathy of uremic HPT is characterized by decreased strength especially of the shoulder and pelvic girdles, muscle aching upon fatigue and proximal wasting. Pruritus affects more than half of uremic patients and can be unbearable in some. The cause of itching is unknown, and it may be ameliorated with UV light therapy. It seems to be related to extensive PTH excess as well as abnormal skin reactions to histamine and cutaneous calcium accumulation.[96] Motor and sensory neuropathy is frequent in long-standing uremia and may contribute to the skin condition.[97]

Ectopic calcification may occur in a variety of locations in patients with uremic HPT. Periarticular deposits may attain extensive proportions and particularly occur in the shoulder, elbow, hip and knuckles. Such extensive masses may hamper joint mobility and cause acute inflammation. Other sites for calcareous deposition include tunica media of vessels, lung, heart, kidney, gastrointestinal tract etc. Progressive ecchymotic necrosis of skin and muscles (calciphylaxis) with ischemia and vascular calcification may develop very rarely and constitutes a condition of considerable mortality.[98-100] The pathogenesis of extraosseous calcium-containing deposits remains to be clarified, but generally has been related to complex interactions between calcium, phosphate, PTH, aluminum, alkalosis, mechanical trauma, lipid disturbances and perhaps PTH-related peptide.[21,101,102] Therapy with vitamin D, especially calcitriol has also been coupled to this potentially severe complication.[103]

Surgical Aspects on Medical Treatment of Uremic HPT

Patients with renal failure generally are recommended for parathyroid operation when satisfactory attempts at medical therapy have failed to control symptoms and signs of HPT. Although this central dogma appears adequate in the vast majority of patients, it has not been adequately challenged during recent years. A common consequence of this strategy seems to be a restrictive of surgery among individuals with biochemically severe HPT. It should also be that currently prevailing modes of medical treatment for uremic HPT are by no means devoid of complications, and that the frequency and seriousness of these complications should be weighed against the comparatively well-documented risks and benefits of parathyroid surgery.

The medical treatment of uremic HPT primarily aims at reducing hyperphosphatemia, supporting serum calcium, decreasing serum PTH, and improving skeletal turnover. Vitamin D_3 sterols should be expected to significantly reduce intact and to lesser extents carboxyterminal and midregional serum PTH levels.[17,20,33,55,104] However the extent of reduced intact PTH values differs considerably between patients and seems be less clinically relevant in those with biochemically more marked HPT. In the most favorable cases, however, setting the intact PTH level slightly above the upper normal range has been considered optimal. Over longer periods of time these sterols might participate in reducing parathyroid cell mass, which probably constitutes a very slow process involving programmed cell death (apoptosis) by free radical and calcium dependent activation of DNA degrading nucleases. Through direct actions possibly on osteoblasts and via improved regulation of PTH secretion, the vitamin hormone also exerts favorable influences on morphology and symptoms associated with renal osteodystrophy.[20,42,80] These improvements seem to encompass pure or mixtures of osteitis fibrosa and aluminum-unrelated osteomalacia, but not the low bone turnover associated with aluminum accumulation. Moreover serum levels of alkaline phosphatases and osteocalcin generally decrease as a result of the more favorable bone turnover. Vitamin D_3 also exerts desirable influences on the glucose responsiveness of insulin secretion, thyroid hormone release, as well as activities of the immune system and reproductive organs in uremic patients.

Calcitriol therapy increases serum calcium in a largely dose-dependent fashion and tends to elevate serum phosphate through enhanced intestinal absorption.[17,20,42,105,106] Adequate phosphate control appears important, otherwise paradoxical stimulation of serum PTH may occur. These actions may lead to frank hypercalcemia especially during concomitant administration of phosphate binding calcium salts in conjunction with the severely reduced calcium clearance in uremia, in patients with aluminum accumulation, and in those with biochemically severe HPT. This complication may be reduced by altering the route, time, pace and dose of calcitriol administration, by reducing dialysate calcium content, and by the application of vitamin D metabolites elevating serum calcium to lesser degree. Hypercalcemia and hyperphosphatemia nevertheless account for important adverse effects in modern modes of uremic therapy and may enhance the risk of calcium precipitation, nephrocalcinosis and progression of renal impairment. Patients exhibiting these biochemical disturbances prior to intiation of therapy generally are difficult to manage adequately.[107-109] Indeed it has been suggested that the currently recommended therapy for secondary HPT might comprise an important cause for the increasing incidence of adynamic renal osteodystrophy through the induction of insufficient PTH levels in relation to the increased requirements in uremia.[110] Moreover calcitriol per se has been suggested to accelerate renal dysfunction, but this effect may relate to tubular creatinine transport rather than to effects on GFR, and to participate in progression of atherosclerosis. Taken together these findings are a strong indication for calcitriol and calcium salts in most stages of uremic HPT, and support that parathyroid surgery may constitute an important measure facilitating the application of such a regimen in the more severe stages of this disease.

Pediatric Aspects of Uremic HPT

Children with progressive renal insufficiency have substantially elevated intact serum PTH values, common osteitis fibrosa—even in the absence of radiological signs of bone involvement, and virtually unmeasurable values of circulating calcitriol.[111] Prominent growth retardation comprises a distinct feature especially in individuals affected very early in life. Many uremic children also display skeletal deformities with epiphysiolysis, avascular necrosis and asymptomatic fracture. It is a clinical impression that patients suffering from uremia during childhood not only develop a generally more serious bone involvement, but also biochemical signs of HPT as well as degrees of parathyroid gland enlargement. Adynamic bone disease seems uncommon in children, and despite suggestions regarding the risk of certain infant formulas,[112] aluminum accumulation largely appears related to phosphate binders especially upon administration with buffered citric acid preparations. However, osteomalacia or mixtures of osteomalacia and osteitis fibrosa may be rather prevalent in pediatric uremia, and this circumstance may relate to suggestions of unusual susceptibility of the growing skeleton to vitamin D deficiency.[113]

In conjunction with their adult counterparts, the extent of hyperparathyroid bone involvement of uremic children roughly correlates to the intact serum PTH level. The more advanced stages of osteitis fibrosa in children seem to respond less favorably to oral calcitriol treatment. This observation emphasizes the importance of early treatment in which case calcium salts alone may comprise a natural choice despite the necessity for induction of mild hypercalcemia and the less satisfactory phosphate binding ability of these therapeutics in substantial proportions of uremic adults.[114,155] Moreover intraperitoneal calcitriol administration has been attempted in pediatric uremics conventionally subjected to cyclic or continuous peritoneal dialysis, although calcitriol demonstrates an unusual propensity to adhere to plastic.[116]

Regarding survival among pediatric patients, what are the risks of iatrogenic hypercalcemia. Even mild elevations of serum calcium have been accompanied by premature death due mainly to cardiovascular disorders.[117-119] Although an unequivocal relationship between serum calcium and the mortality remains to be established and there exist vast discrepancies in the clinical characteristics of primary and uremic HPT, there currently is no reason to believe that elevated serum calcium values might be less lethal in uremic than in primary HPT. Serious efforts must be focused on assessing the long-term benefits from medical treatment of uremic HPT, since hypercalcemia may be necessary in order to satisfactorily suppress PTH secretion and to moderate skeletal influences especially in clinically severe HPT of both children and adults with uremia. Although parathyroid surgery is accompanied by modest morbidity and mortality, therapeutic value might be underrated in extensive uremic HPT.

Renal Transplantation

Successful renal transplantation generally ameliorates several derangements of uremic HPT. The recovery characteristically is slow and incomplete, and rare patients actually suffer from rapidly progressing HPT after transplantation. The rapid improvment in creatinine clearance in transplant recipients generally is accompanied by decreases in serum calcium, phosphate, intact PTH, alkaline phosphatase and osteocalcin values as well as elevation of circulating calcitriol.[39,120-122] Reversal of alkaline phosphatase levels, however, may be unreliable predictors of decreased bone resorption, since this may depend on the direct effects of steroid medication.[123] Patients maintaining normocalcemia after transplantation often display long-standing elevations of serum PTH. This has been associated with reduced sensitivity of the parathyroid glands to alterations in the extracellular calcium concentration and decreased suppressibility of the secretion due to the generally slow involution of the parathyroid cell mass.[124-126] Such derangements in the relationship between calcium and PTH are manifestations persisting defects not only in calcium sensitivity of the parathyroid gland secretion but also in the calcemic action of PTH.[127] These derangements may produce highly variable indices of the calcium homeostasis, such that normocalcemia may be accompanied by substantial PTH excess and modestly elevated PTH values can contribute to unequivocal hypercalcemia. Other evidences for partially recovered HPT in transplant recipients with normocalcemia and satisfactory renal function include persistent increases in bone turnover on radiographic, scintigraphic and histological evaluation as well as tendencies for serum osteocalcin and alkaline phosphatase elevations.[120,128,129] Moreover these patients commonly display hypophosphatemia, which may be related to a variety of factors including persistent HPT, decreased intestinal phosphate uptake, and defective tubular phosphate handling of the grafted kidney.[124,130] It should also be remembered that the currently prevailing immunosuppressive therapy contributes significantly to bone loss and also may aggravate reductions in serum phosphate levels.

Hypercalcemia of highly variable duration and intensity may occur after renal transplantation. This complication should be expected in about 20-35% of the patients, who generally display higher alkaline phosphatase and lower serum phosphate values in comparison to their normocalcemic counterparts.[120,124,130-132] Such hypercalcemia has been found to occur mainly in patients with extensive biochemical indices of HPT, particularly hypercalcemia, as well as severe uremia and a long course of dialysis prior to transplantation. A small proportion of these individuals display rapidly progressing hypercalcemia, the incidence of which seems to decrease with the use of modern medical treatment regimens in uremic HPT. The hypercalcemia usually is substantial in such patients, generally occurs within the first weeks after transplantation, and sometimes is accompanied by at least transient signs of graft dysfunction. The detailed cause of this derangement is unknown, but it possibly relates to combinations of persistently severe PTH excess and improved peripheral sensitivity to its calcemic actions, reversal of hyperphosphatemia, and enhanced calcitriol synthesis.

In more than half the patients with elevated hypercalcemia, after transplantation the disorder is self-limiting.[120,124,130-132] In most of these instances the level of serum calcium is mildly to moderately elevated and resolves within the first year after transplantation. Some patients, however, may have very elevated calcium levels usually during the first few months after transplantation. It is difficult to determine if the condition is reversible. It is essential to analyze intact serum PTH levels in relation to the temporal course and extent of calcium elevation. Moreover, currently very few of these patients suffer from iatrogenic phosphate depletion due to the extensive use of phosphate binders, vitamin D overdosage, persistent hyperphosphatemia from resorption of extraskeletal calcium-phosphate deposits, as well as adrenocortical insufficiency from rapid reduction of extensive corticosteroid therapy. Finally hypercalcemia of moderate severity may persist for more than a year after renal grafting. This type of hypercalcemia currently is the most common in renal graft recipients, frequently resolves within 2-6 years, and rarely may persist considerably longer. Providing that the serum calcium level is stable or slowly decreasing and accompanied by elevated levels of intact serum PTH, insufficient regression of HPT should be expected to prevail in these instances. However late occurrence or progression of hypercalcemia should be examined for other causes, particularly malignancy and granulomatous diseases.

LITHIUM-INDUCED HYPERPARATHYROIDISM

Long-term oral lithium therapy is commonly employed in unipolar and bipolar affective disorders. This monovalent cation influences several physiologic functions including parathyroid and thyroid gland secretion and growth, as well as intestinal and renal fluid and electrolyte balances.[133-135] Moreover it may reduce bone mineral content and induce irreversible renal damage. Experimental and clinical studies on the human parathyroid demonstrate that lithium diminishes the effects of extracellular calcium on the PTH release, so that enhanced hormone output will occur during both acute and chronic exposure.[136-138] This is possibly mediated through interference with the calcium receptor on the parathyroid cell surface leading to insufficient calcium-mediated increases in the cytoplasmic calcium concentration.[139] Furthermore lithium may enhance replication of human parathyroid cells, although this effect has only been dmonstrated in in vitro studies involving pathological glands alone.[137,140]

Against this background it is not surprising that lithium exposure is accompanied by elevation of serum calcium in many individuals and that long-term therapy should be expected to cause hypercalcemia in about 10% of patients.[134,141] This may be an underestimate. It also is pertinent to note that the incidence of hypercalcemia may increase with duration of the lithium therapy. The elevation of serum calcium usually is mild and accompanied by inappropriately elevated values of intact serum PTH thereby making diagnosis relatively uncomplicated. Hypercalcemia may be reversible, however, upon lithium withdrawal at least after limited exposure[142] and urinary calcium output may be decreased prior to the development of a renal calcium leak. It also is apparent that some patients develop hypercalcemia after only a few weeks of therapy, whereas the lithium-associated elevation of serum calcium characteristically develops during years of treatment. Interestingly it has been suggested that hypercalcemia in patients with short-term lithium exposure may represent unmasking of primary HPT, while chief cell hyperplasia otherwise should be expected to occur in lithium-associated secondary HPT.[133,143]

Primary HPT has been demonstrated to be accompanied by frequent psychic symptoms, which generally are affective in character and which commonly go unnoticed unless specifically searched for, and associated with alterations in cerebrospinal fluid monoamine and calcium metabolism.[144,145] Moreover cardiovascular disturbances may be overrepresented in affective disorders, a circumstance which significantly contributes to the increased mortality of untreated primary HPT.[118,119,146] Unless lithium treatment may be permanently interrupted and normocalcemia attained within a few months of observation, most patients with HPT from long-standing lithium treatment should benefit from parathyroid surgery. The actual number of such operations, however, suggests that most of these patients remain unrecognized or are improperly handled in this respect.

Primary parathyroid surgery in lithium-associated secondary HPT usually is uncomplicated despite the divergent theories on pathogenesis. Patients with possibly shorter duration of lithium therapy generally display the classical parathyroid adenoma accompanied by three grossly normal glands, while chief cell hyperplasia rarely involving enlargement of four parathyroids may dominate in those with perhaps at least 3 years of such exposure.[133,143] As in sporadic primary HPT, excision of the enlarged glands alone seems uncontroversial, although universal application of subtotal resections has been suggested.[135] The rarity of reported cases and the limited duration of follow-up, however, generally prevent critical evaluation in this respect. Subtotal parathyroid resection, however, may be necessary in the exceptional patients demonstrating macroscopic signs of four gland enlargement. Postoperative analyses are unusually meager in these individuals, but normocalcemia invariably has been reported during short-term follow-up.[133,135] Postoperative lithium therapy seems inadvisable, continuation of therapy does not invariably lead to recurrence of HPT. Parathyroid reoperations have generally not been described in lithium-associated HPT.

PARATHYROID REOPERATION IN SECONDARY HYPERPARATHYROIDISM

Only a very limited number of studies are available regarding the indications, strategy, findings, and outcome of parathyroid reoperation in secondary HPT. This possibly reflects the generally guarded view of parathyroid surgery which internists handling these patients tend to favor. Successful parathyroid operation especially in uremic individuals receiving no functioning kidney graft should be considered as one of several options in the continuous struggle to ameliorate secondary HPT rather than to provide a definitive cure for this therapy-resistant condition. Conversely recurrence of HPT after previous surgery comprise an equivocal failure. The most important basis for this line of reasoning is the observation that the operation, whether it is performed as subtotal or total parathyroidectomy with or without autotransplantation, should be expected to be accompanied by considerable risks of time-dependent rises in serum PTH levels during longer-term follow-up of patients with persistent uremia.[147-150]

The following discussion on parathyroid re-exploration will deal with patients suffering from uremic HPT alone, since reoperative data essentially is lacking in other causes of secondary HPT and since renal dysfunction by far comprises the most common cause of secondary HPT. Consistent with these observations, during the last decade we have handled only a few individuals with recurrent HPT and gastrointestinal disturbances and none with chronic lithium therapy. In order to appreciate several aspects of reoperative parathyroid surgery in uremic HPT, circumstances associated with the initial operative procedure should be clarified.

Technical Aspects of Primary Parathyroid Operation

Primary parathyroid operation in most patients with secondary HPT of renal or intestinal disturbances may be performed either by subtotal resection or total parathyroidectomy. The technical refinements of these strategies have been described and will only be briefly discussed here. Subtotal resection usually aims at leaving in situ a well vascularized parathyroid remnant of about 50-60 mg, although size ranges of 30-150 mg have been suggested.[7,10,131,151-156] This remnant should be selected from the least enlarged and nodular of the parathyroids preferentially from the inferior glandular pair. It should be marked by an nonabsorbable suture with the ends positioned ventrally to the thyroid lobe in order to facilitate later re-excision. Immediate or deferred autotransplantation during total parathyroidectomy classically involves grafting into brachioradial pockets of the non-dominant forearm carrying no site of long-term vascular access;[11,149-151,155,156,159-164] (for earlier references see 157,158). The size and number of the transplanted pieces have varied and usually encompass 50-80 mg parathyroid tissue divided into 15-40 slivers of approximately 0.5-3 mm^3. Others, however, have utilized a single pocket and few slices weighing up to altogether 200 mg.[150,161,165] In order to facilitate graft excision, each pouch containing the grafted tissue is closed by a nonabsorbable suture and kept within an area covering approximately 2 x 3 cm. Other sites of autotransplantation mainly encompass a single or few pockets in the sternocleidomastoid or other muscles and subcutaneous fat.[157,158,160,166-168] Moreover all identified parathyroid glands should be verified by intraoperative histology, and the tissue selected for subsequent transplantation as well as a remnant left in situ during subtotal resection should be weighed. Both subtotal and total parathyroidectomy should include excision of periparathyroid fat and bilateral cervical thymic resection in order to remove parathyroid tissue islands comprising sites of potential growth and recurrence.

Cryopreservation of parathyroid tissue has been recommended during total parathyroidectomy in order to perform complementary transplantation for advertent and inadvertent hypoparathyroidism.[158,169-173] This strategy might also be considered upon during subtotal resection due to the associated risk of inducing postoperative hypoparathyroidism (for references see 152,156,157). Technical details associated with the technique of graded decrease in temperature, optimal cryoprotectants, and conditions of thawing for the small tissue pieces have been evaluated elsewhere.[157,158,172-175] These studies have supported retained ability to secrete PTH with an essentially unaltered sensitivity to external calcium for at least a portion of the cryopreserved cells upon dispersion after thawing. Tissue necrosis with increasing duration (years) of storage have been reported. Since fresh tissue generally provides better graft survival,[157,158,173,174,176,177] we rarely have utilized delayed transplantation unless inadvertent hypoparathyroidism occurs postoperatively. In such situations slightly larger amounts of tissue (about 150 mg) should be implanted to reduce insufficient graft function, which nevertheless may occur in up to about 40% of the patients.

Delayed autografting is based on the idea of establishing hypoparathyroidism during the first 4-9 postoperative months in order to avoid unnecessary complications from autotransplantation of patients with clinically detectable amounts of residual parathyroid tissue in the neck.[173,178,179] In contemporary patients receiving vitamin D and perhaps also oral calcium as postoperative treatment of HPT, the diagnosis of hypoparathyroidism essentially relies solely upon immeasurable values of intact serum PTH. Delayed autotransplantation rarely is advocated during primary exploration for secondary HPT, which is consistent with the unfavorable influence of cryopreservation on graft function, the generally low incidence of persistent HPT after primary explorations for secondary HPT, and the diagnostic and therapeutic difficulty in determining low normal PTH values. Moreover there are indications for at least short-term influences of parathyroidectomy on tissue aluminum accumulation, whereby transient and complex interaction with parathyroid gland secretion may be encountered.[90,180] In our experience it is essentially impossible to predict the recurrence of HPT from levels of PTH shortly after parathyroidectomy for uremic HPT.

The choice of subtotal or total parathyroidectomy with autotransplantation during primary explorations for secondary HPT generally is related more to personal preference than objective criteria.[152,157,158] However, subtotal resection may be prevented by difficulties to identify, without damage, the vascular pedicle of the gland to be transected. Such damage cannot be dtermined from the color of the gland alone, but relies on the presence of which hemorrhage from multiple small cut surfaces, which coagulate spontaneously. Unequivocal arterial bleeding during transection, however, indicates damage to the vascular supply and should be dealt with accordingly. The vascular supply mainly seems to arise from the inferior thyroid artery sending off a macroscopically recognizable branch along the thyroid capsule to both the inferior and superior glandular pair.[181-185] Parathyroids located close to or in clefts of the thyroid gland and those exhibiting more conspicuous enlargement may pose particular problems in this regard. Moreover, the glands located below the thyreothymic ligament should be expected to be vascularized from above, so that distal resection of the ipsilateral cervical thymus may be attainable. Taken together these circumstances indicate that trimming of a subtotally resected gland should commence prior to extirpation of the other parathyroid glands. Other difficulties in this respect relate to the few patients requiring concomitant thyroid procedures. It has also been suggested that noncompliant individuals, who cannot be relied on to follow medical treatment of secondary HPT, may have increased risk of recurrence and should undergo total parathyroidectomy.[154]

We tend to favor subtotal parathyroid resection during primary operation of secondary HPT in individuals suitable for or scheduled to receive a renal transplant, children, patients with considerable operative risk, and those with less severe biochemical and clinical signs of HPT. Although the last criterion is by no means well-defined, patients with severe HPT tend to exhibit larger glands with usually marked signs of nodular hyperplasia.[8,9,11,186,187] Their parathyroid disease can be difficult to handle with respect to the aquisition of optimal parathyroid gland remnants. Such parathyroid disease seems to be accompanied by an increased risk of recurrence,[71,72,150,188] which possibly is treated more effectively by total than subtotal parathyroidectomy.[152,156,157,174] Moreover, limited follow-up comparing subtotal resection and total parathyroidectomy with immediate autotransplantation suggests the favorable influences of the latter procedure on at least some symptoms associated with pronounced secondary HPT.[156] On the other hand short-term postoperative hypocalcemia is substantially less pronounced after subtotal resection, which might be advantageous especially in children and individuals suffering from unusually increased operative risk. Patients scheduled for their first renal transplantation may be supplied with comparatively large remnants of subtotally resected glands in conjunction with the healing effect of reversed renal dysfunction particularly with moderate HPT.[39,120-122,128,129] In borderline cases, however, intraoperative findings may contribute to a decision regarding the extent of parathyroid extirpation. It should be emphasized that the outcome of all operative procedures for secondary HPT remains to be established.

Total parathyroidectomy without autotransplantation comprises yet another rarely applied surgical therapy in uremic HPT, which has received renewed attention recently.[148,149,189] Proponents of this strategy argue that recurrences are common after operation for secondary HPT particularly among individuals with persistent uremia. Only recurrences attributed to the graft per se, however, would distinguish this operation from the more conventional mode of total parathyroidectomy. Although such proliferations may comprise an underestimated number of individuals with persistent renal insufficiency on the long-term postoperative follow-up, the incidences of graft-dependent elevations of intact serum PTH and calcium exceeding 20% in restricted patient materials has to be verified both with respect to frequency and clinical significance.[148,149,162,190,191] Since this rate of PTH elevation also may occur after subtotal resection as well as from sites other than the grafted tissue,[149,150] parathyroid surgery should not be expected to provide a definite biochemical cure of uremic Total parathyroidectomy without autotransplantation furthermore assumes that several years of PTH deficiency exerts no major adverse impact, a circumstance which contradicts much of the current efforts in preventing postoperative states of low or aplastic bone turnover.[49,89,90,93]

Results of Primary Exploration in Uremia

It should be borne in mind that the outcome of parathyroid surgery in uremia largely depends on successful renal transplantation either prior to or after parathyroidectomy. Serum calcium, intact PTH and alkaline phosphatase values might be expected to normalize promptly in these patients, although comprehensive analysis on the longer-term outcome of parathyroidectomy essentially is lacking in renal transplant recipients.[3,11,132,149,192,193] Moreover the selection of patients undergoing parathyroid operation largely influences the postoperative outcome. A striking example in this respect involves the sometimes unexplored admixture of patients with low bone turnover, who suffer the risk of devastating effects of parathyroidectomy. Failure to recognize these individuals will diminish the results of the operation, so that other subgroups of patients with uremic HPT might not be reccommended for surgery.

Biochemical variables

The serum calcium value generally decreases within the first hours after parathyroid surgery, although the decline must be adjusted to the concomitant decrease in serum albumin. This hypocalcemia should be expected to be deeper and more protracted in patients subjected to total in comparison with subtotal parathyroidectomy.[154,165,194] Moreover the severity of postoperative hypocalcemia and associated calcium requirements have been correlated to the degree of preoperative bone involvement and preoperative vitamin D therapy.[161,180,195-197] The hypocalcemic response to parathyroidectomy is treated by intravenous and oral calcium supplementation together with increased dosages of vitamin D,[198] so that the condition rarely poses an immediate problem. Injections of calcium usually can be withdrawn within a week after total parathyroidectomy provided that sufficient supplementation is instituted on the first postoperative day. Moreover some patients maintain normocalcemia even after total parathyroidectomy. This condition is incompletely understood and naturally may relate to unsuccessful operation. Despite the presence of negligible values of intact PTH mid-normal serum calcium concentrations may occur in some patients with extensive soft tissue calcification and low turnover bone disease.

Analysis of multiple patient series with highly variable postoperative follow-up reveals that subtotal parathyroid resection and total parathyroidectomy with autotransplantation should be expected to be accompanied by a 5-10% incidence of both postoperative hypo- and hyperparathyroidism.[152,156,157] More recent measurements of intact serum PTH, however, have suggested considerably higher rates of biochemical and essentially asymptomatic recurrence.[149,150] PTH elevation above the normal range occurs in essentially half the patients subjected to either operative method, and the proportional incidence of such elevations increases with time from the operation. Moreover the preoperative extent of HPT seems to relate to this biochemical abnormality,[150] which parallels findings on recurrence of sporadic primary HPT due both to adenoma and chief cell hyperplasia.[199] Histological signs of intensely elevated bone turnover, more substantially elevated PTH values, and nodular parathyroid hyperplasia consequently might comprise unsatisfactory prognostic variables in terms of the rate of postoperatively elevated serum PTH values in uremic HPT. Yet other series demonstrate normal serum PTH levels in virtually all patients early after subtotal resection.[10] After total parathyroidectomy with autotransplantation sufficient graft function usually is obtained within 4-9 months, whereby the peroperatively instituted vitamin D treatment frequently can be withdrawn.[152,157,197]

Parathyroidectomy in uremic HPT has been accompanied by transient elevation of alkaline phosphatase but not serum osteocalcin levels.[180] This elevation subsequently falls into the normal range in most patients without recurrent HPT, so that a substantial reduction in comparison with the preoperative level should be expected to occur.[150,151,155,156] The extent of this normalization might be less prominent after subtotal than total parathyroidectomy. Small but in some studies clinically significant reductions in serum phosphate may also occur postoperatively.[10,151,155] Circulating levels of calcitriol have been suggested to decrease in response to parathyroid surgery[180] and conflicting data has been presented as regards any improvement in blood pressure.[200-202]

Bone biopsies in a few series at various times after surgery have demonstrated substantial improvement or complete disappearance of osteitis fibrosa.[10,151,155,203] Moreover subperiosteal erosions should be expected to disappear in essentially half the individuals and to decrease in many of the others.[10,151,155,203] If patients with biochemical indices of severe osteitis fibrosa are considered alone, however, this improvement essentially seems to include every one of them.[10] Bone fractures are truly rare after parathyroidectomy in patients with high bone turnover. However these observations do not include patients with low bone turnover, in whom parathyroid operation may be accompanied by repeated fractures and considerable mortality.[10,81,89,93] Despite selection of patients, various poorly understood unraveled circumstances may favor the development of osteomalacia in 5-15% of patients subjected to parathyroidectomy due to apparent osteitis fibrosa, and this development has been attributed partly to absolute or relative PTH deficiency.

Calcifications of small and medium-sized vessels rarely should be expected to improve after parathyroid surgery even in presence of substantial reductions in serum PTH and calcium-phosphate products, and careful control of serum phosphate levels has been suggested to comprise a decisive factor in the postoperative development of such deposits.[151,155] Other soft tissue calcifications sometimes decrease very dramatically after parathyroidectomy, although persistence in up to half the patients have been found.[151,155] Calciphylaxis frequently responds very favorably to parathyroid operation, although mortality is considerable.[99,204-206] The postoperative improvement of calciphylaxis also has been suggested to occur mainly patients with more distally located ulcerations.[207]

Symptoms, morbidity and mortality

Truly rare deaths have been reported in association with parathyroidectomy in uremia, and these mainly has been attributed to cardiac arrhythmias associated with preoperative cardiovascular disturbances and very early but transient perioperative hyperkalemia. Morbidity also is exceptionally modest considering the pronounced multiple organ systems disturbances of severe and longstanding renal insufficiency. In the rare contemporary analyses available, occasional wound hematoma and infection, pneumonia and below 1% permanent vocal cord paralysis should be expected to occur. In our series of 85 patients undergoing parathyroidectomy in uremia there have been no early (within 30 days) deaths, three temporary but no permanent vocal cord paralyses, one reoperation for hemorrhage and four pyrexias of unknown cause (unpublished data). Despite recent suggestions,[208] hypocalcemic seizures accompanied by fractures at variable sites have not been reported.

Improvement in bone pain usually is appreciable early after parathyroidectomy, and should be expected to include approximately 85% of the patients suffering from this disturbance.[156] This seems to also include symptoms from periarticular soft tissue calcifications, although the radiological signs of these deposits may be ameliorated in fewer patients.[156,161,195,203,209] Some series have demonstrated impressive relief of proximal myopathy and muscular weakness by parathyroidectomy, although this has been less consistent in other analyses.[156,161,200,209] Pruritus seems to be alleviated to a highly variable extent, and hitherto any favorable response in this respect cannot be predicted preoperatively.[156,195,209-211] General symptoms like fatigue, nausea, lethargy and depression generally improve but rarely disappear completely after parathyroid surgery. The single randomized comparison available reveals significantly more improvement in pruritus, muscle weakness and radiological signs of osteitis fibrosa after total parathyroidectomy with immediate autotransplantation than after subtotal resection.[156]

Occasional reports have suggested more functional renal impairment in after parathyroid surgery, which has been attributed principally to the institution of vitamin D and calcium supplementation.[212,213] In our experience this complication is rare,[11] but close observation of urinary output and renal function as well as the application of pertinent therapeutic actions are mandatory, especially in conservatively treated uremia. Adjustment of vitamin D dosages necessitates surveillance especially after total parathyroidectomy, where initial requirements are pronounced and commonly transient due to gradual increases in graft function. Long-term survival has been evaluated in uremic patients undergoing parathyroidectomy.[164] Although patients with renal transplants demonstrate more advantageous actuarial survival rates during

10 year follow-up, there exist no differences with respect to parathyroid operation both among those with persistent or reversed uremia. This message might be important to deliver outside the innermost circle of endocrine surgeons, since misinformation in this respect might unnecessarily prevent timely primary and reoperative parathyroid surgery in uremic HPT.

Causes of Failed Primary Exploration in Uremic HPT

Identification of less than four parathyroid glands during subtotal or total parathyroidectomy essentially comprises a surgical failure.[214,215] It increases the risk but not necessarily leads to postoperative persistence or recurrence of HPT even without reversing the cause of the parathyroid disease. This concept underlies the general recommendation to avoid autotransplantation or partial removal of any gland in primary operations revealing three or fewer parathyroids, which seems to occur in about 10% of either procedure.[11,154,159,216,217] Cryopreservation of parathyroid tissue, however, seems mandatory in this instance. On the other hand secondary HPT should be expected to be accompanied by supernumerary parathyroid glands to an extent which remains to be comprehensively evaluated in autopsy studies, but possibly includes at least 10-15% of the patients.[159,171,215,218,219] Failure to excise such glands theoretically should be accompanied by persistent disease or HPT possibly recurring within the first postoperative years. Although combinations of primary and early re-explorations for secondary HPT have not been analyzed in this respect, failure to excise four parathyroids as well as the expected number of supernumerary glands leads to persistent or recurrent disease in a substantially smaller proportion of patients than anticipated from these calculations.[11] This circumstance possibly relates to the difficulties in sensitive determination of such recurrences due to the generally equivocal criteria for their recognition, the essentially slow reversal of clinical signs of secondary HPT,[150,180] widespread application of reliable PTH determinations only during later years, and a gradually increasing proportion of patients undergoing renal transplantation.

Gland size frequently varies in patients with uremic HPT, and the extent seems to be pronounced in nodular hyperplasia and to increase with the severity and duration of HPT.[8,11,187,220,221] At least one normal-sized gland consequently should be expected to occur in patients with HPT-dependent spontaneous hypercalcemia prior to surgery, and these might be difficult to identify due to the frequent richness of brownish fat in some individuals. In experienced hands, the greatest long-term risk of recurrence after primary and secondary operations nevertheless seems associated with inconspicuous accumulations (<20 mg) of parathyroid tissue exhibiting a virtually unknown prevalence in secondary HPT.[215,222] Analysis with monoclonal antibodies recognizing the functionally critical calcium receptor of parathyroid cells suggests that such islands can be sites of unequivocal derangement in secretory regulation[223,224] which should be expected to be coupled to enhanced rates of cell proliferation and enhanced risk of attaining a cell mass compatible with clinically detectable recurrence of HPT. This line of reasoning is supported by observations on measurable and time-dependent increases in serum PTH levels after total parathyroidectomy without autotransplantation,[147,148] as well as the generally disappointing rate of postoperative cure upon long-term follow-up of patients with persistent pathogenesis of secondary HPT.[149,150]

The selection of parathyroid tissue for autotransplantation has attracted interest due to the risk of graft-dependent recurrence, which generally occurs in about 5-10% of patients operated for secondary HPT.[152,156-158,174] Any clinical importance of selection criteria, however, has not been unequivocally established, and the main support for this hypothesis principally relies on the apparent discrepancy in propensity and signs of tissue differentiation between graft-related recurrences of different sources.[11,72,156,162,163,187,225] Nevertheless studies of PTH secretion as well as indices of parathyroid cell proliferation and histology suggest that preferentially glands of diffuse hyperplasia, low weight, scarce mitoses, and high fat cell content should be selected for autotransplantation.[69,71-73,187,226] Moreover a similar line of reasoning applies the selection of residual tissue during subtotal resection. Nodular hyperplasia thus has been accompanied by increased rates of recurrence after these operations as well as with possible graft-independent elevations in PTH values after total parathyroidectomy.[73,150,187] Appreciation of these tissue characteristics, however, might be more difficult during subtotal resection. The nodular, enlarged and virtually fat-cell free parathyroid glands frequently are unusually firm, grayish and slightly irregular giving the impression of focal tissue expansions. These nodules may be clearly evident upon transection and inspection usually even without low level magnification.

Diagnosis of Uremic HPT after Parathyroid Surgery

In conjunction with the generally complex clinical, biochemical and radiological signs of uremic HPT prior to primary exploration, postoperative parathyroid disease might be difficult to diagnose particularly among patients with persistent or recurrent uremia. Serum calcium has been utilized to describe the proportion of failures from parathyroid exploration (for references see 151,156-158), although such an elevation prior to surgery rarely occurs in a majority of the patients.[3,11,131,151] Under these circumstances, serum calcium as a principal indicator of postoperative HPT should be expected to substantially underestimate the rate of recurrent HPT. On the other hand this criterion seems relevant in the subjects with adequate renal function after successful renal transplantation.[3,132,192,227] The interpretation of serum calcium values in patients with persistent renal insufficiency also is complicated by the necessity of maintaining vitamin D and calcium salt therapy even after reversal of temporary postoperative hypoparathyroidism. The development of hypercalcemia under such circumstances generally indicates unequivocal HPT, although reduction of dosages and an altered route of vitamin D administration should be considered before the elevation of serum calcium is ascribed to parathyroid hyperfunction. Moreover the aluminum load should be evaluated, since an accumulation may increase the tendency for hypercalcemia in association with medical therapy of HPT. This derangement classically is combined with moderate PTH excess, and it has been suggested to increase and to respond less favorably to therapeutic mobilization after parathyroid operation.[93,180,228]

Elevated values of intact serum PTH constitute another biochemical sign which has been used to define postoperative HPT.[149,150,187,217] Moderately elevated PTH excess may not necessarily be harmful but rather an expected counter regulatory reaction in uremic patients; such elevations seem to be less relevant clinically considering the resistance to its peripheral calcium mobilizing actions.[20,49,108,110,229,230] Mild elevations of serum PTH indeed have been reported in variable numbers of patients in long-term follow-up after surgery for primary HPT,[231,232] and constitutes a poorly understood phenomenon not necessarily coupled to increased risk of recurrence. The use of serum PTH as an indicator of postoperative HPT in patients with persistent uremia consequently suggests an unnecessarily high rate of recurrence. It also is pertinent to note that analysis of intact PTH values in antecubital blood of arms bearing parathyroid autografts cannot be utilized to establish the presence or absence of HPT, although measurable levels should be expected to occur even in postoperative hypoparathyroidism.[187,191,233-235]

Several factors thus have to be considered regarding the diagnosis of HPT after parathyroid surgery. Apart from calcium and intact PTH assessments—with respect to temporal trends and in relation to renal function as well as prevailing medications—serum osteocalcin and alkaline phosphatase values, as well as skeletal radiology and bone biopsy should be considered. Findings must be interpreted with respect to clinical symptoms and soft tissue calcifications and must be related to expectations of these variables after successful parathyroid surgery. Most patients being referred for reoperation due to persistent or recurrent uremic HPT usually exhibit indisputable hypercalcemia, impressive PTH excess, overt osteitis fibrosa on skeletal radiology and multiple symptoms of parathyroid disease. It consequently appears that not only primary but also reoperative parathyroid surgery may be an underrated mode of treatment in patients with uremic HPT.

Indication for Parathyroid Reoperation in Uremia

Systematic evaluation of the indications for primary and reoperative parathyroid surgery is lacking in uremic HPT patients. Current policies for regarding parathyroid reoperation are based on lessons from primary explorations. Due to the technical difficulties associated with multiple sites of pathologic parathyroid tissue and the frequent necessity of reoperations for short-term cure,[171,216-218,233] biochemical evidence of severe HPT invariably comprises a requisite for operative reintervention in patients with uremia. Hypercalcemia constitutes a generally undisputed cause for parathyroid reoperation in secondary HPT, which dominates in some[216,233,236,237] but not other series.[159,187,190,225,234] The substantial variation in the relative frequency of hypercalcemia as indication for reoperation and indeed also for primary parathyroid surgery in uremic HPT, suggests interesting and essentially unexplored differences in medical treatment regimens and perhaps also in the natural course of the parathyroid disease. The elevation of serum calcium should be unequivocal upon repeated analysis, and should be verified by concomitant ionized plasma calcium measurements due to the tendency for temporally increasing degrees of dysionization after surgery for uremic HPT.[151] Moreover the serum calcium concentration should be evaluated prior to dialysis, since this procedure may cause elevated values. When medical treatment regimens are suspected of causing elevated values, oral calcium and vitamin D supplementation should be substantially reduced or withdrawn at least temporarily. Among other biochemical signs of secondary HPT, elevated intact serum PTH values are an indication for parathyroid reoperation. This elevation should be considerable, i.e. in the range of at least 400-700 ng/L (reference range 12-55 ng/L) in uremics, since such elevated values demonstrate the futility of conventional medical therapy in uremic HPT. Parathyroid reoperation should never be considered in patients with biochemically equivocal HPT.

Osteitis fibrosa is another prominent indication for reoperation of uremic HPT. In all instances this should be verified by bone biopsy, which also includes patients with radiological signs of subperiostal resorption and elevated alkaline phosphatase values in order to demonstrate the unlikelihood of low bone turnover. Osteomalacia and aplastic bone involvement thus constitute contraindications for parathyroid surgery. Calciphylaxis strongly supports the necessity of reoperation, and both this condition and osteitis fibrosa support the requirements of surgery even in the absence of hypercalcemia. Other frequent symptoms and signs of uremic HPT may only reinforcethe necessity for parathyroid reoperation, although combinations of pruritus, myopathy, nonvascular tissue calcifications, lethargy, and nausea comprise no unequivocal indication for such intervention. It must be recognized, however, that severe symptoms may be devastating to the patient's quality of life. Given the option individuals with even high operative risks thus frequently prefer even a limited chance of postoperative improvement. Small or large vessel calcium deposits in absence of calciphylaxis essentially can be disregarded as an indication for reoperation in uremic HPT.

Patients with a functioning kidney graft rarely are considered for parathyroid reoperation. Yet insertion of such a graft, even prior to primary parathyroid surgery, reduces but not necessarily prevents the development of recurrent HPT nor does it alter the frequent presence of multiple sites of PTH hypersecretion. Hypercalcemia in these instances should be treated surgically provided it is progressive, stable above 2.9-3.0 mmol/l (reference range 2.20-2.60 mmol/l) or accompanied by deteriorating renal function. Intact serum PTH naturally must be evaluated, although the values of patients with a satisfactorily functioning graft are substantially less impressive than in uremics. A complex situation, however, may occur in patients with partial graft function, in whom parathyroid reoperation might alleviate graft dysfunction. Biopsy of the transplanted kidney and analysis of calcium precipitation can be helpful in these instances. Osteopathy after renal transplantation should be carefully evaluated for signs of low bone turnover especially in diabetics and normocalcemic patients with low to moderate PTH excess.

Clarification of Excess Sites before Parathyroid Reoperation in Uremic HPT

Consistent with the routine handling of patients undergoing reoperation for primary HPT, all available modes of nonsurgical localization might be attempted prior to re-exploration for secondary HPT. It should be emphasized, however, that controlled studies on the outcome of such operations in terms of reversed HPT and perioperative complications remains to be performed. Knowledge on PTH excess sites nevertheless should reduce operating time considerably and contribute to cost-effectiveness. There exist important differences between reoperative findings in patients with primary and uremic HPT. The latter patient group, which essentially comprises individuals with hereditary and water-clear cell hyperplasia of primary HPT alonealmost invariably undergo a classical subtotal resection or total parathyroidectomy with autotransplantation. Moreover it is apparent that neither the presence of a functioning parathyroid autograft nor a subtotally resected parathyroid gland remnant in the neck should be expected to prevent concomitant growth of other residual parathyroid tissues, which suggests an unusually complicated situation especially in the patients with renal insufficiency. Consistent with the experience of others,[171,216,217,225,237] we expect to reveal multiple sites of microscopically hyperfunctioning parathyroid tissue in one of about four patients undergoing parathyroid reoperation for uremic HPT.

Surgical history

Findings during previous parathyroid operation(s) as well as the postoperative biochemical variables are essential prior to parathyroid reoperation. Failure of serum calcium and intact PTH values to fall substantially after subtotal resection and, to an even greater extent, after total parathyroidectomy for uremic HPT indicates persistent disease. Supernumerary parathyroids generally may be expected to occur in 15-20% of those subjected to microscopic identification of less than four proper (≥20 mg) parathyroid glands. However among patients requiring reoperation in this context, a >40% incidences of supernumerary parathyroids occasionally has been reported.[171] The risk of inadequate glandular identification should be expected to increase if nodular hyperplasia with its characteristically asymmetric increase in glandular size occurs. An indication of the location of an unidentified fourth parathyroid gland usually can be obtained from the symmetry in glandular anatomy across the midline within essentially 80% of all individuals.[215] There have been suggestions on increased incidence of ectopic glandular locations in individuals with recurrence,[225,237] although our impression is that vast majorities of these specimens are located in or close to anatomically normal positions in both primary and uremic HPT.[238] Consistent with this line of reasoning, a fourth parathyroid gland should be expected to be accessible from a collar incision in at least about 90% of reoperative patients with uremic HPT despite the fact that up to 29% mediastinotomies have been reported in such patient groups.[225]

Individuals, in whom histological verification of at least four completely excised parathyroids has been established, naturally exhibit enlarged supernumerary gland(s) provided that the presence of HPT is satisfactorily substantiated. Although the time necessary for growth of residual parathyroid tissue islands seems to be highly variable, recurrence of unequivocal uremic HPT usually includes considerably longer than the 6 months conventionally utilized to distinguish between persistence and recurrence of primary HPT. This line of reasoning also seems to apply to growth of optimally sized remnants of subtotal resections.[10,154] Moreover we have the distinct impression that individuals displaying a history of one supernumerary gland have considerably increased risk of harboring or developing other such glands provided sufficient time is given and even in the event of successful renal transplantation. The location of supernumerary glands causing persistent uremic HPT is considerably more difficult to determine prior to reoperation. Our impression substantiates that most of these patients have not undergone bilateral thymic resection or sufficient excision of fat surrounding the parathyroid glands. In these instances most causes of HPT are associated with parathyroid specimens located in the vicinity of previously excised glands and in cervically accessible portions of the thymus. It also is worth mentioning that include cervical thymic resection might extirpation of pre- or paratracheal fat rather than the thymus, and that this distinction may be difficult to ascertain in retrospect even on analysis of pathology reports. Also supernumerary glands generally should be expected to reside in regions accessible from the neck,[10,161,216] although very limited series of patients have indicated a mediastinal location for 40% or more of them.[154,163,239] In this context it is woth mentioning, that sternotomy and other procedures of direct access to the mediastinum sometimes are employed with unnecessary liberality during parathyroid surgery, and that many of the glands excised during such procedures actually could have been retrieved from the neck.

Known sites of residual parathyroid tissue naturally should be suspected to cause postoperative HPT; accordingly parathyroid autotransplants invariably are subjected to close scrutiny. Although few series have suggested recurrences of common HPT from brachioradial autografts,[162,190,191] considerably more series report such recurrences in only about 5-10% of the patients (for references see 152,156-158,174) particularly if pertinent measures on tissue selection have been applied.[11,72,73,156,187,225,226] A similar rate of such recurrences is expected to occur at other sites of parathyroid transplantation, although there is currently no evaluation in this respect. It also is noteworthy that the brachioradial transplants generally require 4-8 months to develop sufficient PTH secretion, and that recurrence of HPT due to proliferation of this tissue usually,[73,157,216,217] but not invariably,[162,190,191] should take years to become clinically relevant. Moreover insufficient excision of a subtotally resected gland must be considered due mainly to a partially intrathyroidal location, when more than 80 mg of tissue has been left in situ, and when the estimate of remnant is uncertain. This circumstance seems to be a rare complication to subtotal resection[10,154,156,217,225,237] especially when serum calcium is utilized to verify the presence of postoperative disease. It nevertheless seems to be an underrated consequence of primary exploration in less experienced hands, when persistent and early as well as late recurrence of HPT may be encountered.

Technical aspects of preoperative localization

Patients with clinical and biochemical signs of uremic HPT requiring reoperation usually harbor a substantial amount of pathologic parathyroid tissue, such that radiological and other means of nonsurgical localization should be expected to be truly positive for one such glandular specimen in a majority of individuals. This circumstance, however, generally applies only to larger parathyroid tissue accumulations; normal-sized glands as well as small tissue islands never can be visualized preoperatively. Moreover only very few patient series have been analyzed for the effectiveness of currently available means of localization,[152,171,217,225,237,239] so no unequivocal recommendation on their practical applicability prior to reoperation in uremic HPT can be made. Consistent with previous notions on the pre-reoperative examination of patients with primary HPT, we subject these patients to ultrasound, positron emission tomography with ^{11}C-labeled methionine and computed tomography,[240] magnetic resonance tomography, technetium-thallium scintigraphy, and infrequently venous sampling for measurement of intact serum PTH. This investigation generally is interrupted after consistent findings with two of the modalities, so the complete arsenal only rarely has to be applied. It should be borne in mind, however, that true positive localizations virtually never are accomplished for more than a single pathological parathyroid specimen in each individual.

Particular circumstances apply to the recognition of recurrent uremic HPT due to brachioradial parathyroid autografts. Most of these actually may be recognized on mere palpation and others seem to be demonstrated by ultrasound and thallium scanning,[73,191,234,239,241] so negative findings on both of these examinations strongly support that the cause of HPT is located elsewhere. Moreover functional characterization of these grafts may be obtained by comparing local venous effluents with the systemic circulation. This comparison should yield ratios of intact serum PTH values exceeding 2.0 in virtually all patients with a functioning autograft[239] and in many cases this quotient amounts to 5 or more (unpublished data). It also has been convincingly demonstrated that analysis of intact serum PTH is superior to assays recognizing carboxyterminal domains of the peptide.[239,242] Few overtly normoparathyroid patients nevertheless may be unsuitable for this examination due to the lack of recognizable subcutaneous veins or graft drainage into deep muscular veins. Lack of intact PTH gradients between cubital venous blood of the grafted arm and the systemic circulation thus cannot be completely relied on in the complex assessment of parathyroid hyperfunction after brachioradial transplantation.[241] This problem may be partly overcome by hypocalcemic stimulation, whereby the elevation of intact serum PTH usually is greater upstream to the graft than systemically. Moreover direct axillary vein puncture or sampling during regular venous catherization may solve this difficulty, but this measure has been necessary only very rarely in clinical practice. Assessment of graft function nevertheless is important prior to reoperation for uremic HPT not only to demonstrate a possible source to PTH excess but also to demonstrate the presence of a functional graft precluding further grafting during the subsequent reoperation.

Intact serum PTH values proximal to parathyroid transplants regularly are clearly above the normal range and sometimes exceed this range more than tenfold even in patients without signs of postoperative HPT.[239] Although recurrence from graft proliferation almost invariably is accompanied by unusually high intact serum PTH levels, the numerical extent of this elevation alone never can be utilized to prove the existence of graft-related HPT. It also has become increasingly evident that the ratio of intact serum PTH between the grafted arm and the systemic circulation might be the highest in normoparathyroid individuals, which possibly relates to the concomitant increase in the systemic PTH level of the patients with recurrent HPT. In our hands the systemic PTH value is utilized as one factor contributing to the determination whether or not postoperative HPT exists, while the level in the grafted arm and its ratio with regard to the systemic circulation help to distinguish between PTH excess from the graft or the neck-mediastinum. Moreover graft recurrences invariably have been accompanied by radiologically demonstrable parathyroid tissue expansions at the site of transplantation, although focal thallium accumulation may occur also in overt normoparathyroidism. By use of this concept unnecessary resections of the grafted tissue has been prevented, while such operations seem more or less prevalent in other series.[171,191,217,225,233,237,239,243] Recently vascular occlusion of the grafted arm has been suggested to improve identification of PTH excess sites.[234] This procedure involves 30 minute arterial ischemia of the arm by means of a tourniquet under regional intravenous anesthesia. In conjunction with the short half-life of intact serum PTH, more than about 40% decrease in these values were obtained in patients with graft-related recurrence. Although those with HPT due to parathyroid tissue in the neck demonstrated less serum PTH decrease, the discrepancy has been rather small and requires further examination.

Intraoperative Strategy and Outcome of Reoperation in Uremic HPT

Details on technical measures and practical refinements of parathyroid reoperation in uremic HPT are similar to those in primary HPT, and will be dealt with in a separate chapter. Certain aspects of parathyroid reoperation, however, are rather unique for patients with uremic HPT. Moreover it should be noted that only a limited number of reports have focused on large numbers of patients undergoing parathyroid reoperation for uremic HPT.[163,171,191,216,217,219,225,237,254] In our hands patients with recurrent uremic HPT in the neck regularly undergo bilateral exploration involving excision of not only all macroscopically visible parathyroid tissue but also accessible portions of residual thymic tissue as well as peri-parathyroid fat. Independent of the findings, these procedures regularly involve incision of the carotid sheaths as well as exploration of the peripharyngeal and periesophageal spaces. The rationale for this strategy relates to expectations on the presence of multiple sites of parathyroid tissue which might contibute to HPT at the time of surgery or contribute to recurrent disease after reoperation. Although the true prevalence of parathyroid tissue islands and macroscopically enlarged parathyroid glands remains to be established in postoperative uremic HPT, the necessity of more than one reoperation in 15-30% of patients suggests that this problem might be rewarding to analyze.[171,216,217,237,254]

For the above mentioned reasons we feel uncomfortable with subtotal parathyroid resection during most reoperations for uremic HPT. Patients who have undergone previous subtotal resection thus already have manifested the inadequacy of this method, and there exists a definite risk that the parathyroid gland remnant may consist of suboptimally selected tissue exhibiting increased propensity for proliferation. Although this tissue also is suboptimal for grafting during reoperation, review of patient experience suggests somewhat lower rates of recurrence after total than after subtotal parathyroidectomy.[152,156-158] Moreover patients already having undergone total parathyroidectomy almost invariably have at least some degree of clearly functioning graft tissue, so an additional remnant in the neck comprises a definite disadvantage. A possible exception to the idea of limited applicability of subtotal resection might involve patients who have undergone inadequate previous procedures involving identification of e.g. only two or fewer parathyroid glands, especially if they are scheduled for their first renal transplantation or underwent their previous parathyroid exploration prior to the insertion of a satisfactorily functioning graft. The strategy of reoperative total parathyroidectomy invariably involves decisions on immediate or deferred autotransplantation. Additional grafting rarely is necessary in patients subjected to previous brachioradial transplantation provided that intact serum PTH gradients ≥1.5 between the grafted arm and the systemic circulation can be obtained prior to reoperation. Doubts in this respect, however, primarily should be met by cryopreservation with the option of grafting at least 3 months after the reoperation.

In patients who have undergone previous subtotal resection we currently prefer immediate autotransplantation, since this procedure involves more well characterized amounts of graft tissue and somewhat higher expectations of sufficient function. Others, however, advocate general use of deferred transplantation in order to establish the absence of persistent HPT for 6 months of observation after reoperation.[171]

Recurrence in parathyroid autografts might be handled by subtotal or total extirpation. Any general recommendation in this respect seems difficult to propose, since there obviously exist histories of locally aggressive parathyroid tissue proliferations.[162,190,191] In such instances total excision indeed has been claimed to be arduous but probably highly advantageous. Our experience indicates that HPT from brachioradial grafts is characterized by presence of multiple accumulations of macro- and microscopically well circumscribed parathyroid tissue islands. Consistent with other observations,[73,216,226] these accumulations vary in size. In the most favorable instances incision of the brachioradial muscle parallel to the grafts enables inspection of the parathyroid tissue accumulations and careful selection of those displaying substantial degrees of enlargement. In other instances of primarys and all re-excisions of these transplantss less precise resection of muscle tissue together with about two-thirds of the nonabsorbable sutures demonstrating the pockets of incision have proven to be successful. Intraoperative ultrasound at high frequency may contribute to the identification of enlarged tissue islands in these patients.

Inadvertent implants of parathyroid tissue may cause recurrent HPT of uremia. This occurs in less than 5-10% of patients. The rarity of these implants actually is intriguing in view of the marked ability of the uremic parathyroid tissue to survive intentional grafting into muscle and fat. Subtotal parathyroid resection generally involves intraoperative glandular transection with the possibility of local tissue implantation. Patients with recurrent HPT due to such implants nevertheless may be exceptionally difficult to handle during reoperation. The primary issue is to recognize the presence of the condition. During reoperation these implants regularly appear as multiple brownish nodules varying from less than one to several millimeters in diameter. Most frequently they occur at or close to the thyroid lobe, where they may cover few square centimeters. Another difficulty involves radical resection, since delineation is difficult and the recurrent nerve might be involved. Secondary re-exploration for persistent disease nevertheless is rare and re-recurrence of HPT has not been reported in these patients, which naturally may relate to the adequacy of follow-up.

In general consistency with the variable indication, operative tactics and criteria for recognition of postoperative normoparathyroidism, the outcome of parathyroid reoperation has been highly variable in uremic HPT. Altogether 74% of currently reviewed patients (150) display reversed HPT after a mean 1.5 reoperations.[162,171,190,191,216,217,234,237,239,244,254] There exist, however, considerable differences between series. Patients undergoing graft resection after total parathyroidectomy thus have demonstrated 0-100% cure.[190,234,239] Many failures seem related to combinations of graft proliferations and unexplored residual parathyroid tissue in the neck, so they cannot be interpreted to support notions on the local difficulty handling such recurrences. On the other hand 84% cure has been reported in series exceeding 15 patients and consisting of individuals harboring completely evaluated parathyroid disease and a variety of primary procedures.[171,216,217]

References

1. St Goar WT. Case records of the Massachusetts General Hospital. N Engl J Med 1963; 268: 943-53.
2. Williams ED. Pathology of the parathyroid glands. Clin Endocrinol Metab 1974; 3: 285-303.
3. Diethelm AG, Edwards RP, Whelchel JD. The natural history and surgical treatment of hypercalcemia before and after renal transplantation. Surg Gynecol Obstet 1982; 154: 481-90.
4. Brown EM, Wilson RE, Eastman RC et al. Abnormal regulation of parathyroid hormone release by calcium in secondary hyperparathyroidism due to chronic renal failure. J Clin Endocrinol Metab 1982; 54: 172-9.
5. Wallfelt C, Gylfe E, Larsson R et al. Relationship between external and cytoplasmic calcium concentrations, parathyroid hormone release and weight of parathyroid glands in human hyperparathyroidism. J Endocrinol 1988; 116: 457-64.
6. Mori S. Parenchymal weight of parathyroid gland and the kidney in chronic glomerulonephritis. Tohoku J Exp Med 1978; 125: 85-91.
7. Delmonico FL, Wang CA, Rubin NT et al. Parathyroid surgery in patients with renal failure. Ann Surg 1984; 200: 644-7.
8. Malmaeus J, Grimelius L, Johansson H et al. Parathyroid pathology in hyperparathyroidism secondary to chronic renal failure. Scand J Urol Nephrol 1984; 18: 157-66.
9. Åkerström G, Malmaeus J, Grimelius L et al. Histological changes in parathyroid glands in subclinical and clinical renal disease. Scand J Urol Nephrol 1984; 18: 75-84.
10. Johnson WJ, McCarthy JT, van Heerden JA et al. Results of subtotal parathyroidectomy in hemodialysis patients. Am J Med 1988; 84: 23-32.
11. Hellman P, Åkerström G, Ljunghall S et al. Surgical findings and results of subtotal and total parathyroidectomy in hypercalcemic patients with uremic hyperparathyroidism. Acta Chir Scand 1989; 155: 573-82.
12. Hellman P, Backman U, Danielson BG et al. Values of intact serum parathyroid hormone in different stages of renal insufficiency. Scand J Urol Nephrol 1991; 25: 227-32.
13. Delmez JA, Tindira C, Grooms P et al. Parathyroid hormone suppression by intravenous 1,25 dihydroxyvitamin D. A role for increased sensitivity to calcium. J Clin Invest 1989; 83: 1349-55.
14. Mai ML, Emmett M, Sheikh MS et al. Calcium acetate, an effective phosphorus binder in patients with renal failure. Kidney Int 1989; 36: 690-5.
15. Slatopolsky E, Weerts C, Norwood K et al. Long-term effects of calcium carbonate and 2.5 mEq/liter calcium dialysate on mineral metabolism. Kidney Int 1989; 36: 897-903.
16. Trompeter SE, Mujais SK. Parathyroidectomy: The diminshing role of surgery. Int J Artifical Organs 1991; 14: 133-5.
17. Ritz E, Matthias S, Seidel A et al. Disturbed calcium metabolism in renal failure—Pathogenesis and therapeutic strategies. Kidney Int 1992; 42 (Suppl 38): S37-42.
18. Delmez JA, Slatopolsky E. Recent advances in the pathogenesis and therapy of uremic secondary hyperparathyroidism. J Clin Endocrinol Metab 1991; 72: 735-9.
19. Portale AA, Morris RC. Pathogenesis of secondary hyperparathyroidism in chronic renal insufficiency. Miner Electrolyte Metab 1991; 17: 211-20.
20. Goodman WG, Coburn JW. The use of 1,25 dihydroxyvitamin D_3 in early renal failure. Ann Rev Med 1992; 43: 227-37.
21. Massry SG, Fadda GZ. Chronic renal failure is a state of cellular calcium toxicity. Am J Kidney Dis 1993; 21: 81-6.
22. Bricker NS. On the pathogenesis of the uremic state. An exposition of the "trade off" hypothesis. N Engl J Med 1972; 286: 1093-9.
23. Delmez JA, Slatopolsky E. Hyperphosphatemia: Its consequences and treatment in patients with chronic renal disease. Am J Kidney Dis 1992; 19: 303-17.
24. Lopez-Hilker S, Galceran T, Chan Y-L et al. Hypocalcemia may not be essential for the development of secondary hyperparathyroidism in chronic renal failure. J Clin

Invest 1986; 78: 1097-1102.
25. Lopez-Hilker S, Dusso AS, Rapp NS et al. Phosphorus restriction reverses hyperparathyroidism in uremia independent of changes in calcium and calcitriol. Am J Physiol 1990; 259: F432-7.
26. Bichara M, Mercier O, Borensztein P et al. Acute metabolic acidosis enhances circulating parathyroid hormone, which contributes to the renal response against acidosis in the rat. J Clin Invest 1990; 86: 430-43.
27. Reichel H, Deibert B, Geberth S et al. Frusemide therapy and intact parathyroid hormone plasma concentrations in chronic renal insufficiency. Nephrol Dial Transplant 1992; 7: 8-15.
28. Nygren P, Larsson R, Johansson H et al. $1,25(OH)_2D_3$ inhibits hormone secretion and proliferation but not functional dedifferentiation of cultured bovine parathyroid cells. Calif Tissue Int 1988; 43: 213-8.
29. Shvil Y, Naveh-Many T, Barach P et al. Regulation of parathyroid cell gene expression in experimental uremia. J Am Soc Nephrol 1990; 1: 99-104.
30. Szabo A, Merke J, Beier E et al. $1,25(OH)_2$ vitamin D_3 inhibits parathyroid cell proliferation in experimental uremia. Kidney Int 1989; 35: 1049-56.
31. Schaefer F, Mehls O, Ritz E. New insights into endocrine disturbances of chronic renal failure. Miner Electrolyte Metab 1992; 18: 169-73.
32. Eisman JA. Vitamin D and cancer: New insight into vitamin D physiology and potential for cancer therapy. In: Heersche JNH, Kanis JA, eds. Bone and Mineral Research. Amsterdam: Elsevier. 1994; 8: 45-76.
33. Massry SG. Role of $1,25(OH)_2D$ in the genesis of secondary hyperparathyroidism of early renal failure and its use in the prevention of this abnormality. Metabolism 1990; 39: 13-7.
34. Seidel A, Stein G, Schneider S et al. Do limited changes in phosphate intake modulate $1,25(OH)_2D_3$ levels in early renal failure? Clin Nephrol 1991; 36: 274-80.
35. Dusso AS, Finch J, Brown A et al. Extrarenal production of calcitriol in normal and uremic humans. J Clin Endocrinol Metab 1991; 72: 157-64.
36. Reichel H, Deibert B, Schmidt-Gayk H et al. Calcium metabolism in early chronic renal failure: Implications for the pathogenesis of hyperparathyroidism. Nephrol Dial Transplant 1991; 6: 162-9.
37. Dusso A, Lopez-Hilker S, Rapp N et al. Extrarenal production of calcitriol in chronic renal failure. Kidney Int 1988; 34: 368-75.
38. Wilson L, Felsenfeld A, Drezner MK et al. Altered divalent ion metabolism in early renal failure: Role of $1,25(OH)_2D$. Kidney Int 1985; 27: 565-73.
39. Lucas PA, Woodhead JS, Brown RC. Vitamin D3 metabolites in chronic renal failure and after renal transplantation. Nephrol Dial Transplant 1988; 3: 70-6.
40. Ritz E, Seidel A, Ramisch H et al. Attenuated rise of $1,25(OH)_2$ vitamin D_3 in response to parathyroid hormone in patients with incipient renal failure. Nephron 1991; 57: 314-8.
41. Bonjour JP. 1,25-dihydroxyvitamin D and phophate homeostasis in early chronic renal failure: The "trade off" hypothesis revisited. In: Davison AM, ed. Nephrology. London: Ballière Tindall. 1988: 1059-66.
42. Malluche HH, Monier-Faugere M-C. Uremic bone disease: Current knowledge, controversial issues, and new horizons. Miner Electrolyte Metab 1991; 17: 281-96.
43. St John A, Thomas MB, Davies CP et al. Determinants of intact parathyroid hormone and free 1,25-dihyroxyvitamin D levels in mild and moderate renal failure. Nephron 1992; 61: 422-7.
44. Ashby JP, Newman DJ, Rinsler MG. Is intact PTH a sensitive biochemical indicator of deranged calcium homeostasis in vitamin D deficiency? Ann Clin Biochem 1989; 26: 324-7.
45. Llach F, Massry SG. On the mechanism of secondary hyperparathyroidism in moderate renal insufficiency. J Clin Endocrinol Metab 1985; 61: 601-6.
46. Galceran T, Martin KJ, Morrissey JJ et al. Role of 1,25-dihydroxyvitamin D on the skeletal resistance to parathyroid hormone. Kidney Int 1987; 32: 801-7.
47. Urena P, Kubrusly M, Mannstadt M et al. The renal PTH/PTHrP receptor is downregulated in rats with chronic renal failure.

Kidney Int 1994; 45: 605-11.
48. McCarron DA, Muther RS, Lenfesty B et al. Parathyroid function in persistent hyperparathyroidism: Relationship to gland size. Kidney Int 1982; 22: 662-70.
49. Felsenfeld AJ, Rodriguez M, Dunlay R et al. A comparison of parathyroid-gland function in haemodialysis patients with different forms of renal osteodystrophy. Nephrol Dial Transplant 1991; 6: 244-51.
50. Dunlay R, Rodriguez M, Felsenfeld AJ et al. Direct inhibitory effect of calcitriol on parathyroid function (sigmoidal curve) in dialysis. Kidney Int 1989; 36: 1093-8.
51. Ljunghall S, Althoff P, Fellström B et al. Effects on serum parathyroid hormone of intravenous treatment with alphacalcidol in patients on chronic hemodialysis. Nephron 1990; 55: 380-5.
52. Sprague SM, Moe SM. Safety and efficacy of long-term treatment of secondary hyperparathyroidism by low-dose intravenous calcitriol. Am J Kidney Dis 1992; 19: 532-9.
53. Slatopolsky E, Weerts C, Thielan J et al. Marked suppression of secondary hyperparathyroidism by intravenous administration of 1,25-dihydroxy-cholecalciferol in uremic patients. J Clin Invest 1984; 74: 2136-43.
54. Slatopolsky E, Berkoben M, Kelber J et al. Effects of calcitriol and non-calcemic vitamin D analogs on secondary hyperparathyroidism. Kidney Int 1992; 42 (Suppl 38): S43-9.
55. Malberti F, Surian M, Cosci P. Improvement of secondary hyperparathyroidism and reduction of the set point of calcium after intravenous calcitriol. Kidney Int 1993; 43 (Suppl 41): S125-30.
56. Korkor AB. Reduced binding of [^{3}H]1,25-dihydroxyvitamin D_3 in the parathyroid glands of patients with renal failure. N Engl J Med 1987; 316: 1573-7.
57. Merke J, Hügel U, Zlotkowski A et al. Diminished parathyroid 1,25$(OH)_2D_3$ receptors in experimental uremia. Kidney Int 1987; 32: 350-3.
58. Brown AJ, Dusso A, Lopez-Hilker S et al. 1,25-$(OH)_2D$ receptors are decreased in parathyroid glands from chronically uremic dogs. Kidney Int 1989; 35: 19-23.
59. Fukuda N, Tanaka H, Tominaga Y et al. Decreased 1,25-dihydroxyvitamin D_3 receptor density is associated with a more severe form of parathyroid hyperplasia in chronic uremic patients. J Clin Invest 1993; 92: 1436-43.
60. McCarthy JT, Klee GG, Kao PC et al. Serum bioactive parathyroid hormone in hemodialysis patients. J Clin Endocrinol Metab 1988; 68: 340-5.
61. Nagode LA, Chew DJ. Nephrocalcinosis caused by hyperparathyroidism in progression of renal failure: Treatment with calcitriol. Sem Vet Med Surg 1992; 7: 202-20.
62. Morrissey J, Slatopolsky E. Effect of aluminium on parathyroid hormone secretion. Kidney Int 1986; 29 (Suppl 18): S41-4.
63. Cannata JB, Lopez JBD, Fernandez Menéndez MJ et al. The parathyroid gland and aluminium overload: An overview. Contr Nephrol 1988; 64: 113-9.
64. Zelikovic I, Dabbagh S, Friedman AL et al. Severe renal osteodystrophy without elevated serum immunoreactive parathyroid hormone concentrations in hypomagnesemia due to renal magnesium wasting. Pediatrics 1987; 79: 403-9.
65. Hsiao RJ, Mezger MS, O'Connor DT. Chromogranin A in uremia: Progressive retention of immunoreactive fragments. Kidney Int 1990; 37: 955-64.
66. Fasciotto BH, Gorr S-U, Bourdeau AM et al. Autocrine regulation of parathyroid secretion: Inhibition of secretion by chromogranin-A (secretory protein-I) and potentiation of secretion by chromogranin-A and pancreastatin antibodies. Endocrinology 1990; 127: 1329-35.
67. Nygren P, Larsson R, Gylfe E et al. Development of abnormal parathyroid cell function during monolayer culture and its relation to cellular hypertrophy and proliferation. Acta Pathol Microbiol Immunol Scand, A 1987; 95: 207-14.
68. Nygren P, Larsson R, Johansson H et al. Inhibition of cell growth retains differentiated function of bovine parathyroid cells in monolayer culture. Bone Miner 1988; 4: 123-32.

69. Lloyd HM, Parfitt AM, Jacobi JM et al. The parathyroid glands in chronic renal failure: A study of their growth and other properties made on the basis of findings in patients with hypercalcemia. J Lab Clin Med 1989; 114: 358-67.
70. Mendes V, Jorgetti V, Nemeth J et al. Secondary hyperparathyroidism in chronic haemodialysis patients: A clinico-pathological study. Proc EDTA 1983; 20: 731-8.
71. Wallfelt CH, Larsson R, Gylfe E et al. Secretory disturbance in hyperplastic parathyroid nodules of uremic hyperparathyroidism: Implication for parathyroid autotransplantation. World J Surg 1988; 12: 431-8.
72. Niederle B, Hörandner H, Roka R et al. Morphologic and functional studies to prevent graft-dependent recurrence in renal osteodystrophy. Surgery 1989; 106: 1043-8.
73. Tominaga Y, Tanaka Y, Sato K et al. Recurrent renal hyperparathyroidism and DNA analysis of autografted parathyroid tissue. World J Surg 1992; 16: 595-603.
74. Sakaguchi K, Santora A, Zimering M et al. Functional epithelial cell line cloned from rat parathyroid glands. Proc Natl Acad Sci (USA) 1987; 84: 3269-73.
75. Kremer R, Bolivar I, Goltzman D et al. Influence of calcium and 1,25 dihydroxycholecalciferol on proliferation and protooncogene expression in primary cultures of bovine parathyroid cells. Endocrinology 1989; 125: 935-41.
76. Fukagawa M, Okazaki R, Takano K et al. Regression of parathyroid hyperplasia by calcitriol-pulse therapy in patients on long-term dialysis. N Engl J Med 1990; 323: 421-2.
77. Falchetti A, Bale AE, Amorosi A et al. Progression of uremic hyperparathyroidism involves allelic loss on chromosome 11. J Clin Endocrinol Metab 1993; 76: 139-44.
78. Eguchi S, Hirata Y, Imai T et al. Endothelin receptors in human parathyroid gland. Biochem Biophys Res Commun 1992; 184: 1448-55.
79. De Feo ML, Bartolini O, Orlando C et al. Natriuretic peptide receptors regulate endothelin synthesis and release from parathyroid cells. Proc Natl Acad Sci, USA 1991; 88: 6496-500.
80. Sutton RAL, Cameron EC. Renal osteodystrophy: Pathophysiology. Semin Nephrol 1992; 12: 91-100.
81. Llach F, Felsenfeld AJ, Coleman MD et al. The natural course of dialysis osteomalacia. Kidney Int 1986; 29 (suppl 18): S74-9.
82. Sherrard DJ. Renal osteodystrophy. Semin Nephrol 1986; 6: 56-67.
83. Ito M, Hayashi K, Ito M. Vertebral density distribution pattern: CT classification of patients undergoing maintenance hemodialysis. Radiology 1991; 180: 253-7.
84. Ott SM, Maloney NA, Coburn JW et al. The prevalence of bone aluminium deposition in renal osteodystrophy and in its relation to the response to calcitriol therapy. N Engl J Med 1982; 307: 709-13.
85. Kanis JA, Brown CB, Cameron EC et al. The role of vitamin D metabolites in the osteomalacia of renal disease. Curr Med Res Opin 1981; 7: 294-315.
86. Malluche HH, Faugere M-C, Smith AJ et al. Aluminium intoxication of bone in renal failure—fact or fiction? Kidney Int 1986; 29 (suppl 18): S70-3.
87. Parfitt AM. The localization of aluminium in bone: Implications for the mechanism of fixation and for the pathogenesis of aluminium-related bone disease. Int J Artif Organs 1988; 11: 79-90.
88. Van de Vyver FL, Visser WJ, D'Haese PC et al. Iron overload and bone disease in chronic dialysis patients. Nephrol Dial Transplant 1990; 5: 781-7.
89. Andress DL, Ott SM, Maloney NA et al. Effect of parathyroidectomy on bone aluminium accumulation in chronic renal failure. N Engl J Med 1985; 312: 468-73.
90. de Vernejoul MC, Marchais S, London G et al. Increased bone aluminium deposition after subtotal parathyroidectomy in dialyzed patients. Kidney Int 1985; 27: 785-91.
91. Carney SL. Ionized calcium concentration in maintenance hemodialysis patients. Clin Nephrol 1992; 38: 167-70.
92. Salusky IB, Goodman WG. Renal bone disease in pediatric patients receiving treatment with maintenance peritoneal dialysis. Child Nephrol Urol 1991; 11: 165-8.
93. Felsenfeld AJ, Harrelson JM, Gutman RA et al. Osteomalacia after parathyroidectomy

in patients with uremia. Ann Int Med 1982; 96: 34-9.
94. McCarthy JT, Milliner DS, Johnson WJ. Clinical experience with desferrioxamine in dialysis patients with aluminium toxicity. Quart J Med 1990; 74: 257-76.
95. Pei Y, Hercz G, Greenwood C et al. Noninvasive prediction of aluminium bone disease in hemo-and peritoneal dialysis patients. Kidney Int 1992; 41: 1374-82.
96. Ståhle-Bäckdahl M. Pruritus in hemodialysis patients. Skin Pharmacol 1992; 5: 14-20.
97. Fraser CL, Arieff AI. Nervous system complications in uremia. Ann Intern Med 1988; 109: 143-53.
98. Adrogüe HJ, Frazier MR, Zeluff B et al. Systemic calciphylaxis revisited. Am J Nephrol 1981; 1: 177-83.
99. Khafif RA, DeLima C, Silverberg A et al. Calciphylaxis and systemic calcinosis. Arch Intern Med 1990; 150: 956-9.
100. Geffriaud C, Allinne E, Page B et al. Decrease of tumor-like calcification in uremia despite aggravation of secondary hyperparathyroidism: A case report. Clin Nephrol 1992; 38: 158-61.
101. Southwood RL, Mueller BA, Copley JB. Soft tissue calcification in renal failure. Ann Pharmacother 1990; 24: 855-9.
102. Wenzel-Seifert K, Harwig S, Keller F. Fulminant calcinosis in two patients after kidney transplantation. Am J Nephrol 1991; 11: 497-500.
103. Milliner DS, Zinsmeister AR, Lieberman E et al. Soft tissue calcification in pediatric patients with end-stage renal disease. Kidney Int 1990; 38: 931-6.
104. Schaefer K, Umlauf E, von Herrath D. Reduced risk of hypercalcemia for hemodialysis patients by administering calcitriol at night. Am J Kidney Dis 1992; 19: 460-4.
105. Llach F, Nikakhtar B. Current advances in the therapy of secondary hyperparathyroidism and osteitis fibrosa. Miner Electrolyte Metab 1991; 17: 250-5.
106. Brandi L, Daugaard H, Tvedegaard E et al. Long-term suppression of secondary hyperparathyroidism by intravenous 1α-hydroxyvitamin D_3 in patients on chronic hemodialysis. Am J Nephrol 1992; 12: 311-8.
107. Andress DL, Norris KC, Coburn JW et al. Intravenous calcitriol in the treatment of refractory osteitis fibrosa of chronic renal failure. N Engl J Med 1989; 321: 274-9.
108. Mornière P, Maurouard C, Boudailliez B et al. Prevention of hyperparathyroidism in patients on maintenance dialysis by intravenous 1-alpha-hydroxyvitamin D_3 in association with $Mg(OH)_2$ as sole phosphate binder. Nephron 1992; 60: 154-63.
109. Fournier A, Morinière P, Hamida FB et al. Use of alkaline calcium salts as phophate binder in uremic patients. Kidney Int 1992; 42 (Suppl 38): S50-61.
110. Cohen-Solal ME, Sebert JL, Boudailliez B et al. Non-aluminic adynamic bone disease in non-dialyzed uremic patients: A new type of osteopathy due to overtreatment? Bone 1992; 13: 1-5.
111. Salusky IB, Goodman WG. Renal osteodystrophy in dialyzed children. Miner Electrolyte Metab 1991; 17: 273-80.
112. Freundlich M, Zilleruelo G, Abitbol C et al. Infant formula as a cause of aluminium toxicity in neonatal uraemia. Lancet 1985; ii: 527-9.
113. Langman C. Childhood uremic bone disease. Pediatr Ann 1987; 16: 974-8.
114. Fournier A, Morinière P, Sebert JL et al. Calcium carbonate, an aluminium-free agent for control of hyperphosphatemia, hypocalcemia and hyperparathyroidism in uremia. Kidney Int 1986; 29 (Suppl 18): S114-9.
115. Jüppner H, Hoyer PF, Latta K et al. Efficacy of calcium carbonate and low-dose vitamin D/1,25 $(OH)_2D_3$ in reducing the risk of developing renal osteodystrophy in children on continuous ambulatory peritoneal dialysis. Pediatr Nephrol 1990; 4: 614-7.
116. Salusky IB, Goodman WG, Horst R et al. Pharmacokinetics of calcitriol in continuous ambulatory and cycling peritoneal dialysis patients. Am J Kidney Dis 1990; 16: 126-32.
117. Ljunghall S, Jakobsson S, Joborn C et al. Longitudinal studies of mild primary hyperparathyroidism. J Bone Miner Res 1991; 6 (Suppl 2): S111-6.
118. Hedbäck G, Tisell LE, Bengtsson BÅ et al. Premature death in patients operated on for primary hyperparathyroidism. World J Surg

1990; 14: 829-35.
119. Hedbäck G, Odén A, Tissell LE. Parathyroid adenoma weight and the risk of death after treatment for primary hyperparathyroidism. Surgery, in press.
120. Cundy T, Kanis JA, Heynen G et al. Calcium metabolism and hyperparathyroidism after renal transplantation. Quart J Med 1983; 52: 67-78.
121. Boiskin I, Epstein S, Ismail F et al. Serum osteocalcin and bone mineral metabolism following successful renal transplantation. Clin Nephrol 1989; 31: 316-22.
122. Vlcek J, Binswanger U, Keusch G et al. Hyperparathyroidism after kidney transplantation: A retrospective case controlled study. Klin Wochenschr 1991; 69: 669-73.
123. Cundy T, Kanis JA. Rapid suppression of plasma alkaline phosphatase activity after renal transplantation in patients with osteodystrophy. Clin Chim Acta 1987; 164: 285-91.
124. Parfitt AM. Hypercalcemic hyperparathyroidism following renal transplantation: Differential diagnosis, management, and implications for cell population control in the parathyroid gland. Miner Electrolyte Metab 1982; 8: 92- 112.
125. Pabico RC, McKenna BA. Metabolic problems in renal transplant patients. Persistent hyperparathyroidism and hypophosphatemia: Effects of intravenous calcium infusion. Transplant Proc 1988; 20 (suppl 1): 438-42.
126. Mitlak BH, Alpert M, Lo C et al. Parathyroid function in normocalcemic renal transplant recipients: Evaluation by calcium infusion. J Clin Endocrinol Metab 1991; 72: 350-5.
127. Kleerekoper M, Bernstein RS, Cruz C et al. Parathyroid hormone resistance in renal allograft recipients. Adv Exp Med Biol 1982; 151: 185-7.
128. Schmidt H, Stracke H, Schatz H et al. Osteocalcin serum levels in patients following renal transplantation. Klin Wochenschr 1989; 67: 297-303.
129. Katz IA, Epstein S. Posttransplantation bone disease. J Bone Miner Res 1992; 7: 123-6.
130. Julian BA, Quarles LD, Niemann KMW. Musculoskeletal complications after renal transplantation: Pathogenesis and treatment Am J Kidney Dis 1992; 19: 99-120.
131. Sitges-Serra A, Caralps-Riera A. Hyperparathyroidism associated with renal disease. Pathogenesis, natural history, and surgical treatment. Surg Clin North Am 1987; 67: 359-77.
132. D'Alessandro AM, Melzer JS, Pirsch JD et al. Tertiary hyperparathyroidism after renal transplantation: Operative indications. Surgery 1989; 106: 1049-56.
133. Mallette LE, Eichhorn E. Effects of lithium carbonate on human calcium metabolism. Arch Intern Med 1986; 146: 770-6.
134. McIntosh WB, Horn EH, Mathieson LM et al. The prevalence, mechanism and clinical significance of lithium-induced hypercalcaemia. Med Lab Sci 1987; 44: 115-8.
135. McHenry CR, Rosen IB, Rotstein LE et al. Lithiumogenic disorders of the thyroid and parathyroid glands as surgical disease. Surgery 1990; 108: 1001-5.
136. Birnbaum J, Klandorf H, Giuliano A et al. Lithium stimulates the release of human parathyroid hormone in vitro. J Clin Endocrinol Metab 1988; 66: 1187-91.
137. Mallette LE, Khouri K, Zengotita H et al. Lithium treatment increases intact and midregion parathyroid hormone and parathyroid volume. J Clin Endocrinol Metab 1989; 68: 654-9.
138. Seely EW, Moore TJ, LeBoff MS et al. A single dose of lithium carbonate acutely elevates intact parathyroid hormone levels in humans. Acta Endocrinol 1989; 121: 174-6.
139. McHenry CR, Racke F, Meister M et al. Lithium effects on dispersed bovine parathyroid cells grown in tissue culture. Surgery 1991; 110: 1061-6.
140. Saxe AW, Gibson G. Lithium increases tritiated thymidine uptake by abnormal human parathyroid tissue. Surgery 1991; 110: 1067-77.
141. Toffaletti J, McComb RB, Bowers GN. Increase in dialyzable calcium associated with therapy with lithium. Clin Chem 1979; 25: 1806-9.
142. Dubovsky SL, Franks RD. Intracellular calcium ions in affective disorders: A review and a hypothesis. Biol Psychiatry 1983; 18:

781-97.
143. Nordenström J, Strigård K, Perbeck L et al. Hyperparathyroidism associated with treatment of manic-depressive disorders by lithium. Eur J Surg 1992; 158: 207-11.
144. Joborn C, Hetta J, Johansson H et al. Psychiatric morbidity in primary hyperparathyroidism. World J Surg 1988; 12: 476-81.
145. Rastad J, Joborn C, Åkerström G et al. Incidence, type and severity of psychic symptoms in patients with sporadic primary hyperparathyroidism. J Endocrinol Invest 1992; 15 (Suppl 6-9): 149-56.
146. Palmér M, Adami HO, Bergström R et al. Survival and renal function in untreated hypercalcaemia: Population-based cohort study with 14 years of follow-up. Lancet 1987; i: 59-62.
147. Farrington K, Varghese Z, Chan MK et al. How complete is a total parathyroidectomy in uraemia? Br Med J 1987; 294: 743.
148. Kaye M, D'Amour P, Henderson J. Elective total parathyroidectomy without autotransplant in end-stage renal disease. Kidney Int 1989; 35: 1390-9.
149. Higgins RM, Richardson AJ, Ratcliffe PJ et al. Total parathyroidectomy alone or with autograft for renal hyperparathyroidism? Quart J Med 1991; 79: 323 32.
150. Gagné E-R, Urena P, Leite-Silva S et al. Short- and long-term efficacy of total parathyroidectomy with immediate autografting compared with subtotal parathyroidectomy in hemodialysis patients. J Am Soc Nephrol 1992; 3: 1008-17.
151. De Francisco AM, Ellis HA, Owen JP et al. Parathyroidectomy in chronic renal failure. Quart J Med 1985; 55: 289-315.
152. Rothmund M. Surgical treatment of secondary hyperparathyroidism: Indication, operative management and results. Prog Surg 1986; 18: 186-205.
153. Leapman SB, Filo RS, Thomalla JV et al. Secondary hyperparathyroidism. The role of surgery. Am Surg 1989; 55: 359-65.
154. Demeure MJ, McGee DC, Wilkes W et al. Results of surgical treatment for hyperparathyroidism associated with renal disease. Am J Surg 1990; 160: 337-40.
155. Nichols P, Owen JP, Ellis HA et al. Parathyroidectomy in chronic renal failure: A nine-year follow-up study. Quart J Med 1990; 77: 1175-93.
156. Rothmund M, Wagner PK, Schark C. Subtotal parathyroidectomy versus total parathyroidectomy and autotransplantation in secondary hyperparathyroidism: A randomized trial. World J Surg 1991; 15: 745-50.
157. Niederle B, Roka R, Brennan MF. The transplantation of parathyroid tissue in man: Development, indications, technique, and results. Endocrine Rev 1982; 3: 245-79.
158. Saxe A. Parathyroid transplantation: A review. Surgery 1984; 95: 507-26.
159. Kinnaert P, Vanherweghem J-L, Fuss M et al. Total parathyroidectomy and parathyroid autograft for renal osteodystrophy: Analysis of the cause of failure. World J Surg 1985; 9: 500-6.
160. Kinnaert P, Salmon I, Decoster-Gervy C et al. Total parathyroidectomy and presternal subcutaneous implantation of parathyroid tissue for renal hyperparathyroidism. Surg Gynecol Obstet 1993; 176: 135-8.
161. Levitt MD, Vivian AB, Saker BM. Parathyroidectomy in chronic renal failure. Aust N Z J Surg 1986; 56: 233-9.
162. Korzets Z, Magen H, Kraus L et al. Total parathyroidectomy with autotransplantation in haemodialysed patients with secondary hyperparathyroidism-should it be abandoned? Nephrol Dial Transplant 1987; 2: 341-6.
163. Tominaga Y, Tanaka Y, Sato K et al. Surgical treatment of secondary hyperparathyroidism. J Bone Miner Metab 1991; 9: 56-62.
164. Botha JR. Renal hyperparathyroidism. Surg Ann 1992; 24: 43-57.
165. Welsh CL, Taylor GW, Cattell WR et al. Parathyroid surgery in chronic renal failure: Subtotal parathyroidectomy or autotransplantation? Br J Surg 1984; 71: 591-2.
166. Jansson S, Tisell L-E. Autotransplantation of diseased parathyroid glands into subcutaneous abdominal adipose tissue. Surgery 1987; 101: 549-56.
167. Lando MJ, Hoover LA, Zuckerbraun L et al. Autotransplantation of parathyroid tissue into sternocleidomastoid muscle. Arch

Otolaryngol Head Neck Surg 1988; 114: 557-60.
168. Funahashi H, Satoh Y, Imai T et al. Our technique of parathyroid autotransplantation in operation for papillary thyroid carcinoma. Surgery 1993; 114: 92-6.
169. Wells SA, Stirman JA, Bolman RM. Parathyroid transplantation. World J Surg 1977; 1: 747-56.
170. Brennan MF, Brown EM, Spiegel AM et al. Autotransplantation of cryopreserved parathyroid tissue in man. Ann Surg 1979; 189: 139-42.
171. Dubost C, Kracht M, Assens P et al. Reoperation for secondary hyperparathyroidism in hemodialysis patients. World J Surg 1986; 10: 654-60.
172. Wagner PK, Rumpelt HJ, Krause U et al. The effect of cryopreservation on hormone secretion in vitro and morphology of human parathyroid tissue. Surgery 1986; 99: 257-64.
173. Herrera M, Grant C, van Heerden JA et al. Parathyroid autotransplantation. Arch Surg 1992; 127: 825-30.
174. Wagner PK. Autotransplantation of fresh and cryopreserved human parathyroid tissue. Prog Surg 1986; 18: 206-20.
175. Herrera MF, Grant CS, van Heerden JA et al. The effect of cryopreservation on cell viability and hormone secretion in human parathyroid tissue. Surgery 1992; 112: 1096-102.
176. Romanus ME, Farndon JR, Wells SA. Transplantation of the parathyroid glands. In: Johnston I, Thompson N, eds. Endocrine Surgery. London: Butterworth. 1983: 25-40.
177. Basile C, Drüeke T, Lacour B et al. Total parathyroidectomy and delayed parathyroid autotransplantation using a simplified cryopreservation technique. Human and animal studies. Am J Kidney Dis 1984; 3: 366-70.
178. Saxe AW, Spiegel AM, Marx SJ et al. Deferred parathyroid autografts with cryopreserved tissue after reoperative parathyroid surgery. Arch Surg 1982; 117: 538-43.
179. Rothmund M, Wagner PK. Assessment of parathyroid graft function after autotransplantation of fresh and cryopreserved tissue. World J Surg 1984; 8: 527-33.
180. Urena P, Basile C, Grateau G et al. Short-term effects of parathyroidectomy on plasma biochemistry in chronic uremia. Kidney Int 1989; 36: 120-6.
181. Daseler EH, Anson BJ. Surgical anatomy of the subclavian artery and its branches. Surg Gynecol Obstet 1959; 108: 149-74.
182. Doppman JL, Hammond WG, Melson GL et al. Staining of parathyroid adenomas by selective arteriography. Radiology 1969; 92: 527-30.
183. Doppman JL, Marx SJ, Brennan MF et al. The blood supply of mediastinal parathyroid adenomas. Ann Surg 1977; 185: 488-90.
184. Jelenko C, Teeslink CR, Herndon JR et al. Localization of parathyroid adenomata by selective arteriography. Am Surg 1971; 37: 25-33.
185. Kuntz CH, Goldsmith RE. Selective arteriography of parathyroid adenomas. Radiology 1972; 102: 21-8.
186. Harach HR, Jasani B. Parathyroid hyperplasia in tertiary hyperparathyroidism: A pathological and immunohistochemical reappraisal. Histopathology 1992; 21: 513-9.
187. Tanaka Y, Seo H, Tominaga Y et al. Factors related to the recurrent hyperfunction of autografts after total parathyroidectomy in patients with severe secondary hyperparathyroidism. Jpn J Surg 1993; 23: 220-7.
188. Tominaga Y, Grimelius L, Falkmer UG et al. DNA ploidy pattern of parathyroid parenchymal cells in renal secondary hyperparathyroidism with relapse. Analyt Cell Pathol 1991; 3: 325-33.
189. Ogg CS. Total parathyroidectomy in treatment of secondary (renal) hyperparathyroidism. Br Med J 1967; 4: 331-4.
190. Klempa I, Frei U, Röttger P et al. Parathyroid autografts—Morpholgy and function: Six years' experience with parathyroid autotransplantation in uremic patients. World J Surg 1984; 8: 540-6.
191. Hampl H, Steinmüller T, Stabell U et al. Recurrent hyperparathyroidism after total parathyroidectomy and autotransplantation in patients with long-term hemodialysis. Miner Electrolyte Metab 1991; 17: 256-60.
192. Sitges-Serra A, Gores P, Hesse U et al.

Serum calcium as an early indicator for surgical treatment of hyperparathyroidism after renal transplantation. World J Surg 1986; 10: 661-7.
193. Dotzenrath C, Goretzki PE, Röher HD. Operative therapie des sekundären hyperparathyreoidismus nach nierentransplantation. Langenbecks Arch Chir 1993; 378: 121-4.
194. Takagi H, Tominaga Y, Uchida K et al. Subtotal versus total parathyroidectomy with forearm autograft for secondary hyperparathyroidism in chronic renal failure. Ann Surg 1984; 200: 18-23.
195. Dawborn JK, Brown DJ, Douglas MC et al. Parathyroidectomy in chronic renal failure. Nephron 1983; 33: 100-5.
196. Felsenfeld AJ, Gutman RA, Llach F et al. Postparathyroidectomy hypocalcemia as an accurate indicator of preparathyroidectomy bone histology in the uremic patient. Miner Electrolyte Metab 1984; 10: 166-72.
197. Litchman MB, Kinder BK, Johnson BM. Calcium requirements with ESRD patients after total parathyroidectomy with autotransplantation. Dial Transplant 1987; 16: 611-21.
198. Clair F, Leenhardt L, Bourdeau A et al. Effect of calcitriol in the control of plasma calcium after parathyroidectomy. Nephron 1987; 46: 18-22.
199. Wallfelt C, Ljunghall S, Bergström R et al. Clinical characteristics and surgical treatment of sporadic primary hyperparathyroidism with emphasis on chief cell hyperplasia. Surgery 1990; 107: 13-9.
200. Rothmund M, Wagner PK. Total parathyroidectomy and autotransplantation of parathyroid tissue for renal hyperparathyroidism. A one- to six-year follow-up. Ann Surg 1983; 197: 7-16.
201. Zucchelli P, Santoro A, Zucchelli A et al. Long-term effects of parathyroidectomy on cardiac and autonomic nervous system functions in haemodialysis patients. Nephrol Dial Transplant 1988; 3: 45-50.
202. Pizzarelli F, Fabrizi F, Postorino M et al. Parathyroidectomy and blood pressure in hemodialysis patients. Nephron 1993; 63: 384-9.
203. Malmaeus J, Åkerström G, Johansson H et al. Parathyroid surgery in chronic renal insufficiency. Acta Chir Scand 1982; 148: 229-38.
204. Gipstein RM, Coburn JW, Adams DA et al. Calciphylaxis in man. A syndrome of tissue necrosis and vascular calcification in 11 patients with chronic renal failure. Arch Intern Med 1976; 136: 1273-80.
205. Mehregan DA, Winkelmann RK. Cutaneous gangrene, vascular calcification and hyperparathyroidism. Mayo Clin Proc 1989; 64: 211-5.
206. Duh Q-Y, Lim RC, Clark OH. Calciphylaxis in secondary hyperparathyroidism. Diagnosis and parathyroidectomy. Arch Surg 1991; 126: 1213-9.
207. Chan YL, Mahony JF, Turner JJ et al. The vascular lesions associated with skin necrosis in renal disease. Br J Dermatol 1983; 109: 85-95.
208. Llach F. Parathyroidectomy in chronic renal failure: Indications, surgical approach and the use of calcitriol. Kidney Int 1990; 38 (Suppl 29): S62-8.
209. Mallette LE, Eisenberg KL, Schwaitzberg SD et al. Total parathyroidectomy and autogenous parathyroid graft placement for treatment of hyperparathyroidism due to chronic renal failure. Am J Surg 1983; 146: 727-33.
210. Diaz-Buxo JA, Geissinger WT, Walker PJ et al. Total parathyroidectomy and autotransplantation. Clin Nephrol 1981; 16: 276-82.
211. Hayes JF, Gross GF, Schuman ES. Surgical management of renal hyperparathyroidism in the dialysis patient. Am J Surg 1982; 143: 569-71.
212. Collier VU, Mitch WE. Accelerated progression of chronic renal insufficiency after parathyroidectomy. JAMA 1980; 244: 1215-8.
213. Chan YL, Posen S, Savdie E et al. Total parathyroidectomy and renal function in patients with chronic renal failure. Miner Electrolyte Metab 1983; 9: 57-61.
214. Alveryd A. Parathyroid glands in thyroid surgery. I. Anatomy of parathyroid glands. Acta Chir Scand 1968; 389: 1-120.
215. Åkerström G, Malmaeus J, Bergström R. Surgical anatomy of human parathyroid

glands. Surgery 1984; 95: 14-21.
216. Rothmund M, Wagner PK. Reoperations of persistent and recurrent secondary hyperparathyroidism. Ann Surg 1988; 207: 310-14.
217. Henry J-FR, Denizot A, Audiffret J et al. Results of reoperations for persistent or recurrent secondary hyperparathyroidism in hemodialysis patients. World J Surg 1990; 14: 303-7.
218. Edis AJ, Levitt MD. Supernumerary parathyroid glands: Implications for the surgical treatment of secondary hyperparathyroidism. World J Surg 1987; 11: 398-401.
219. Proye C, Carnaille B, Sautier M. Hyperparathyroidie chez l'insuffisant rénal chronique: Parathyroidectomie subtotale ou parathyroidectomie totale avec autotransplantation? J Chir 1990; 127: 136-40.
220. McCarron DA, Lenfesty B, Narasimhan N et al. Anatomical heterogeneity of parathyroid glands in posttransplant hyperparathyroidism. Am J Nephrol 1988; 8: 388-91.
221. Oka T, Yoshioka T, Shrestha GR et al. Immunohistochemical study of nodular hyperplastic parathyroid glands in patients with secondary hyperparathyroidism. Virchows Arch A Pathol Anat 1988; 413: 53-60.
222. Reddick RL, Costa JC, Marx SJ. Parathyroid hyperplasia and parathyromatosis. Lancet 1977; i: 549.
223. Juhlin C, Holmdahl R, Johansson H et al. Monoclonal antibodies with exclusive reactivity against parathyroid cells and tubule cells of the kidney. Proc Natl Acad Sci, USA 1987; 84: 2990-4.
224. Juhlin C, Rastad J, Klareskog L et al. Parathyroid histology and cytology with monoclonal antibodies recognizing a calcium sensor of parathyroid cells. Am J Pathol 1989; 135: 321-8.
225. Alexander PT, Schuman ES, Vetto RM et al. Repeat parathyroid operation associated with renal disease. Am J Surg 1988; 155: 686-9.
226. Ellis HA. Fate of long-term parathyroid autografts in patients with chronic renal failure treated by parathyroidectomy: A histopathological study of autografts, parathyroid glands and bone. Histopathology 1988; 13: 289-309.
227. Garvin PJ, Castaneda M, Linderer R et al. Management of hypercalcemic hyperparathyroidism after renal transplantation. Arch Surg 1985; 120: 578-83.
228. Weinstein RS. Decreased mineralization in hemodialysis patients after subtotal parathyroidectomy. Calcif Tissue Int 1982; 34: 16-20.
229. Rodriguez M, Martin-Malo A, Martinez ME et al. Calcemic response to parathyroid hormone in renal failure: Role of phosphorus and its effect on calcitriol. Kidney Int 1991; 40: 1055-62.
230. Rodriguez M, Felsenfeld AJ, Llach F. Calcemic response to parathyroid hormone in renal failure: Role of calcitriol and the effect of parathyroidectomy. Kidney Int 1991; 40: 1063-8.
231. Duh QY, Arnaud CD, Levin KE et al. Parathyroid hormone: Before and after parathyroidectomy. Surgery 1986; 100: 1021-31.
232. Lundgren E, Rastad J, Ridefelt P et al. Long-term effects of parathyroid operation on serum calcium and parathyroid hormone values in sporadic primary hyperparathyroidism. Surgery 1992; 112: 1123-9.
233. Baker LRI, Otieno LS, Brown AL et al. Pitfalls after total parathyroidectomy and parathyroid autotransplantation in chronic renal failure. Am J Nephrol 1991; 11: 186-91.
234. Casanova D, Sarfati E, De Francisco A et al. Secondary hyperparathyroidism: Diagnosis of site of recurrence. World J Surg 1991; 15: 546-50.
235. Hellman P, Skogseid B, Juhlin C et al. Findings and long-term results of parathyroid surgery in multiple endocrine neoplasia type 1. World J Surg 1992; 16: 718-23.
236. Niederle B, Hörandner H, Roka R et al. Parathyreoidektomie und autotransplantation beim renalen hyperparathyreoidismus. I. Klinische und laborchemische untersuchungen nach gewebeauswahl. Chirurg 1989; 60: 665-70.
237. Kessler M, Avila JM, Renoult E et al. Reoperation for secondary hyperparathyroidism in chronic renal failure. Nephrol

Dial Transplant 1991; 6: 176-9.
238. Åkerström G, Rudberg C, Grimelius L et al. Causes of failed primary exploration and technical aspects of re-operation in primary hyperparathyroidism. World J Surg 1992; 16: 562-9.
239. Takagi H, Tominaga Y, Tanaka Y et al. Total parathyroidectomy with forearm autograft for secondary hyperparathyroidism in chronic renal failure. Ann Surg 1988; 208: 639-44.
240. Hellman P, Ahlström H, Bergström R et al. Positron emission tomography with ^{11}C-methionine in hyperparathyroidism. Surgery, in press.
241. Karsenty G, Petraglia A, Bourdeau A et al. Evaluation of parathyroid autograft growth and function in hemodialysis patients. Am J Kidney Dis 1986; 8: 43-50.
242. Parnham AJ, Wijeyesingh ECR, Tarbit IF et al. Intact parathyroid hormone assay offers increased sensitivity over C-terminal assays in the study of parathyroid graft function. Nephron 1986; 44: 8-10.
243. Krutak-Krol H, Mace C, Nichols WK et al. Diagnostic dilemma of an unsuspected hyperfunctioning accessory parathyroid gland after total parathyroidectomy with autotransplantation in a peritoneal dialysis patient. Am J Nephrol 1989; 9: 495-8.
244. Niederle B, Roka R, Hörandner H. Rezidivierender renaler hyperparathyroidismus: Reoperationen am autotransplantat. Wien Klin Wochenschr 1988; 100: 369-72.

CHAPTER 10

Parathyroid Carcinoma

Göran Åkerström, Claes Juhlin, Henry Johansson

Parathyroid carcinoma is a rare, comparatively indolent malignancy with a great tendency to recur after surgery. Improvement in therapy is likely to result from a more general appreciation of the diagnosis, whereby radical primary surgery may successfully remove the lesion. Repeated procedures will, however, frequently be required in order to deal with recurrence or metastases.

Surgery constitutes the appropriate therapy for parathyroid carcinoma, and is generally accepted also as the most efficient therapy even in cases of local recurrence or metastases. Surgical intervention will therefore frequently include repeated procedures aiming at prevention of fatal hypercalcemia.

The diagnosis of parathyroid carcinoma has entailed problems and it may still be difficult to establish the diagnosis by histopathology, so recurrence or metastases sometimes heralds the presence of the malignancy. The histopathology, including modern methods of nuclear DNA cytometry should, however, generally raise suspicion regarding the diagnosis, and these methods have also been important for prognosis. Advances in operative technique combined with imaging procedures have furthermore improved the efficacy of surgical treatment in parathyroid carcinoma, such that a radical en-bloc procedure at the primary operation offers the best chance for cure. Since parathyroid carcinomas are slow-growing neoplasms, repeated resections of recurrence are often beneficial, and generally the only possibility to deal effectively with severe hypercalcemia. Even if cure by subsequent operations is rare, palliative resections are strongly recommended even for distant metastases. Only when hypercalcemia is refractory to surgical treatment will other treatment modalities be considered for long-term therapy.

The first description of a malignant parathyroid tumor was given by de Quervain in 1909, but not until 1948 before Norris reported on a series of some 40 collected cases.[1-3] More detailed histopathological and clinical characteristics of parathyroid carcinoma were later described by Black and Ackerman in 1950, Woolner et al in 1952 and Black in 1954.[4-6] Some 70 years after de Quervain's original paper Schantz

Current Controversy in Parathyroid Operation and Reoperation,
edited by Göran Åkerström.

and Castleman contributed an extensive review of 70 patients with parathyroid carcinoma, in which they outlined the classical histological criteria for this disease.[7] Recently Sandelin et al presented a worldwide study of parathyroid carcinoma including 95 cases where clinical, histopathological and cytometric variables were assessed in relation to prognosis.[8,9]

INCIDENCE

Parathyroid carcinoma remains a rare cause of sporadic primary HPT, but has occasionally also been described in HPT secondary to uremia and as isolated cases in familial and MEN-1 associated HPT.[10-15] A few decades ago parathyroid carcinoma was reported to account for up to 5% of patients with primary HPT,[7,16] but at that time primary HPT was a comparatively rare disease. Subsequently have the classical histological criteria for the carcinoma diagnosis, defined by Schantz and Castleman, have been seriously debated, even if the contribution of these authors in its essence is considered of indisputable value for our present knowledge of the disease.[17-19] More recently the difficulties in distinguishing between benign "atypical" parathyroid adenoma and parathyroid carcinoma have been further appreciated and this have led to the formulation of more strict criteria for the malignant diagnosis.[9,17-22] A concommitant increased recognition of primary HPT in general has resulted in a decreased proportional incidence for parathyroid carcinoma. Currently this entity thus appears to comprise less than 1% of contemporary patients with primary HPT and in our own experience no more than 0.4%.[1,23-26] A higher proportional incidence around 5% is, however, still reported from Japan.[27,28] This could represent a variable geographical distribution of the histological entities of HPT, since the overall prevalence of the disease has been significantly lower in Japan as compared to the Western world.[27] Only occasional case reports have indicated a possible relationship between external irradiation and parathyroid carcinoma.[29]

CLINICAL FEATURES

Parathyroid carcinoma has been recognized with equal frequency in males and females, and the average patient age at diagnosis has usually been 45-55 years.[7,8,21,22,24,28,30] Occasionally the disease has occurred in children.[27,28,30,31] The reported sex and age distribution contrasts with that normally encountered in patients with primary HPT due to adenoma, who are normally at least one or two decades older and predominantly females.

The serum calcium values have generally been higher in patients with parathyroid carcinoma than in individuals with benign parathyroid disease.[7,19,21,27-34] Earlier patient series reported average initial values of around 3.8 mmol/l, while more recent reports demonstrate lower but still generally markedly raised serum calcium values in these patients.[8,24,28,33-35] A considerable proportion of patients has presented with hypercalcemic crisis or has developed such crisis during progression of the disease.[27,28,32-34] Accordingly the levels of parathyroid hormone (PTH) have with few exceptions been markedly elevated, and during follow-up many patients have exhibited a continuous rise, sometimes to extremely high values, due to progression to more advanced stages of the disease.[34]

The symptoms of patients with parathyroid carcinoma have often been pronounced and related to the generally prevailing severe hypercalcemia.[27,28,32-34] Common complaints have been polyuria, polydipsia, weakness, fatigue, anorexia and some patients have even suffered from vomiting, dehydration, weight loss and anemia. Consistent with the significant metabolic disturbances, the patients of the older series have more or less invariably displayed a remarkably high incidence of bone and renal complications[7,19,21,24,30,34] (Table 10.1). Skeletal abnormalities, consisting of severe osteoporosis, subperiostal bone resorption or advanced osteitis fibrosa cystica, have been encountered in up to 50-90% of the patients. Presentation with bone pain, markedly elevated alkaline phosphatases and pathological fractures has not been un-

Table 10.1. Clinical manifestations of functioning parathyroid carcinoma

	Author, Reference, Year		
	Holmes et al[30] 1969	**Shane and Bilezikian[21] 1982**	**Obara and Fujimoto[34] 1991**
Period of review	1933-1968	1968-1981	1981-1989
Number of cases	46	62	163
Female:male ratio	0.8:1	1.2:1	1.2:1
Average age in yr (range)	44 (12-72)	48 (18-73)	46.6 (13-78)
Manifestations (%):			
Serum calcium (mg/dl)	15.9	15.5	15.0
>14 mg/dl	75	70	65
Bone disease	73	70	39
Palpable neck mass	52	48	34
Renal involvement	32	60	48
Pancreatitis	15	10	5.5
Hypercalcemic crisis			12
No symptoms		2	2
Local recurrence following surgery	65	47	36
Lymphatic metastasis	32	11	17
Distant metastasis	21	24	25

Reprinted with permission from Obara T et al.[34]

common.[28,34] Renal complications have occurred in 50-80%, and these have consisted of nephrolithiasis in approximately 70%, nephrocalcinosis in 20% and more or less severely impaired renal function in 50% of the patients.[24,30] A combination of skeletal and renal abnormalities was reported in up to 50% of the patients in earlier series but seems to occur somewhat more infrequently today.[21,24,28,30,33,34] Complicating acute and occasionally recurrent pancreatitis, as well as peptic ulcer or dyspeptic symptoms, have been described in up to 10-15% of the patients.[7,21,30,33-35] This pattern of pronounced symptomatology is currently rare in association with benign primary HPT and comparable symptomatology is essentially only encountered when these patients present with hypercalcemic crisis.[22] However, consistent with more efficient and earlier recognition of parathyroid carcinoma recent series report patients with moderate hypercalcemia and less severe complications. Some patients suffer merely from weakness, fatigue or psychiatric disability but few are still asymptomatic.[27,28,36]

A palpable neck mass is a conspicuous feature which should arouse suspicions about the carcinoma diagnosis and has been reported in 30-50% of the patients. This is in contrast to the patients with benign HPT where a tumor is rarely or ever palpable.[7,19,21,26-28,30-37] The palpable carcinomas are generally firm and adherent to surrounding neck structures. Occasional patients have demonstrated vocal cord paralysis prior to surgery.[22,28,30]

DIAGNOSIS

Due to the rarity of parathyroid carcinoma the diagnosis is seldom apparent prior to surgery. The possibility needs to be appreciated, however, especially in the younger individual with HPT who presents with marked hypercalcemia and severe symptoms.[28,34] If not recognized before surgery the malignant diagnosis should at least be evident peroperatively if the surgeon is experienced enough to recall the characteristic features of parathyroid carcinoma.[28,34] The tumor is typically large, multilobulated, white or tan-greyish and often hard to palpation. It may also have a conspicuously thick capsule with adherence to the surrounding muscles, the thyroid, the trachea or to the esophagus.[7,18,26,27,33,38,39] Only occasionally is the thyroid gland totally replaced by tumor.[22] These typical characteristics should distinguish carcinoma from a benign parathyroid adenoma, being of soft consistency and a more brown-reddish color. The adenoma typically is loosely connected to the surrounding tissues and easily delivered at operation.[19] The distinction is not always easy, however, since the benign parathyroid tumor may sometimes also be adherent to the surroundings possibly as a result of capsular bleeding. Occasionally the carcinoma is of softer consistency and exhibits the brown-reddish color typical of adenoma.[19,36,40] Although a parathyroid tumor should never be transected within the operative field, the fibrosis and the hard consistency of the tumor may be even more apparent when the cut surface is inspected, and it may then also reveal a typical lobulated texture.[40] Often the presence of malignancy has not been apparent until the disease has recurred during follow up, and some patients have even undergone reoperation before the malignant diagnosis was recognized.[19,28] Recurrence after removal of a single, unusually large parathyroid tumor should in this respect be particularly suspicious for malignancy. Parathyroid carcinoma has occasionally also been present in multiglandular parathyroid disease, and it has then coexisted with both adenoma and hyperplasia and the tumor has also been reported to develop within an originally hyperplastic gland.[8,40-43] Generally, however, the parathyroid glands associated with carcinoma have been described as normal or atrophic.[7,28,30]

The histopathological diagnosis of parathyroid carcinoma is known to be exceptionally difficult, essentially because more general histopathological criteria for malignancy tend to be insufficient in association with endocrine tumors and particularly in the diagnosis of parathyroid lesions.[25] According to the classical histological descriptions of parathyroid carcinoma the tumor is characteristically an unusually large parathyroid tumor, surrounded by a *thick fibrotic capsule* with broad, acellular fibrous-hyalinie bands, which often tend to divide the parenchyma into lobules of variable size[4,5,7,20] (Fig. 10.1). The classical criteria of parathyroid carcinoma have furthermore comprised a trabecular or rosette-like pattern of the parenchymal cells, as well as invasive growth into the tumor capsule and a high mitotic index.[4,5,7,20] In addition to these criteria the characteristic gross features of a tan, gray tumor, with hard consistency and lobulated cut surface have been considered to support the carcinoma diagnosis.[20] However, the significance of these criteria have been considerably debated and several authors claim that only the presence of metastases or demonstration of clear-cut invasiveness into surrounding tissues validate a carcinoma diagnosis.[17-19,23,25,44,45] The trabecular pattern is probably the least significant of the criteria, as it is apparently relatively uncommon among the carcinomas and may also be present within benign lesions.[9,24] The interpretation of *invasiveness* as a criterion of malignancy has also evoked considerable discussion as nests of parenchymal cells may be present within the tumor capsule or in vessels of the benign parathyroid lesions.[17,18] Only extension beyond the capsule into surrounding tissues or demonstration of tumor emboli in vessels should be interpreted as definite signs of malignancy. In the presence of such criteria invasiveness of the primary lesion has been demonstrated in approximately half of the carcinomas.[9,17-19,40]

It must be emphasized in this respect that ectopic, rudimentary parathyroid glands occur normally in the fat tissue surrounding the parathyroids and also as dispersed microscopic islets of cells within the thymus, and such parathyroid gland rudiments should not be interpreted as invading tumor cells.[46] The carcinoma should also be

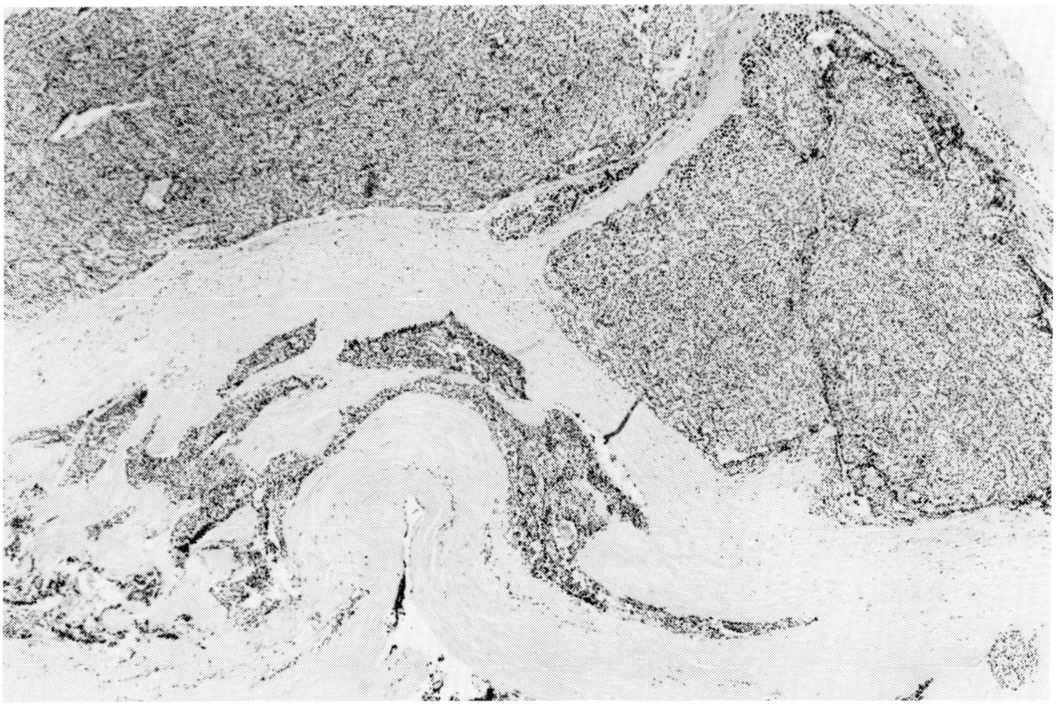

Fig. 10.1. Parathyroid carcinoma with typical fibrosis and capsular invasion. Obtained by the courtesy of Prof. L Grimelius.

distinguished from cases of recurrent HPT due to seeding and implantation of parathyroid cells, which has occasionally occurred when the capsule of benign lesions has been violated during excision.[47-50] Such benign parathyroid implants may have inherited a propensity for growth if they originate from an adenomatous or hyperplastic gland. Since they will also commonly be surrounded by dense fibrosis induced by the previous surgery, it may sometimes be difficult to distinguish them from carcinoma, but generally these implants exhibit clearly benign features.[9] A *high mitotic index* has been claimed as the single, most important of the classical histological criteria for parathyroid carcinoma, and an unusually high frequency of mitoses is indeed a significant feature in many of the malignant tumors.[7,9,20,51] It is not always a valid criterion, however, as approximately half of the carcinomas may exhibit a lower mitotic rate or absence of mitoses even when metastases have occurred. The benign parathyroid lesions, comprising both adenomas and hyperplastic glands may in fact also demonstrate a rather high rate of mitoses.[9,44] Consequently, the discrimination between benign and malignant parathyroid tumors is sometimes not possible with available criteria, and histologically benign "adenomas" have in fact been associated with metastases.[17,18,45,51] Recent studies nevertheless emphasize that if the overall picture is considered the majority of parathyroid carcinomas exhibit relatively distinct and characteristic histological features.[9,40] Thus, even if clearly demonstrated local invasiveness or the presence of metastases are the indisputable criteria for the carcinoma, other signs such as marked increase in cell size, pronounced nuclear pleomorphism, macronucleoli, foci of necrosis and a typical pattern of fibrosis constitute important contributing indications of malignancy.[9,40,52] Unusually marked mitotic activity is present in some carcinomas and this, as well as an aneuploid DNA content strongly support the carcinoma diagnosis.[7,9,53-55] These features have also been demonstrated to influence the prognosis in parathyroid carcinoma.[9,54] Since there has previously been a general tendency to histologically overdiagnose parathyroid carcinoma many current pathologists designate a gland with equivocal features as *atypical* adenoma rather than carcinoma. However, in some cases the malignant potential becomes evident during long term follow-up where the patient experiences local recurrence or metastases.[6,16,32,43,44,56,57] The same course of events has occured in circumstances when the carcinoma has never been suspected. Emphasizing these difficulties associated with the histopathological evaluation, an intraoperative frozen section can often only demonstrate signs that are suspicious for carcinoma. The appropriate diagnosis, however, generally has to await proper examination of paraffin-embedded sections.

TREATMENT

Primary Surgery

Surgery still remains the sole possibility to cure patients with parathyroid carcinoma, and the foremost opportunity for this should be at the time of the initial operation.[14,27,28,30-32,36,58] If a surgeon thus comes across a multilobulated, gray, firm and densely adherent tumor during an operation for primary HPT the carcinoma diagnosis definitely needs to be entertained. On the basis of these gross findings the surgeon should directly perform an en-bloc excision of the lesion and include any infiltrated adjacent tissue with the resected specimen.[21,28,30-32,58] If the diagnosis is highly suspicious the procedure should neither be preceded by biopsy nor by any more limited tumor excision for frozen section examination. The radical initial surgery has been clearly demonstrated to reduce the risk of local dissemination from parathyroid carcinoma, and will consequently also minimize the incidence of persistent or recurrent disease.[34,36] Similar reasoning may in fact also be valid even for some large, benign parathyroid tumors, which may occasionally be extraordinarily fragile, so that dissection close to the tumor risks violation of the tumor capsule, spillage of cells and the recurrence by implantation. Moreover, some carcinomas may lack the characteristic gross features of malignancy and appear most adenoma-like, and therefore hemithyroidectomy is generally recommended for removal of any thyroid-adjacent, parathyroid lesion with suspicious features.[36]

The procedure for *primary en bloc removal of parathyroid carcinoma* has been previously detailed by Fujimoto et al.[28,31] As initial part of the radical excision these authors recommend that the lateral border of the en bloc specimen is outlined by exposure of the carotid artery along its extension in the neck.[28] The strap muscles are thereafter transected or removed in order to obtain better exposure and complete tumor excision. The recurrent laryngeal nerve is identified close to its caudal origin in the neck. The nerve is followed in the cranial direction and dissected from the tumor mass, if necessary with the aid of magnifying glasses.[28] However, if the nerve is firmly adherent to the tumor, or its preservation will jeopardize radical tumor excision it will generally be sacrificed and removed with the tumor specimen. The en bloc resection also requires that the thyroid lobe on the tumor side is excised together with para- and pretracheal areolar fat and the ipsilateral thymus.[28] The trachea and the esophageal wall are carefully skeletonized in order to remove all fat and lymph nodes between the trachea and the vascular sheath. Special care is taken to include lymph nodes in the tracheoesophageal groove with the resected specimen. After excision of the tumor the vascular sheath is opened and carefully explored, and any suspicious lymph node is excised and subjected to frozen section examination. Since regional lymph node metastases have been infrequently demonstrated in parathyroid carcinoma and have generally appeared late in the disease, the requirement for routine prophylactic neck dissection is moot and is not often recommended in association with the primary surgery.[7,14,27,32] However, a modified neck dissection is performed if grossly enlarged or histologically positive nodes have been revealed during central neck dissections or have been detected by intraoperative palpation of the lateral neck compartment.[28,32]

Occasionally a parathyroid carcinoma has occurred within the mediastinal thymus, and it has even been found within a fifth, supernumerary gland in this location.[59] Such tumors are removed via sternotomy and the operation should include complete excision of the thymus together with adjacent tissues of both the upper mediastinum and the lower neck.

If the malignant diagnosis has been incidentally revealed by histological examination of a parathyroid tumor which has been simply excised at surgery it may be difficult to decide if reoperation is required.[28] The absence of typical gross features or histological invasiveness as well as a low rate of mitoses indicate a less aggressive tumor so reoperative surgery may be postponed until the serum calcium and PTH values rise.[28] However, signs of local invasiveness as well as persistent or recurrent hypercalcemia during follow-up will indicate the need for localization studies and reoperative surgery.[28]

Follow Up

Long term cure after the primary surgery has been reported in 30-50% of patients with histologically verified parathyroid carcinoma and seems to depend largely on the adequacy of the initial operative management.[7,21,24,28,30,36] As an indication of successful surgery the serum calcium values will rapidly be normalized postoperatively, and many patients will even require oral calcium and vitamin D supplementation because of coexistent severe bone disease and ensuing "bone hunger."[28]

Recurrence of parathyroid carcinoma will occur in 50-70% of the patients after initially apparently successful surgery.[7,19,21,24,28,30,36] If the tumor has been grossly removed at operation there is an approximate 50% chance that the patient will remain disease-free after 5 years. A variable recurrence rate in different series seems to reflect a discrepancy in histological criteria and tumor stage. An apparently higher cure rate in recent series could reflect both early diagnosis and more effective therapy.[8] The vast majority comprising up to 70% of recurrences, occurs locally in the neck, and many are thought to result from violation of the tumor capsule and implantation of tumor cells.[7,21,28,30] In up to 45% of the patients with recurrent carcinoma the tumor has been palpable in the neck and tumor implants have occurred in the previous operative incision, subcutaneously or within the strap muscles. Lymph node metastases and particularly distant metastases to the lungs, liver or bone have generally appeared as late manifestations of the disease.[28,34]

The outcome, with respect to rate and time to recurrence seems to be strongly related to inherent biological properties of individual tumors. In patients with clinically unequivocal parathyroid carcinoma, displaying typical gross features, histological signs of local invasiveness and high mitotic index, the majority of recurrences has been encountered already within 2 to 3 years after the primary surgery.[7,18,21,28] Among patients with tumors having less obvious histological characteristics, fewer have experienced recurrence and some tumors have been found to progress very slowly, so that recurrence may have been delayed up to 10 years after the primary surgery[7,16,32,34,58] (Fig. 10.2). Unusual patients have distant metastases as a cause of recurrent disease soon after surgery.[27,28,34] In a review comprising 167 patients reported in the English literature between 1981-1989 Obara and Fujimoto reported persistent disease in 4% and recurrence in 37%.[34] The recurrences were encountered with an average delay of 2.6 years after surgery, but in occasional patients they were delayed and occurred more than 7 years postoperatively.[34] In their recent study Sandelin et al reported recurrence in altogether 42% of patients with parathyroid carcinoma.[8] The majority of the tumors recurred locally in the neck and with a median delay from the primary surgical procedure of 33 months.[8] The authors emphasized that the DNA content as well as other histological features of the tumors were related to the risk for recurrence[8] (Figs. 10.3 and 10.4).The DNA determinations were therefore considered useful both as support for the carcinoma diagnosis but also as meaningful estimates of the prognosis.[8]

A majority of the patients with recurrent parathyroid carcinoma has exhibited slow, but continuous rise in serum calcium values, and it has generally been considered wise to postpone treatment until the serum calcium concentration has risen to values around 3.0 mmol/l or more. Moderate hypercalcemia has often been well tolerated—the effect of presently available antihypercalcemic agents is still variable, and has a limited duration of time. Occasionally a more rapid rise in serum calcium and development of hypercalcemic crisis will dictate more aggressive treatment, comprising various forms of medication to ameliorate the symptoms of severe hypercalcemia. Generally, however, when the hypercalcemia becomes marked, surgery remains the only efficient means to alleviate the hypercalcemia, and patients will ultimately have to undergo reoperation. Since the best results of reoperation in parathyroid carcinoma will be obtained if the tumor is preoperatively localized, efforts are often made to manage the patient medically until the site of the tumor mass has been radiologically visualized.[28] Not unusually, however, the patient will become resistant to medical therapy or experience such rapid progression of hypercalcemia that reoperation is urgently called for and has to be performed blindly.[32]

Radiological Localization

In patients with recurrent parathyroid carcinoma serious efforts should always be made to localize the site of recurrence with radiology.[27,28] Fujimoto and Obara have emphasized the value of reviewing operative notes and histopathological findings in order to predict the site of recurrence.[28] If en bloc resection was not performed initially tumor recurrence should be expected at the site of the original lesion. In contrast, carcinomas with markedly invasive features and with histopathological specimens showing frequent mitoses are likely to recur with metastases to regional lymph nodes or with hematogenous spread.[28]

The noninvasive methods for tumor localization consisting of ultrasonography (US), computed tomography (CT), magnetic resonance imaging (MRT) and technetium/thallium scintigraphy are additive in effect and should therefore be used in combination in order to increase the precision of the diagnosis.[60,61] US may sometimes demonstrate signs of gross invasion and irregular tumor margins in parathyroid carcinoma and may also be of considerable val-

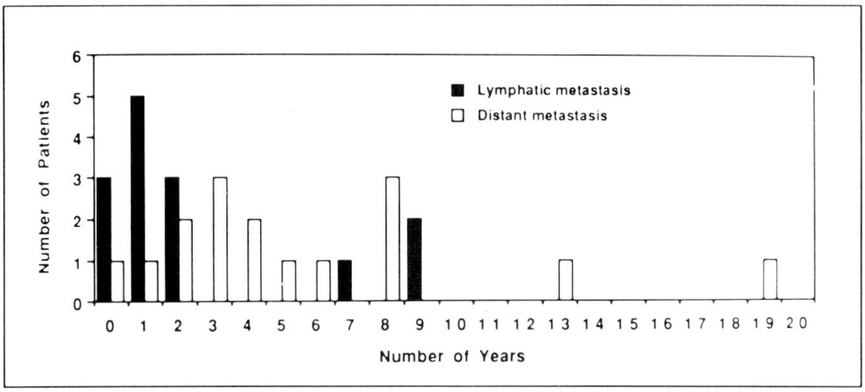

Fig. 10.2. Interval between the initial operation and the first clinical manifestation of metastasis in patients with parathyroid carcinoma. Reprinted with permission from Obara T et al.[34]

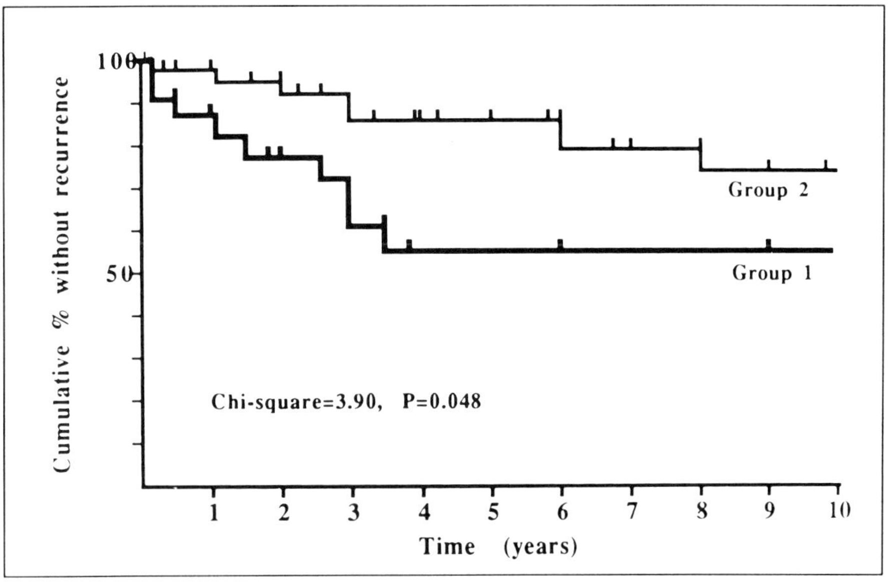

Fig. 10.3. Kaplan-Meier plot of freedom from recurrence in patients with unequivocal parathyroid carcinoma. Group 1 represents patients with clear histopathological criteria for carcinoma, Group 2 those with less obvious histological signs of malignancy. (log rank test) Reprinted with permission from Sandelin K et al.[8]

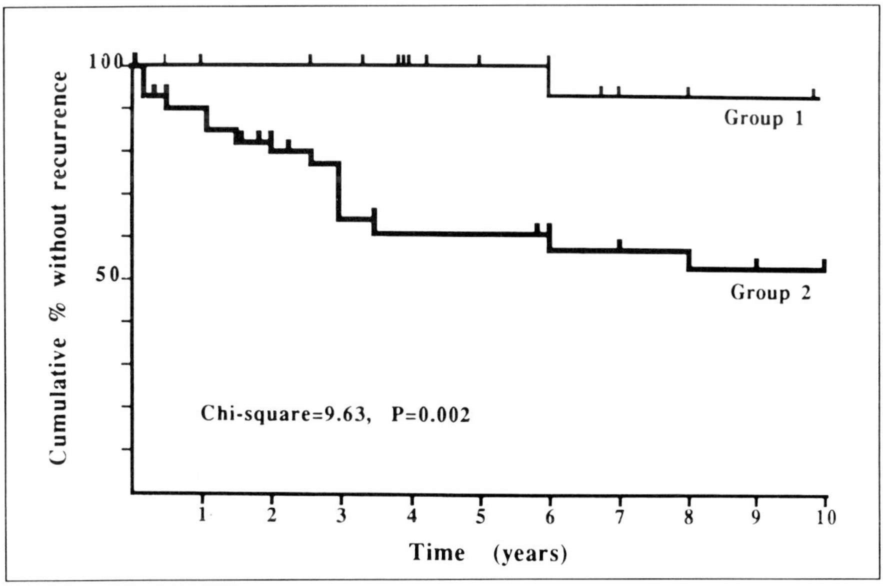

Fig. 10.4. Kaplan-Meier plot of freedom from recurrence in patients with unequivocal parathyroid carcinoma in relation to DNA cytometry. Group 1 represents patients with euploid DNA pattern, Group 2 those with aneuploidy (log rank test) Reprinted with permission from Sandelin K et al.[8]

ue for detection of cervical lymph gland metastases prior to surgery.[61-63] Fine needle aspiration biopsy may diagnose the carcinoma but should probably be applied cautiously since it may theoretically result in seeding of tumor cells.[34,64-66] Both the CT and the MRT investigation should include examination of the lungs in order to detect pulmonary metastases prior to a second operation.[28,58,60,67] If noninvasive radiological studies are negative, selective venous sampling and measurements of intact PTH may be undertaken. This investigation may determine whether the recurrence is likely to be in the neck or at a distant site. It may also localize a neck recurrence to a specific side, which may be important since local spread of parathyroid carcinoma does not necessarily respect the midline but can occur contralaterally.[28,34,60] Selective angiography has been claimed to be efficient in localizing parathyroid carcinoma, and may be considered if other localization studies are negative.[28,34,60] Especially when dealing with repeated recurrence later in the course, the search for distant metastases is more crucial and the investigation should include also bone scintigraphy, CT of the liver and selective venous sampling for PTH determination in hepatic and other distant veins.[26]

If localization studies are negative it is considered wise to sometimes postpone surgery and repeat the localization studies after a few months if the progression of hypercalcemia allows delay.

REOPERATIVE SURGERY

Parathyroid carcinoma is generally a comparatively indolent malignancy and aggressive surgery is strongly recommended for control of tumor recurrence until there are unequivocal signs of wide dissemination.[28,58] The surgical treatment also constitutes more or less the only effective means by which long term amelioration of the hypercalcemia can be achieved. It is therefore important to adopt liberal indications for operation, and patients with slowly progressive disease are often good candidates even for repeated surgery.[28,30,58,67] It needs to be emphasized, however, that parathyroid carcinoma is generally an unusually tenacious tumor and the possibility to cure a patient by repeated surgery is virtually nil or restricted to few patients who have undergone inadequate primary operations.[28] Considerable palliation of the hypercalcemia of even long duration may nevertheless be achieved by a second operation in up to 70% of the patients, and a third operative procedure may still palliate a further 55%.[24] Even subsequent surgery is thus recommended and many series report patients who have undergone several, even up to ten subsequent operations for parathyroid carcinoma.[7,21,28,30,32,34] Autopsy studies have furthermore demonstrated that there often remains only few surgically well accessible residual tumors in patients who die from parathyroid carcinoma after having undergone repeated surgery for the disease.[28] The first reoperation provides the next best opportunity to obtain long term palliation of the hypercalcemia. Due to subsequent progressive development of massive adhesions in the neck further surgery will become increasingly difficult and will ultimately be associated with risks of higher complication. The periods of normocalcemia will also have a tendency to become shorter after the repeated surgery. Reoperation in parathyroid carcinoma will, however, have to lean heavily on localization studies, both with respect to indications and strategy, and in the absence of positive localization re-repeated surgery frequently fail.

It is thus essential that the first reoperation successfully reveals all locally residing gross tumor and that this operation not result in unnecessary recurrent laryngeal nerve injury, which may complicate or even contraindicate further surgery. Although this may be achieved via a neck incision only, *a combined neck and mediastinal exploration* is more effective and safe in this context. This approach provides a superior possibility for identification of the recurrent laryngeal nerve close to its origin in the lower neck before it enters the residual scar tissue after previous surgery. The nerve may be followed rostrally and possibly dissected from the tumor. As parathyroid carcinoma implants may occur also contralaterally to the original lesion, this safe preservation of the recurrent nerve greatly simplifies further handling of the patient. The mediastino-cervical exploration also provides exposure of the areas around the origin of the vessels to the neck and the upper mediastinum, which are difficult to reach from the neck during reoperation, and the procedure also minimizes the risk for unexpected bleeding from the inominate vein or the neck arteries.

After an extended Kocher incision and electrocautery dissection of a platysma/skinflap up to the level of the mandible the neck is entered via incisions along the anterior border of both sternocleidoid muscles, after which the carotid arteries and the jugular veins are dissected bilaterally. The strap muscles are transversally divided and frequently removed below the thyroid, in order to expose the pre- and paratracheal areas which have to be carefully cleared bilaterally. Having dissected the trachea, the esophagus and perhaps a remaining thyroid lobe from the vascular sheath bilaterally, a median sternotomy is performed after which the thymus, the lymph glands as well as fat in the anterior superior mediastinum are cleared out. The thyroid lobe on the side of the original lesion is ectomized, so the trachea can be skeletonized of areolar fat. The vascular sheath is explored ipsilaterally along its total extension in the neck. Reoperation will generally also involve clearance of lymph nodes and fat from the ipsilateral neck compartment by modified neck dissection preserving the sternocleidoid muscle and the accessory nerve.

Residual tumor may be retrieved as subcutaneous or strap muscle implants in a considerable proportion of patients. Persistent tumor is also frequently found at the site of the original lesion, where it may also extend into the pre- and paratracheal fat if this was not removed at the initial surgery. Such tumors should be removed by wide excision including involved neighboring structures. Recurrent tumor may also be located near the laryngeal nerve entrance, because this area may have been cautiously approached at the initial surgery. In such cases the nerve may be dissected with magnifying glasses or resected. Residual tumor can be found in the tracheoesophageal groove, between the esophagus and the trachea, behind the esophagus or in the upper anterior mediastinum.[7,28,30,36,57,58,67] The areas behind the clavicles and around the origin of the carotid arteries may harbor metastases, impossible to reach via the neck incision, but may be readily accessible via the mediastinotomy. Tumor recurrence has also been encountered within the carotid sheath as well as lateral to or behind the vessels. In advanced cases the tumor may encase the vessels, but can usually be dissected from the carotid artery implying that an arterial graft substitute should only rarely be required.[68] The jugular vein may, however, have to be resected and this may be performed unilaterally without risk, though bilateral vein resection is not recommended. Occasionally the tumor infiltrates the esophagus, in which case its outer muscle layer can be excised. In case of tracheal invasion limited tracheal resection has occasionally been employed.[69]

Examination with intraoperative US should be of considerable value during reoperative surgery for parathyroid carcinoma because of the possibility of guiding the exploration directly to sites of residual tumor.

Further reoperative surgery in the neck will become considerably more difficult once this thorough exploration has been performed, and such operations will rarely be undertaken as extensively as the first reoperation. Also in such subsequent operations a lateral approach will generally be utilized in order to obtain a dissectable cleavage plain, in which case the carotid artery and jugular veins are dissected as first steps. Thereafter the exploration is directed towards the sites of preoperatively localized lesions, and complete, bilateral exploration of the neck and mediastinum is avoided as far as possible.

Lymph node metastases occurs in 20-35% of patients, with parathyroid carcinoma.[7,21,30,34] Some series report lower incidence, but it has often been difficult to decide whether locally recurrent disease represented implantation or node metastases.[34] In their review of 167 cases Obara and Fujimoto reported lymph node metastases in 17% of the patients, two-thirds of these residing in the neck and the remainder in the upper mediastinum.[34] This lends considerable support to the recommendation that a combined neck and mediastinal exploration and modified neck dissection be undertaken in association with the first reoperation in parathyroid carcinoma, as this procedure should offer optimal chance to retrieve these node metastases.[27,28,34,36,70] Demonstration of contralateral metastases or implants supports bilateral, modified neck dissection.

Distant metastases have been reported to ultimately occur in around 30% of the patients, with spread to the lung (12-40%), liver (8%) and bone (8%), and more rarely to the adrenal glands, pancreas and brain.[7,18,21,30,34] Only occasionally have distant metastases been demonstrated at time of diagnosis.[28,34,55,71] The exact incidence of distant metastases should, however, be cautiously interpreted as these may be minute and difficult to detect, even in patients dying from parathyroid carcinoma. Recent series demonstrate that the lungs should be the earliest and definitely the most common location for the distant spread.[8] Several authors have reported considerable palliation of hypercalcemia by resection of solitary or multiple, unilateral and even bilateral lung metastases.[27,28,30,32,54,57] If such metastatic lesions are localized and few, they can be excised by conventional lateral thoracotomy and limited wedge resections of the lung parenchyma. Even if such excision should definitely be attempted the experience is that half of the operations will fail to affect the hypercalcemia and only occasionally will resection of the metastases result in substantial normocalcemia.[27,28,30,32,43,57,72] However, Fujimoto et al have reported apparent cure in a single patient and have also obtained long disease-free intervals after this surgery.[27,28,34] Beneficial excision of liver metastases has not been described in parathyroid carcinoma. Bone metastases occur more frequently, with tumor deposits in ribs, spine or pelvis, and occasionally resection of such metastases has provided short term alleviation of hypercalcemia.[26]

Medical Management of Severe Hypercalcemia

Management of hypercalcemia by medical means will be needed when patients with parathyroid carcinoma experience recurrent disease. Such treatment should be considered when the serum calcium value rises above 3.2 mmol/l, especially if surgery is not possible or has to await positive localization. The response to this therapy varies between patients, and a number of drugs or combination of drugs often have to be utilized. The most important, and generally the initial measure in the acute situation, is to ensure adequate rehydration by liberal saline infusion, together with requirements of electrolytes, particularly sodium which increases the propensity for Ca^{2+} excretion in the kidney tubule. Loop diuretics may also be used to augment calcium excretion if the patient is rehydrated. Calcitonin, 1-2 IE/kg/hour, is generally effective in lowering serum calcium values, but the effect is of limited duration even if it may be prolonged by simultaneous steroid administration.[21,73,74] Pamidronate (APD) and other bisphosphonates are usually efficient if high doses are given and since APD has few side effects, this drug presently constitutes the principle basis of the therapy together with calcitonin and measures to restore the fluid and electrolyte balance.[75-79] Even if the serum calcium often remains moderately elevated, this treatment may provide considerable palliation in patients with advanced parathyroid carcinoma. Other agents recommended in this context, including WR 2721, gallium nitrate and estrogens, seem to have limited efficacy.[80-84]

Radiation and Chemotherapy

When carcinoma invades the neck structures or is widely disseminated and

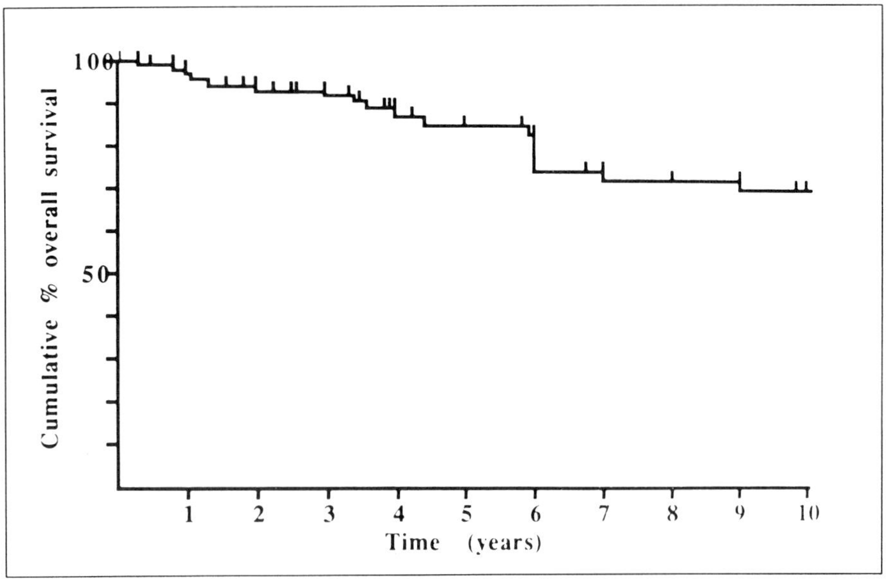

Fig. 10.5. Kaplan-Meier plot of actuarial survival in 95 patients with parathyroid carcinoma Reprinted with permission from Sandelin K et al.[8]

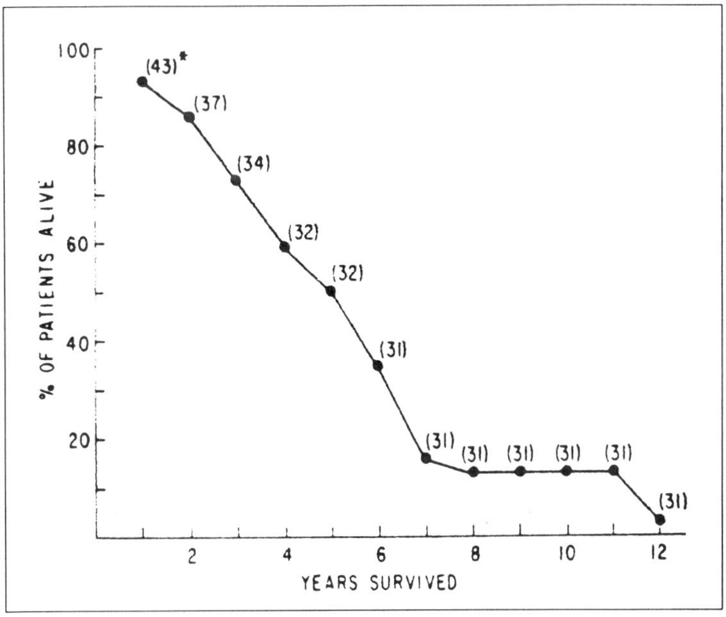

Fig. 10.6. Survival following surgical treatment of parathyroid carcinoma. Reprinted with permission from Holmes EC et al.[30]

surgery ultimately fails to control the hypercalcemia, other treatment modalities will have to be employed, but are generally only occasionally effective. Radiation is often recommended but has only exceptionally been beneficial.[21,24,28,30,32] The majority of patients with parathyroid carcinoma will also fail to benefit from chemotherapy. Occasional reports describe positive responses, however, to a combined regimen of cyclophosphamide, fluorouracil and dakarbacine; to dakarbacine alone, or to the combination of metotrexate, doxorubicin, cyclophosphamide and lomostine.[22,24,85,86] In our limited experience chemotherapy as well as interferon, and somatostatin have been without effect. Mithramycin has more frequently been beneficial, but the doses have to be carefully tritrated because of considerable risk of inducing renal failure and of compromising liver and bone marrow function.[24,70,87] These inherent risks have restricted or prevented the use of this drug.

PROGNOSIS

Patients with recurrent parathyroid carcinoma will ultimately succumb from metabolic complications of hypercalcemia, such as uremia, pancreatitis and cardiac arrhythmia, or from thrombosis and pulmonary embolism. In the end the patients may suffer pathological fractures, and are often bedridden in a miserable condition during the last days of their lives. The prognosis depends largely on the biological behavior of the tumor and some patients may survive for several years or even decades with metastases, and have then undergone frequent surgery.[6,18,21,24,28,34-36,58] The reported 5-year survival has varied between 30-70%, and the 10-year survival between 10-50%.[7,8,21,24,28,30,34,36] These differences reflect variable diagnostic criteria, discrepancies in disease stage as well as variably effective operative treatment. Thus, aggressive surgery seems to result in longer survival.[28,36] In patients in whom hypercalcemia persists after the primary surgery 60% will be dead within 3 years. Recurrence within 2 years or earlier after surgery has also been associated with a worse prognosis.[24,27,28] Tumors with advanced histopathological features, invasive growth and a high rate of mitoses tend to have considerably less favorable survival.[7,32,43,58] The value of DNA determination in the diagnosis of parathyroid carcinoma has been debated, as benign parathyroid tumors may indeed contain aneuploid cells.[53-55] The most recent series of parathyroid carcinoma comprising 95 patients with unequivocal diagnosis demonstrated a 5-year survival of 70% and 10-year survival of 50%, being considerably more favorable than the survival reported in older series[8,21,30] (Figs. 10.5 and 10.6).

NON-FUNCTIONING PARATHYROID CARCINOMA

There are few cases of non-functioning parathyroid carcinoma reported in the literature.[21,30,88-93] Histologically these tumors must be differentiated from thyroid carcinoma or other neck tumors, as well as from metastases to the parathyroid from other organs. Immunostaining for PTH may be used to confirm the diagnosis.[93] The presence of mRNA for PTH and concomitant absence of secretory granules have suggested impairment of hormone synthesis in the non-functioning parathyroid carcinoma.[90]

The non-functioning parathyroid carcinomas tend to be considerably larger at diagnosis than their functioning counterpart. In half of the reported cases metastases to the lungs, bone, brain and liver have occurred already at the time of diagnosis and lymph node involvement has been present at a similar rate.[88-93] In the presence of metastases the reported survival for this tumor has generally been less than 3 years. Presumably is the unfavorable prognosis of this carcinoma related to late detection of the disease. US, CT as well as technetium/thallium scintigraphy may be utilized for visualization of the carcinoma and its metastases.

The non-functioning parathyroid carcinoma is treated surgically according to the same principles as outlined for their functioning counterpart, but aggressive surgery is generally less successful.[88-93]

References

1. de Quervain F. Parastruma maligna aberrata. Dtsch Z Chir 1909; 100: 334-53.
2. Norris EH. Carcinoma of the parathyroid glands: With a preliminary report of 3 cases. Int Abstr Surg 1948; 86: 1-21.
3. van Heerden JA, Weiland LH, ReMine WH et al. Cancer of the parathyroid glands. Arch Surg 1979; 114: 475-80.
4. Black BK, Ackerman LV. Tumors of the parathyroid: A review of twenty- three cases. Cancer 1950; 3: 415-44.
5. Woolner LB, Keating FR Jr, Black BM. Tumors and hyperplasia of the parathyroid glands: A review of the pathological findings in 140 cases of primary hyperparathyroidism. Cancer 1952; 5: 1069-88.
6. Black BK. Carcinoma of the parathyroid. Ann Surg 1954; 139: 355-63.
7. Schantz A, Castleman B. Parathyroid carcinoma: A study of 70 cases. Cancer 1973; 31: 600-5.
8. Sandelin K, Auer G, Bondesson L et al. Prognostic factors in parathyroid cancer. A review of 95 cases. World J Surg 1992; 16: 724-31.
9. Bondesson L, Sandelin K, Grimelius L. Histopathological variables and DNA cytometry in parathyroid carcinoma. Am J Surg Path 1993; 17(8): 820-9.
10. Kodama M, Ikegami M, Imanishi M et al. Parathyroid carcinoma in a case of chronic renal failure on dialysis. Urol Int 1989; 44: 110-12.
11. Iwamoto N, Yamazaki S, Fukuda T et al. Two cases of parathyroid carcinoma in patients on long-term hemodialysis. Nephron 1990; 55: 429-31.
12. Mallette LE, Bilezikian JP, Ketcham AS et al. Parathyroid carcinoma in familial hyperparathyroidism. Am J Med 1974; 57: 642-8.
13. Dinnen JS, Greenwood RH, Jones JH et al. Parathyroid carcinoma in familial hyperparathyroidism. J Clin Pathol 1977; 30: 966-75.
14. Streeten EA, Weinstein LS, Norton JA et al. Studies in a kindred with parathyroid carcinoma. J Clin Endocrinol Metab 1992; 75: 362-6.
15. Frayha RA, Nassar VH, Dagher F et al. Familial parathyroid carcinoma. J Med Liban 1972; 25: 299-309.
16. Jarman WT, Myers RT, Marshall RB. Carcinoma of the parathyroid. Arch Surg 1978; 113: 123-25.
17. Kay S, Hume DM. Carcinoma of the parathyroid gland: how reliable are the clinical and histological features? Arch Pathol 1973; 96: 316-19.
18. McKeown PP, McGarity WC, Sewell CW. Carcinoma of the parathyroid glands: Is it overdiagnosed? A report of three cases. Am J Surg 1984; 147: 292-8.
19. Levin KE, Galante M, Clark OH. Parathyroid carcinoma versus parathyroid adenoma in patients with profound hypercalcemia. Surgery 1987; 101: 649-60.
20. Castleman B, Roth SI. Tumours of the parathyroid glands. Atlas of the tumour pathology. Second series, Facicle 14. Washington: Armed Forces Institute of Pathology 1978; 74-82.
21. Shane E, Bilezikian JP. Parathyroid carcinoma: A review of 62 patients. Endocrin Rev 1982; 3: 218-26.
22. Andersson BJ, Samaan NA, Vassilopoulou-Sellin R et al. Parathyroid carcinoma: Features and difficulties in diagnosis and management. Surgery 1983; 94: 906-15.
23. Pyrah LN, Hodgkinsson A, Anderson CK. Primary hyperparathyroidism. Br J Surg 1966; 53: 245-316.
24. Wynne AG, van Heerden J, Carney JA et al. Parathyroid carcinoma: Clinical and pathologic features in 43 patients. Medicine 1992; 71: 197-205.
25. McCance DR, Kenny BD, Sloan JM et al. Parathyroid carcinoma: A review. J Roy Soc Med 1987; 80: 505-9.
26. Sandelin K, Thompson NW, Bondesson L. Metastatic parathyroid carcinoma: Dilemmas in management. Surgery 1991; 110: 978-88
27. Fujimota Y, Obara T, Ito Y et al. Localization and surgical resection of metastatic parathyroid carcinoma. World J Surg 1986; 10: 539-47.
28. Fujimoto Y, Obara T. How to recognize and treat parathyroid carcinoma. Surg Clin North Am 1987; 67(2): 343-57.
29. Christmas TJ, Chapple CR, Noble JG et al.

Hyperparathyroidism after neck irradiation. Br J Surg 1988; 75: 873-4.
30. Holmes EC, Morton DL, Ketcham AS. Parathyroid carcinoma: A collective review. Ann Surg 1969; 169: 631-40.
31. Fujimoto Y, Obara T, Ito Y et al. Surgical treatment of ten cases of parathyroid carcinoma: Importance of an initial en bloc tumor resection. World J Surg 1984; 8: 392-400.
32. Aldinger KA, Hickey RC, Ibanez ML et al. Parathyroid carcinoma: A clinical study of seven cases of functioning and two cases of nonfunctioning parathyroid cancer. Cancer 1982; 49: 388-97.
33. Palnaes Hansen C, Lau Pedersen L, Christensen L. Diagnosis, treatment and outcome of parathyroid cancer, a report of eight patients. Eur J Surg 1991; 157: 517-20.
34. Obara T, Fujimoto Y. Diagnosis and treatment of patients with parathyroid carcinoma: An update and review. World J Surg 1991; 15: 738-44.
35. Cohn K, Silverman M, Corrado J et al. Parathyroid carcinoma: The Lahey Clinic experience. Surgery 1985; 98: 1095-1100.
36. Wang C, Gasz RD. Natural history of parathyroid carcinoma: Diagnosis, treatment and results. Am J Surg 1985; 149: 522-27.
37. Sherril CK, Anderson CH, Phillips CE Jr et al. Carcinoma of the parathyroid gland: A 30-year experience. Surgery 1991; 110: 704-8.
38. Fyfe ST, Hoover LA, Zuckerbraun L et al. Parathyroid carcinoma: clinical presentation and treatment. Am J Otolaryngol 1990; 11: 268-73.
39. Lillemoe K, Dudley NE. Parathyroid carcinoma: pointers to successful management. Ann Roy Coll Surg Engl 1985; 67: 222-4.
40. Smith JF, Coombs RRH. Histological diagnosis of carcinoma of the parathyroid gland. J Clin Pathol 1984; 37:1370-78.
41. Golden A, Canary JJ, Kerwin DM. Concurrence of hyperplasia and neoplasia of the parathyroid glands. Am J Med 1965; 38: 562-78.
42. Shapiro DM, Recant W, Hemmati H et al. Synchronous occurrence of parathyroid carcinoma and adenoma in an elderly woman. Surgery 1989; 106: 929-33.
43. Ellis HA, Floyd M, Herbert FK. Recurrent hyperparathyroidism due to parathyroid carcinoma. J Clin Pathol 1971; 24: 596-602.
44. Snover DC, Focar K. Mitotic activity in benign parathyroid disease. Am J Clin Pathol 1981; 75: 345-7.
45. Altenahr E, Saeger W. Light and electron microscopy of parathyroid carcinoma. Virchows Arch 1973; 360: 107-122.
46. Åkerström G, Malmaeus J, Bergström R. Surgical anatomy of human parathyroid glands. Surgery 1984; 95: 14-21.
47. Rattner DW, Marrone GC, Kadson E et al. Recurrent hyperparathyroidism due to implantation of parathyroid tissue. Am J Surg 1985; 149: 745-8.
48. Åkerström G, Rudberg C, Grimelius L et al. Recurrent hyperparathyroidism due to peroperative seeding of neoplastic or hyperplastic parathyroid tissue. Acta Chir Scand 1988; 154: 549-52.
49. Fitko R, Roth SI, Hines JR et al. Parathyromatosis in hyperparathyroidim. Hum Pathol 1990; 21(2): 234-7.
50. Fraker DL, Travis WD, Merendino JJ Jr et al. Locally recurrent parathyroid neoplasms as a cause for recurrent and persistent primary hyperparathyroidim. Ann Surg 1991; 213(2): 58-65.
51. Rosai J. Ackerman's surgical pathology, 6th Ed. St. Louis: CV Mosby 1981: 392.
52 Jacobi JM, Lloyd HM, Smith JF. Nuclear diameter in parathyroid carcinoma. J Clin Pathol 1986; 39: 1353-4.
53. Levin KE, Chew KL, Ljung BM et al. Deoxyribonucleide acid cytometry helps identify parathyroid carcinomas. J Clin Endocrinol Metab 1988; 67: 779-84.
54. Obara T, Fujimoto Y, Hirayama A et al. Flow cytometric DNA analysis of parathyroid tumors with special reference to its diagnostic and prognostic value in parathyroid carcinoma.Cancer 1990; 65: 1789-93.
55. Obara T, Fujimoto Y, Kanaji Y et al. Flow cytometric DNA analysis of parathyroid tumors: implication of aneuploidy for pathologic and biologic classification. Cancer 1990; 66: 1555-62.
56. Gittler RD, Maier H. Carcinoma of the parathyroid. Arch Intern Med 1972; 130:

413-17.

57. Davies DR, Dent CE, Ives DR. Successful removal of single metastasis in recurrent parathyroid carcinoma. Br Med J 1973; 1: 397-8.
58. Flye MW, Brennan MF. Surgical resection of metastatic parathyroid carcinoma. Ann Surg 1981; 193: 425-35.
59. Kastan DJ, Kottamasu SR, Frame B et al. Carcinoma in a mediastinal fifth parathyroid gland. JAMA 1987; 257: 1218-9
60. Krudy AG, Doppman JL, Marx SJ et al. Radiographic findings in recurrent parathyroid carcinoma. Radiology 1982; 142: 625-9.
61. Daly BD, Coffey SL, Behan M. Ultrasonographic appearances of parathyroid carcinoma. Br J Radiol 1989; 62: 1017-9.
62. Kinoshita Y, Fukase M, Uchihashi M et al. Significance of preoperative use of ultrasonography in parathyroid neoplasms: Comparison of sonographic textures with histologic findings. J Clin Ultrasound 1985; 13: 457-60.
63. Edmonson GR, Charboneau JW, James EM et al. Parathyroid carcinoma: High-frequency sonographic features. Radiology 1986; 161: 65-7.
64. de-la-Garza S, Flores-de-la-Garza, Hernandez-Batres F. Functional parathyroid carcinoma: Cytology, histology and ultrastructure of a case. Diagn Cytopathol 1985; 1: 232-5.
65. Holmquist N. Fine-needle aspiration and parathyroid carcinoma [letter]. Diagn Cytopathol 1986; 2: 179-80.
66. Sulak LE, Brown RW, Butler DB. Parathyroid carcinoma with occult bone metastases diagnosed by fine needle aspiration cytology. Acta Cytol 1989; 33: 645-8.
67. Dubost C, Jehanno C, Lavergne A et al. Successful resection of intrathoracic metastases from two patients with parathyroid carcinoma. World J Surg 1984; 8: 547-51.
68. Qvist N, Kroll L, Ladefoged C et al. Parathyroid carcinoma: A case with recurrence treated with extensive vascular surgery to the neck. Eur J Surg Oncol 1986; 12: 187-91.
69. Inoue H, Ishihara T, Fukai S et al. Parathyroid carcinoma with tracheal invasion and airway obstruction. Surgery 1980; 87(1): 113-17.
70. Trigonis C, Cedermark B, Willems et al. Parathyroid carcinoma problems in diagnosis and treatment. Clin Oncol 1984; 10: 11-19.
71. Iwashita S, Nakajo M, Nakabeppu Y et al. A case of parathyroid carcinoma visualized by 67Ga citrate and 201TI chloride scintigraphy. Radioisotopes 1989; 38: 430-3.
72. Thomas RJ, Bowling T, Cassoni AM et al. Metastatic parathyroid carcinoma: a radiological, biochemical and symptomatic response to metastectomy. J R Soc Med 1992; 85(3): 182.
73. Saunders KB. Carcinoma of the parathyroids. Proc Roy Soc Med 1970; 63: 453-4.
74. Au WY. Calcitonin treatment of hypercalcemia due to parathyroid carcinoma: synergistic effect of prednisone on long term treatment of hypercalcemia. Arch Intern Med 1975; 135: 1594-7.
75. Shane E, Jacobs TP, Siris ES et al. Therapy of hypercalcemia due to parathyroid carcinoma with intravenous dichloromethylene diphosphonate. Am J Med 1982; 72: 939-44.
76. Jungst D. Disodium clodronate effective in management of severe hypercalcaemia caused by parathyroid carcinoma [letter]. Lancet 1984; 2: 1043.
77. Ralston Sh, Alzaid AA, Gardner MD et al. Treatment of cancer associated hypercalcaemia with combined aminohydroxypropylidene diphosphate and calcitonin. Br Med J 1986; 292: 1549-50.
78. Jansson S, Tisell L-E, Lindstedt G et al. Disodium pamidronate in the preoperative treatment of hypercalcemia in patients with primary hyperparathyroidism. Surgery 1991; 110: 480-6.
79. Portmann L, Thiebaud D, Jaeger P et al. Effective control of hypercalcemia of primary hyperparathyroidism by a single infusion or oral administration of the bisphosphonate APD. J Bone Mineral Res 1989; 4: 317.
80. Pollack S, Goldin RR, Cohen M. Parathyroid carcinoma. Arch Intern Med 1961; 108: 583-7.

81. Goepfert H, Smart CR, Rochlin DB. Metastatic parathyroid carcinoma and hormonal chemotherapy. Case report and response to Hexestrol. Am J Surg 1966; 164: 917-20.
82. Warrell RP Jr, Issacs M, Alcock NW et al. Gallium nitrate for treatment of refractory hypercalcemia from parathyroid carcinoma. Ann Intern Med 1987; 107: 683-6.
83. Glover DJ, Shaw L, Glick JH et al. Treatment of hypercalcemia in parathyroid cancer with WR-2721, S-2-3-aminopropylamino)ethyl-phosphorothioic acid. Ann Intern Med 1985; 103: 55-7.
84. Hirschel-Scholz S, Jung A, Fischer J et al. Suppression of parathyroid secretion after administration of WR-2721 in a patient with parathyroid carcinoma. Clin Endocrinol (Oxf)1985; 23: 313-8.
85. Bukowski RM, Sheeler L, Cunningham J et al. Successful combination chemotherapy for metastatic parathyroid carcinoma. Arch Intern Med 1984; 144: 399-400.
86. Calandra DB, Chejfec G, Foy BK et al. Parathyroid carcinoma: Biochemical and pathologic response to DTIC. Surgery 1984; 96: 1132-37.
87. Singer FR, Neer RM, Murray TM et al. Mithramycin treatment of intractable hypercalcemia due to parathyroid carcinoma. N Engl J Med 1970; 283: 634-6.
88. Chahinian AP, Holland JF, Nieburgs HE et al. Metastatic nonfunctioning parathyroid carcinoma: Ultrastructual evidence of secretory granules and response to chemotherapy. Am J Med 1981; 282: 80-4.
89. Yamashita H, Noguchi S, Nakayama I et al. Light and electron microscopic study of nonfunctioning parathyroid carcinoma. Report of a case with a review of the litterature. Acta Pathol Jpn 1984; 34(1): 123-32.
90. Murphy MN, Glennon PG, Diocee MS et al. Nonsecretory parathyroid carcinoma of the mediastinum. Cancer 1986; 58: 2468-76.
91. Manente P, Cecchettin M, Infantolino D et al. Apparently nonfunctioning metastases of parathyroid carcinoma. Tumori 1987; 73: 191-3.
92. Klink BK, Karulf RE, Maimon WN et al. Nonfunctioning parathyroid carcinoma. Am Surg 1991; 57: 463-7.
93. Yamashita H, Noguchi S, Murakami N et al. Immunohistological study of nonfunctional parathyroid carcinoma. Acta Pathol Jpn 1992; 42(4): 279-85.

INDEX

Page numbers in italics denote figures (f) and tables (t).

H

I

J

K

L

M

N

O

P

R